Growth and Development
ACROSS THE LIFESPAN

Growth and Development

ACROSS THE LIFESPAN

3RD EDITION

Gloria Leifer, RN, MA, CNE
Professor, Obstetric and Pediatric Nursing
Riverside City College
Riverside, California

Eve Fleck, MS, ACE GFI, ACE PT, NASM CPT
Lecturer, Kinesiology
California State University, Northridge
Northridge, California

ELSEVIER

Elsevier
3251 Riverport Lane
St. Louis, Missouri 63043

GROWTH AND DEVELOPMENT ACROSS THE LIFESPAN, THIRD EDITION   ISBN: 978-0-323-80940-5

Notice

Practitioners and researchers must always rely on their own experience and knowledge in evaluating and using any information, methods, compounds or experiments described herein. Because of rapid advances in the medical sciences, in particular, independent verification of diagnoses and drug dosages should be made. To the fullest extent of the law, no responsibility is assumed by Elsevier, authors, editors or contributors for any injury and/or damage to persons or property as a matter of products liability, negligence or otherwise, or from any use or operation of any methods, products, instructions, or ideas contained in the material herein.

Previous editions copyrighted 2013 and 2004.

Library of Congress Control Number: 2021932120

Content Strategist: Brandi Graham
Content Development Specialist: Melissa Rawe/Andrew Schubert
Publishing Services Manager: Deepthi Unni
Project Manager: Radjan Lourde Selvanadin
Design Direction: Brian Salisbury

Printed in India

Last digit is the print number: 9 8 7 6 5 4

Working together
to grow libraries in
developing countries

www.elsevier.com • www.bookaid.org

Dedicated to the memory of

Sarah Masseyaw Leifer,
a nurse, humanitarian, and mother

and

Daniel Peretz Hartston, MD,
a pediatrician, husband, and world traveler,

and to the honor of

Heidi, Paul, Ruby
Barnet, Michelle,
Daniel, McKenzie, Tess, and Sofia
Amos, Gina, Spencer, and Ryan
Eve, Zoe, Elliot, and Ian

who acquaint me with the beauty, joys, and challenges of my lifespan voyage.
Gloria Leifer Hartston

Dedicated to my children

Zoe, Elliot, and Ian,
and to my mother, Gloria.

You give my life meaning and purpose, and fill it with love.
Eve Fleck

Dedicated to Dad,
your storytelling brings words to life and I strive to walk in your footsteps,
and to Mom for your gift of quick wit and impish sense of humor.

Special thanks to my amazing husband, Paul, who tolerates my manic creativity,
and my precious daughter, Jessica, who owns my heart entirely.
Janet Servoss

Contributor

Janet Servoss, RN, BS, MSN, CGRN
Clinical Nurse IV, Endoscopy Educator
Endoscopy
St. Jude Medical Center
Fullerton, California

Ancillary Writers

Melanie Richeson, MA
Freelance Medical Editor
Unison Health
Toledo, Ohio
TEACH Lesson Plans

Laura Bevlock Kanavy, MSN, RN
Director
CTC of Lackawanna County Practical Nursing Program
Scranton, Pennsylvania
Test Bank

Liz Summers, MSN, RN, CNE
Coordinator of PN Program
Cass Career Center
Harrisonville, Missouri
Student Review Questions

Reviewers

Amanda Churchman, RN, MSN
Director of Practical Nursing Program
Practical Nursing
Red River Technology Center
Duncan, Oklahoma

Heather Clark, DNP, RN
Director
Penn State Practical Nursing Program
Penn State Lehigh Valley
Center Valley, Pennsylvania

Odelia Garcia, MS, MSN, BSN, RN
Vocational Nurse Instructor
Nursing
Texas State Technical College – Harlingen
Harlingen, Texas

Alice M. Hupp, BS, RN
Lead Instructor
Vocational Nursing
North Central Texas College
Gainesville, Texas

Lorraine Kelley, RN
Faculty
Department of Nursing and Emergency Medical Services
Pensacola State College
Pensacola, Florida

Darla K. Shar, MSN, RN
Associate Director
Nursing
Hannah E. Mullins School of Practical Nursing
Salem, Ohio

Molly M. Showalter, MSN Ed, RN
Interim Vocational Nursing Program Director
Department of Health Professions
Texas Southmost College
Brownsville, Texas

Elaine Kay Strouss
Dean–School of Health Sciences
School of Health Sciences
Community College of Beaver County
Monaca, Pennsylvania

Preface

Understanding growth and development at each age and stage of the life cycle is a valuable tool for the nurse or health-care worker. This knowledge can be useful when assessing, planning, and implementing health care and education for clients. This text enables the student to study growth and development in a continuum across the entire lifespan and integrate the understanding of changes that normally occur in each stage of the life cycle.

The course of growth and development has been charted by many researchers and theorists who formed a framework for understanding lifespan development. This text reviews specific theories and concepts of typical physical and behavioral changes that occur at each stage in the life cycle. When a health-care worker is familiar with normal developmental stages, alterations can be identified, and typical patterns can be noted when designing approaches to care.

Next generation test questions (NGN) at the end of chapters are included to assist with review of the chapter content and familiarize the student with NGN-type questions. This will challenge the reader to evidence understanding of the content as well as familiarize the student with the style of questions that are presented on licensing examinations.

This text provides a comprehensive review of concepts of growth and development from conception to death, integrated with the goals of *Healthy People 2030* that can be utilized by nurses and health-care workers in the achievement of their professional objectives.

Healthy People 2030, officially launched on August 18, 2020, provides a list of national goals to be achieved by the year 2030, related to meeting the needs of a diverse population across the lifespan in a variety of settings. Focusing health care on illness prevention is less costly than focusing on the treatment or cure of an illness after it develops. Research validates the importance of a healthy lifestyle in preventing many types of illnesses.

Learning occurs in all phases of the life cycle, but abilities and individual needs differ at each phase and influence the effectiveness of teaching styles. Each stage of the life cycle involves specific developmental tasks or crises of the individual and the family that must be mastered during life's journey. This text provides an understanding of how physical changes, learning styles, and these developmental tasks affect each other, which is useful in assessing needs and designing a plan to help support family dynamics and empower both the individual and the family to participate in maintaining health.

The twenty-first century brings with it possibilities of increased population growth, intensified international conflict, health challenges, and advanced scientific achievements, all of which can influence the world's social, economic, and health environments. Our abilities to improve health, enrich the quality of life, and lengthen the lifespan may become even more important as the future unfolds. Promoting healthy behaviors and healthy lifestyles is an integral part of improving quality of life.

This text also discusses the emergence of new knowledge and understanding of microbiomes, which offers opportunities to teach healthy behaviors during pregnancy and the newborn phase of the life cycle that can affect the adult health of the newborn and maintain health during various stages of the life cycle.

Today, people want control over their health care and want to be part of the decision-making process concerning their health-care needs. The increasing popularity of complementary and alternative medicine (CAM) reflects trends toward self-management and preventive care. Internet resources that provide evidence-based knowledge and on-demand access to health clubs, gyms, self-help groups, and new exercise options have increased rapidly over the past decade. The reliance on the internet use of Zoom and other online programs, which enabled continuation of education at all levels as well as continuation of many business services and health care via telecommunication during the pandemic of 2020, will continue and be further refined after the crisis passes. This also reflects people's growing concern with health as people grow, mature, and age.

This text explains concepts and theories about physical, cognitive, social, and personality development in each stage of the life cycle, from conception to death. It also provides a discussion of external influences such as culture and environment on normal development. Each chapter provides information that helps the student identify teaching strategies that incorporate personal priorities, skills, and limitations that characterize each stage of life. For example, teaching strategies or techniques that a health-care worker would use for a young child would be different from the strategies used to teach an adolescent. Children learn as adults do, but because they are unencumbered by experiences, their processing and interpretation may be different.

Preventive health care is a vital part of the objectives of *Healthy People 2030*. Understanding how behavior is influenced by heredity, life stage, and environment is critical for the nurse or health-care worker. With this knowledge, they can develop education and care plans designed to meet the unique needs of individual clients. These clients will then have the ability to make sound and healthy lifestyle decisions empowered by information provided in a culturally sensitive, developmentally appropriate manner.

Most health outcomes measured in *Healthy People 2030* data are related to choices made by individuals during each stage of the life cycle. Health-care workers and nurses are well qualified to focus on educating clients about health promotion and healthy lifestyles.

The effective use of every teaching opportunity to educate at-risk populations about healthy diets, exercise, mental health, and lifestyle choices is the heartbeat of preventive care.

Acknowledgments

The birth of a book is a team effort. The authors wish to express sincere appreciation to those who contributed materially, as well as to those whose support and encouragement were vital to the outcome.

Terri Wood, former Senior Nursing Editor at Elsevier, seeded the vision and expressed confidence and support in the efforts of the authors to complete this text. Our sincere appreciation is extended to the many faculty reviewers who shared their expertise and provided constructive comments for this revision. We would also like specially to thank Dr. Marjorie Hardy, Assistant Professor of Psychology at Eckerd College in St. Petersburg, Florida, for her detailed review of Chapter 5 and her helpful suggestions.

Janet Servoss, BS, MSN, RN, CGRN has joined our writing team, and she brings with her a vast amount of clinical expertise in medical-surgical nursing and teaching of preventative health practices to professionals as well as patients. We appreciate her contributions to the front lines working in the hospital during the 2020 COVID-19 pandemic, as well as her contributions to this text as research consultant, editor, and special contributor. She kept the project moving and facilitated the meeting of deadlines in a painless fashion. Jessica Servoss contributed several original illustrations for this edition, and we are proud of her accomplishments.

The able assistance of the Elsevier nursing editorial staff, including Nancy O'Brien and Brandi Graham, Senior Content Strategists, Education Content; Melissa Rawe, Senior Content Development Specialist, Education, Reference, and Continuity; and Andrew Schubert, Content Development Specialist; who provided the necessary tools, expert planning and editing skills, and helpful guidance throughout the publication process.

Professor Barnet Hartston deserves special thanks for his encouragement, support, and motivating ideas. Several of our photographic models add sparkle to many of the illustrations that appear in this text; their patience was appreciated. Amos Hartston deserves special recognition for taking time out of his busy schedule to offer personal assistance and encouragement as well as he and Gina Hartston volunteering to provide comfortable and safe facilities to write the text during the mandated social isolation during the 2020 COVID-19 worldwide pandemic.

The authors express appreciation to each other for the support and mutual respect generated by this collaboration.

We wish to thank the students at Fordham School of Nursing in the Bronx, New York, Hunter College of the City University of New York, California State University at Los Angeles, California State University at Northridge, and Riverside City College for helping us understand their learning needs and inspiring us to continue the professionally challenging and personally rewarding careers of teaching and writing.

The utilization of information contained in this book is not dependent on scope of practice, so the text can be useful to those studying in multidisciplinary health-related fields such as nursing, psychology, counseling, early childhood education, or any field where the understanding of the needs, risks, and challenges of a specific age group influences a positive outcome of the interaction. We hope that the information contained in this text will provide the reader with the tools to enhance communication and develop effective plans of care for individuals and their families.

Gloria Leifer Hartston, RN, MA, CNE
Eve Fleck MS, ACE GFI, ACE CPT, NASM CPT

Contents

Healthy People 2030

http://evolve.elsevier.com/Leifer/growth

OUTLINE

OBJECTIVES

1. Describe what *Healthy People 2030* is and what it is meant to do.
2. List public health issues defined by *Healthy People 2030*.
3. Discuss how the health status of a population is measured.
4. State one health issue or goal for each stage of the life cycle.
5. Discuss the role of the health-care worker in achieving *Healthy People 2030* objectives.
6. Discuss the role of the health-care worker in worldwide health improvement.

KEY TERMS

behaviors
biology
determinants of health
food insecurity

health status
Healthy People 2030
infant mortality rate
Leading Health Indicators

life expectancy
physical environment
social environment

DEFINITION

What *Healthy People 2030* Is

Healthy People 2030 is an evidence-based 10-year report card describing health-care accomplishments within the United States from the years 2010 to 2020. It is also a prescription for what needs to be done between now and the year 2030. The overarching goals of the *Healthy People 2030* plan are to engage leadership; enable the nation to attain health and well-being; eliminate health disparities; and create social and physical environments that promote good health, quality of life, healthy development, and positive health behaviors across all life stages.

Published by the U.S. Department of Health and Human Services (USDHHS) in 2020, *Healthy People 2030* is currently considered by many to be the most important document regarding health in the United States. First written in 1979, *Healthy People* is the work of more than 350 governmental agencies, organizations, and experts in the health-care field. By analyzing current statistics every 10 years, *Healthy People* provides a snapshot of progress, trends, and issues, and it highlights future needs in health care by identifying specific goals. Goals and objectives are revised periodically based on accomplishments and needs.

Healthy People 2030 sought to reduce the overall number of objectives compared to 2020. The list includes 41 topic areas (general categories) with 355 objectives (statements of movement toward targets), to be achieved by the year 2030. Health problems and suggested improvements in health practices are designed according to evidence-based knowledge. The document defines four major age groups: (1) infants, (2) children, (3) teens and young adults, and (4) older adults and the geriatric population.

What *Healthy People 2030* Does

The *Healthy People 2030* guidelines established in 2017 focus on the larger social picture surrounding health-care outcomes compared with those presented in *Healthy People 2020*. While *Healthy People 2020* focused on disease, *Healthy People 2030* has a primary focus on achieving health equity, where every member of the population has an equal opportunity to be healthy. *Healthy People 2030's* vison is to create "a society in which all people can achieve their full potential for health and well-being across the lifespan" (USDHHS, 2030). Given this health equity focus, objectives fall under these primary categories:

1. Remove obstacles to health.
2. Address structural and systematic prejudice and discrimination.
3. Develop policies and practices that promote health equity including preventive care.
4. Give children and youth opportunities to allow attainment of the highest level of health and well-being throughout their lifespan.
5. Create healthy physical, social, and economic environments.

Aspects of the goals and objectives of *Healthy People 2030* will be integrated throughout the chapters in this text. Specific tasks or risk factors will be identified, and health-care interventions such as suggested age-appropriate exercise activities will be presented to promote a healthy lifestyle that leads to normal growth and development throughout the life cycle.

Leading Health Indicators

Health indicators are measurements of health-related concepts across the lifespan. *Leading Health Indicators* are selected high-priority issues for the current 10-year period. The leading health indicators for 2030 are:

1. Access to health services, including increasing the proportion of persons with medical insurance, and preventing hospitalizations through treatment in outpatient settings.

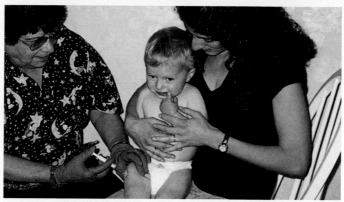

Figure 1.1 A mother holds her child in the "hug position" during immunization. Current immunization schedules for infants and children may be accessed at www.CDC.GOV/vaccines/index.html.

2. Clinical preventive services, including monitoring the population of adults with high blood pressure, tracking children receiving recommended immunizations (Figure 1.1), and monitoring measurements of urban decay and residential segregation or isolation, which can be barriers to receiving care.
3. Environmental quality, including overall environmental qualities (air, water, land, amount and type of buildings), and sociodemographic factors (age, sex, education, migration background, ethnicity, employment, income, etc.), heat vulnerability, and general environmental health-related quality of life (EPA, 2018).
4. Occurrence of injury and violence, including numbers of firearm-related deaths and other all-cause unintentional deaths.
5. Maternal, infant, and child health, including reduction of all infant and maternal deaths.
6. Mental health, including reduction of frequent mental distress and suicide.
7. Obesity, including reduction of children and adolescents with obesity through healthy diets and physical activity (Figure 1.2).
8. Oral health, including increasing the number of people older than 2 years who use the oral-care health system each year.
9. Reproductive and sexual health, including encouraging sexually active adolescents who use any method of contraception at first intercourse, and reducing new HIV diagnoses.
10. Social determinants, including increasing the number of fourth grade students reading at or above proficiency, reducing poverty rates, reducing household food insecurity (the state of being without reliable access to a sufficient quantity of affordable, nutritious food), and reducing proportions of households spending more than 30% of income on housing.
11. Substance abuse, including reducing overall drug overdose death rate, and reducing alcohol use disorders.
12. Tobacco, including reducing use of any tobacco products by adolescents (National Academies of Sciences, Engineering, and Medicine, 2020).

A sample chart showing how the topics, indicators, and objectives of *Healthy People 2030* are integrated and tracked is shown in Table 1.1. Preparedness is not yet listed as a

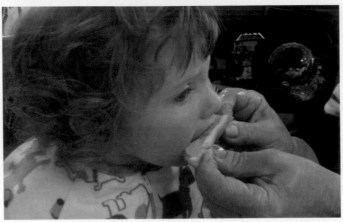

Figure 1.2 A child begins to learn about healthy food and nutrition early in life by developing a taste for fresh vegetables and fruits provided as daytime snacks.

TABLE 1.1   Sample Tracking of Relationships Among *Healthy People 2030* Topics, Indicators, and Objectives

Topic	Indicator	Objectives (for Action Planning)
Access to health care	Actual proportion of population with medical insurance	Increase the number of people with access to medical and preventive care
Injury and violence	Actual proportion of population experiencing injury/violence	Reduce the occurrence of unintentional injury deaths
Social determinants	Proportion of population experiencing a healthy living environment	Reduce frequent mental distress Improve proportion of fourth graders reading at proficiency Increase access to affordable housing and lower the proportion of persons living in poverty
Health-related quality of life	Proportion of population engaging in healthy behaviors, such as good nutrition and physical exercise	Reduce household food insecurity Reduce occurrence of obesity and hypertension Reduce alcohol use disorders, use of tobacco products, and drug overdose deaths

Data from National Academies of Sciences, Engineering, and Medicine 2020. *Leading Health Indicators 2030: Advancing Health, Equity, and Well-Being.* The National Academies Press. https://doi.org/10.17226/25682.

leading health indicator because of a lack of literature in which to identify evidence-based practices, but the topic is listed as a core objective in *Healthy People 2030*.

Determinants of Health

Determinants of health are the range of social, economic, and environmental factors that influence health status. These can include individual behavior and biological and genetic factors.

Behavior and biology are interrelated. A disease affects biology, but behaviors can make a person susceptible or resistant to a disease. Social and physical environments impact behavior. For example, education can motivate healthy behaviors, but toxins in the environment can have a negative impact on biology. Policies and access to health care also figure prominently in this cycle. Therefore, personal health behavior is closely related to the general environment in achieving the *Healthy People 2030* goals (Figure 1.3).

Biology refers to the individual's genetic makeup (those factors with which he or she is born), family history (which may impact risk for disease), and the physical and mental health problems acquired during life. Aging, diet, physical activity, smoking, stress, alcohol or illicit drug abuse, injury or violence, or infectious or toxic agents may result in illness or disability and can produce a "new" biology for the individual.

Behaviors are individual responses or reactions to internal stimuli and external conditions. Behaviors can have a reciprocal relationship to biology (i.e., each can react to the other). For example, smoking (behavior) can alter the cells in the lung and can result in shortness of breath, emphysema, or cancer (biology) that then may lead an individual to stop smoking (behavior). Similarly, a family history that includes heart disease (biology) may motivate an individual to develop good eating habits, avoid tobacco, and maintain

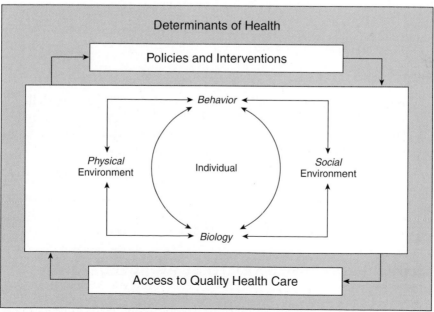

Figure 1.3 Determinants of health. (From U.S. Department of Health and Human Services (2000). *Healthy People 2010.* International Publishing, Inc.)

an active lifestyle (behaviors), which may prevent his or her own development of heart disease (biology).

Personal choices and the social and physical environments surrounding individuals can shape behaviors. The social and physical environments include all factors that affect the life of individuals, positively or negatively, many of which may not be under their immediate or direct control.

Social environment includes interactions with family, friends, coworkers, and others in the community. It also encompasses social institutions, such as law enforcement, the workplace, places of worship, and schools. Housing, public transportation, and the presence or absence of violence in the community are among other components of the social environment. The social environment has a profound effect on the health of the individual and the larger community and is unique because of cultural customs, language, and personal, religious, or spiritual beliefs. At the same time, individuals and their behaviors contribute to the quality of the social environment.

Physical environment is that which can be seen, touched, heard, smelled, and tasted. However, the physical environment also contains less tangible elements, such as radiation, ozone, or chemical toxins. The physical environment can harm individual and community health, especially when individuals and communities are exposed to toxic substances, irritants, infectious agents, and physical hazards in homes, schools, and worksites. The physical environment also can promote good health by providing clean and safe places for people to work, exercise, and play.

Policies and interventions can have a powerful and positive effect on the health of individuals and the community. Examples include health promotion campaigns to prevent smoking, policies mandating child restraints and safety-belt use in automobiles, disease prevention services (e.g., immunization of children, adolescents, and adults), and clinical services (e.g., enhanced mental health care). Policies and interventions that promote individual and community health may be implemented by a variety of agencies (e.g., transportation, education, energy, housing, labor, justice, and other venues), places of worship, community-based organizations, civic groups, and businesses.

Health Status

Evaluating specific details of the *determinants of health* enables understanding of the population's health status, which refers to medical conditions (both physical and mental health), claims experience, receipt of health care, medical history, genetic information, evidence of insurability, and disability. The health status can be measured by birth and death rates, life expectancy, morbidity from specific disease, access to health care, and health-insurance coverage, as well as other factors. These factors are reported in publications such as *Healthy People Review* or *Health, United States*. In these publications, the health status is described for the total population of the United States. The leading causes of death across the lifespan are presented in Box 1.1.

PROGRESS AND GOALS YET TO BE ACHIEVED

Each decade, when the goals and objectives of *Healthy People* are identified, communities and health-care professionals are expected to develop action plans to help achieve and maintain healthy behaviors and lifestyles, thus enabling access to and use of federal, state, and community programs and resources.

BOX 1.1   Leading Causes of Death by Age Group*

YOUNGER THAN 1 YEAR
- Congenital anomalies
- Disorders related to premature birth
- Maternal pregnancy complications
- Sudden infant death syndrome
- Unintentional injury

1–4 YEARS
- Unintentional injuries
- Birth defects
- Cancer
- Homicides
- Heart disease

5–9 YEARS
- Unintentional injuries
- Cancer
- Birth defects
- Homicide
- Heart disease

10–14 YEARS
- Unintentional injuries
- Suicide
- Cancer
- Birth defects
- Homicide

15–24 YEARS
- Unintentional injuries
- Suicide
- Homicide
- Cancer
- Heart disease

25–34 YEARS
- Unintentional injuries
- Suicide
- Homicide
- Heart disease
- Cancer

35–44 YEARS
- Unintentional injury
- Cancer
- Heart disease
- Suicide

45–54 YEARS
- Cancer
- Heart disease
- Unintentional injury
- Suicide

55–64 YEARS
- Cancer
- Heart disease
- Unintentional injury
- Long-term respiratory disease
- Diabetes mellitus

OVER 65 YEARS
- Heart disease
- Cancer
- Long-term respiratory disease
- Stroke
- Dementia

*Listed in order of prevalence within each age group.
Data from National Vital Statistics System, National Center for Health Statistics, Center for Disease Control and Prevention (2017). *10 leading causes of death by age group United States 2017.* Retrieved April 26, 2020, from https://www.cdc.gov/injury/wisqars/pdf/leading_causes_of_death_by_age_group_2017-508.pdf

One example of the goals of *Healthy People 2030* is to increase quality and years of human life. Life expectancy is the average number of years a person born in a given year is expected to live. In 1900, the life expectancy was 47.3 years. In 2019, the life expectancy was 80.3 years. These statistics show definite improvement; however, in 2019, many countries had better life expectancy rates than the United States (Table 1.2).

Life-expectancy statistics can further be analyzed in terms of sex (women live an average of 6 years longer than men), race (White women have a greater life expectancy than other racial groups in the United States), income and education status (increased years of education and income increases life expectancy across all races) (CDC, 2019). Life-expectancy statistics from other countries may reflect the quality of health care

TABLE 1.2   Life Expectancy at Birth by Country

Rank	Country	Life Expectancy in Years
1	Monaco	89.30
2	Japan	86.00
3	Singapore	86.00
4	Macau	84.60
5	San Marino	83.30
6	Canada	83.40
7	Iceland	83.30
8	Hong Kong	83.20
9	Andorra	83.00
10	Israel	83.00
11	Guernsey	82.80
12	Malta	82.80
13	Switzerland	82.80
14	Australia	82.70
15	Korea, South	82.60
16	Luxembourg	82.60
17	Italy	82.50
18	Sweden	82.40
19	France	82.20
20	Jersey	82.20
21	Liechtenstein	82.20
22	New Zealand	82.10
23	Norway	82.10
24	Spain	82.00
25	Austria	81.90
26	Anguilla	81.80
27	Bermuda	81.70
28	Netherlands	81.70
29	Cayman Islands	81.60
30	Isle of Man	81.60
31	Belgium	81.40
32	Slovenia	81.40
33	Finland	81.30
34	Puerto Rico	81.30
35	Denmark	81.20
36	Ireland	81.20
37	Germany	81.10

TABLE 1.2   Life Expectancy at Birth by Country (*Cont.*)

Rank	Country	Life Expectancy in Years
38	Greece	81.10
39	Portugal	81.10
40	United Kingdom	81.10
41	Saint Pierre and Miquelon	81.00
42	Faroe Islands	80.60
43	Taiwan	80.60
44	Turks and Caicos Islands	80.30
45	United States	80.30
46	Saint Barthelemy	80.20
47	Saint Martin	80.20
48	Wallis and Fortuna	80.20
49	Gibraltar	80.00
50	Saint Helena, Ascension, and Tristan da Cunha	80.00

From Central Intelligence Agency. (2020). Country comparison: Life expectancy at birth. *The World Factbook.* Retrieved April 26, 2020, from https://www.cia.gov/library/publications/the-world-factbook/fields/355rank.html.

in that country or the endemic prevalence of high infection, mortality, or HIV/AIDS infections.

Progress toward stated goals has been seen in several areas since the inception of *Healthy People* in 1979, but much remains to be done. Another important indicator that measures the status of the nation's health is the infant mortality (death) rate. The infant mortality rate is the number of deaths that occur before 1 year of age per 1000 live births. In 1975, the infant mortality was 15 per 1000 live births. In 1997, the number decreased to 7.2 deaths per 1000 live births (USDHHS, 2000) and in 2017 the U.S. infant mortality rate was 5.8 per 1000 live births (CDC, 2019).

Addressing issues related to nutrition is another area of focus for *Healthy People 2030*. The Scientific Report of the 2020 Dietary Guidelines Advisory Committee states more than 70% of Americans are overweight or obese, and the prevalence of those who are morbidly obese has increased. Of particular concern is the increasing numbers of obese young people, as this can have persistent effects on health across the lifespan, specifically cardiovascular disease, type 2 diabetes, and some types of cancer. Food insecurity and lack of access to affordable healthy food contributes to this statistic. In 2018, more than 37 million people, including 6 million children, experienced food insecurity.

The 2010–2014 review of the *Healthy People 2020* goals showed that approximately 53.9% of the objectives either met their target or have shown improvement. Fewer adults are smoking cigarettes, fewer children are exposed to secondhand smoke, more adults are meeting physical activity targets, and fewer adolescents are using alcohol or illegal drugs (USDHHS, 2014).

ISSUES AND GOALS RELATED TO PHASES OF THE LIFE CYCLE

Prenatal and Infant Health

Maternal and infant health is the core of the health status of the next generation. The U.S. infant mortality rate has declined steadily since 1979, but as of 2017, 55 countries have a lower infant mortality rate than the United States (CIA, 2020). The leading areas of progress between the years 2010 and 2020 include reducing sudden infant death syndrome (SIDS) with the back-to-sleep educational program that urges parents to place infants on their backs rather than on their abdomen when putting their infants down to sleep, and promoting the use of folic acid supplements early in pregnancy to reduce congenital malformations such as spina bifida. Guidelines for "baby friendly" hospitals have been established to increase breastfeeding during the first days of life.

Childhood Health

The overall goals for this population are to increase the proportion of children who communicate positively with their parents, have parents read to them, and get sufficient sleep. Children with health issues should receive any age-specific treatment and be on track and ready for school. Health issues should be added to school curricula, teachers should be well informed, and school nurses should be available in all schools. Completion of high school should be encouraged to provide the education necessary for understanding the importance of healthy lifestyle choices. The target set is 90% of persons will receive a regular diploma 4 years after entering the ninth grade and that the United States will have the highest proportion of graduates in the workforce by the year 2030 (USDHHS, 2019). Encouraging school attendance, home schooling during prolonged illness, and school counseling services aid in achieving these goals. Increasing access to quality education, preparing students for college, providing early education (in the form of Head Start) programs, helping children with special needs, and using innovative strategies to help achieve positive student outcomes are also current objectives for *Healthy People 2030*. Innovative strategies are particularly imperative in the post–coronavirus disease 2019 (COVID-19) pandemic world, where the roles of educators are being redefined and the power of technology is delivering education in rapidly expanding formats.

School health services were established more than 100 years ago to reduce absenteeism caused by communicable diseases. Current school health programs reflect the concept that physical health and mental health are related to academic and social success. School nurses assess development, screen for specific health problems, refer to community agencies, and provide immunization information.

Adolescent and Young-Adult Health

In 2017, the adolescent death rate was 51.5 per 100,000 (CDC, 2017). The *Healthy People 2030* goal is to reduce the death rate by increasing access to preventive health-care visits, improve school attendance and educational skills in reading and math leading to a regular high school diploma, and improve adolescent's nutritional status through School Breakfast

Programs. Indicators for health in this age group focus on preventing risk behaviors and reducing rates of disease onset rather than reducing the effects of current disease states. Actions such as reducing tobacco and alcohol use, encouraging a healthy diet, increasing physical activity, and preventing risky sexual behaviors can have long-term beneficial effects (Weiss, 2019).

Older Adult Health

Although the life expectancy has increased, the problems related to maintaining an independent lifestyle remain a challenge. Goals for older adults include improving health, function, and quality of life through access to preventive health. Objectives include increasing physical activity, increasing overall heart health, reducing use of inappropriate medications, reduction of hospital admissions for falls, pneumonia, urinary tract infections, and diabetes.

Geriatric Adult Health

Goals for the geriatric phase of life include reducing the number of illnesses and deaths related to vaccine-preventable illnesses by increasing the number of adults over age 65 who receive annual vaccines against influenza and pneumococcal pneumonia, reducing the number of hip fractures (more than 75% of which occur in elderly females), increasing identification and treatment of chronic kidney disease, and increasing the availability of diagnostic tools that can decrease the number of undiagnosed dementia cases.

ROLE OF THE HEALTH-CARE WORKER IN ACHIEVING *HEALTHY PEOPLE 2030* GOALS

Health-care workers play an important role in helping to achieve the goals of *Healthy People 2030* at all phases of the life cycle by:
- Increasing the use of prenatal services, which reduces the occurrence of low-birth-weight newborns and prematurity.
- Promoting breastfeeding, which increases the health of the newborn and bonding between mother and infant.
- Educating the school-age child about nutrition, diet and exercise, smoking and drug use, and healthy lifestyles.
- Promoting health through employer-sponsored programs.
- Providing health-education services to patients in managed-care organizations.
- Identifying health risks through screening programs, which can lead to early diagnosis and treatment of disease.
- Encouraging older adults to participate in at least one organized health-promotion activity.

Recent health-care reforms such as the Affordable Care Act and the Health Care and Education Reconciliation Act of 2010 were enacted in order to enable all people to be covered by some type of health-care insurance to increase accessibility and aid in achieving the stated goals of *Healthy People 2030.* These reforms are subject to continuous political revision.

WORLD HEALTH

At the same time as *Healthy People* was being initiated and developed, efforts toward worldwide health improvement were also initiated by the World Health Organization (WHO). In 1978, the International Conference on Primary Health Care was held in Alma-Ata, Kazakhstan. The world community was urged to protect and promote the health of all people of the world, and a list of world-health goals was developed. A charter for health promotion was adopted at an international conference in 1986 in Ottawa, Canada. This charter defined world-health promotion as "those processes that enable people to increase control over and improve their health" (WHO, 1986). As a result of meetings held in various locations around the world in the 1990s, objectives were developed for improving the environment; eliminating poverty; and providing reproductive health services, adolescent health, women's empowerment, human rights, and tobacco control.

Progress has been made in improving world health by decreasing infant mortality rates, increasing access to immunizations, and providing areas of safer environmental sanitation. However, much work has yet to be completed. In September 2000, the United Nations adopted a "UN Millennium Declaration" that stated a series of goals and targets and indicators related to health and the alleviation of poverty. In 2005, these goals were restated at a meeting with WHO and the World Bank, and again in 2015, where specific steps were recommended to speed achievement of the worldwide sustainable development goals (United Nations, 2020). A core principle of the Millennium Declaration was that human development is a shared responsibility. WHO will monitor the progress, which will be reported by the National Health Information System.

The current global targets to be achieved by the year 2030 include eradicating extreme poverty and hunger; ensuring primary education for all children; promoting gender equity and empowering women; reducing child mortality; improving maternal health; combating the spread of HIV/AIDS, malaria, and other major diseases; ensuring environmental sustainability; and continuing to develop a global partnership to achieve these goals. In developing countries, progress has been slow and education is an important first step. WHO uses these goals and targets to focus on collaborative programs to improve global health care.

An outline of some effective interventions is available on *Evolve*.

Global health efforts are necessary because health problems are no longer confined to local areas. Outbreaks of illness in one area of the world can quickly spread to other areas of the world with the ease of international travel, as seen with the global COVID-19 pandemic of 2020. Improvement in technology is not the key to improvement in health—prevention is. Prevention of illness through education and access to early health care is essential. The cultural competence of health-care workers and their willingness to be change agents for the traditional health-care delivery system is also essential.

Health-care workers must work with the local community and form partnerships for health. Improving prenatal care, nutrition, exercise, and access to children's health care all over the world are important beginning efforts toward improving world health. The health-care team can build a bridge of health that extends around the world. Providing culturally competent care in the local community is the starting point for that bridge. Working with organizations, political groups, and government agencies to help form legislation for policies and practices relating to health care is the responsibility of the individual as a health-care worker, as well as the individual as a citizen.

KEY POINTS

- *Healthy People* is a 10-year report card issued by the USDHHS concerning what has been accomplished in the area of health care in the United States and what is yet to be accomplished.
- *Healthy People 2030* identifies leading health indicators that are of priority concern in health maintenance.
- The *overarching goals* of *Healthy People 2030* are to enable the nation to achieve health equity, to eliminate disparities, and to create social and physical environments that promote good health, quality of life, healthy development, and positive health behaviors across all life stages.
- *Topics* are general categories addressed by *Healthy People 2030*. There are 41 topic areas with 355 related objectives in the current document.
- *Objectives* are statements of movement toward a target, such as "the number of days the air quality index is above 100."
- *Indicators* are high-priority issues that measure progress toward objectives.
- *Determinants of health* are the range of social, economic, and environmental factors that influence the health status, such as genetics, biology, policy, and law.
- *Health status* is measured by statistics, such as birth rates, death rates, and life expectancy.
- Global efforts are necessary to improve health care because problems are no longer confined to local areas.
- The UN Millennium Declaration (updated in 2015) identifies worldwide goals.
- Providing culturally competent health care increases compliance with healthy lifestyles and can help in meeting the goals of *Healthy People 2030*.

Clinical Judgment Case Study

School nurses and health-care workers, working as a team, can contribute to the goals of *Healthy People 2030* by teaching relevant health topics to students. A school nurse or health-care worker is assigned to teach one class to a group of elementary-school children and one class to a group of high-school students. List one topic for each class that would be age appropriate and relevant to the goals of *Healthy People 2030*.

REVIEW QUESTIONS

1. The goals of *Healthy People 2030* include: (select all that apply)
   A. achieving health equity.
   B. removing obstacles to health care.
   C. recommending preventive health care.
   D. increasing research concerning management of common health problems.
   E. improving physical, social and economic environments.

2. Leading health indicators of *Healthy People 2030* list high priority issues for the next 10 years and include: (select all that apply)
   A. improved access to health care.
   B. providing preventative services such as immunizations.

C. encouraging outdoor activities.

D. reducing gun violence and deaths.

E. increasing publications concerning health status of populations.

3. Worldwide health improvement goals are monitored by:

    A. coordinated WHO meetings.

    B. health-care providers.

    C. a National Health Organization system.

    D. the American National Health Association.

4. *Healthy People 2030* is: (select all that apply)

    A. a report card on the progress of health care and identification of priority future needs.

    B. a report of new laws that concern health-care requirements.

C. a list of mandates related to medical practice.

D. a list of health-care facilities that should be available by the year 2030.

E. published by the U.S. Department of Health and Human Services.

5. Health-care workers play an important role in helping to achieve the goals of *Healthy People 2030* by:

    A. treating the poor population who are ill.

    B. promoting breastfeeding and early prenatal care.

    C. agreeing to work overtime to meet patient needs.

    D. working in community-based clinics.

Government Influences on Health Care

http://evolve.elsevier.com/Leifer/growth

OUTLINE

OBJECTIVES

1. Trace the history of government involvement in health care.
2. Analyze health-care legislation and its influence on health-care delivery.
3. List some factors that influence the cost of health care.
4. Describe two types of health-care delivery systems.
5. Discuss current health-care policy issues, including health-care reform.
6. Identify future trends in health care.
7. Discuss the nurse's role in political activity related to health care.

KEY TERMS

accreditation
Federal Register
health maintenance organizations (HMOs)
homeopathy
hydrotherapy
informed consent
managed care organizations (MCOs)

Medicaid
Medicare
nurse practice acts
Nursing Licensure Compact (NLC)
Occupational Safety and Health Act (OSHA)
plan of care
political action committees (PACs)

preferred provider organizations (PPOs)
scope of practice
standards of practice

THE IMPORTANCE OF UNDERSTANDING THE ROLE OF GOVERNMENT IN HEALTH CARE

The government plays a key role in promoting the health and well-being of Americans. Understanding the government's contributions and influences on health care is important (Mason, 2020).

This brief chapter presents a history of government involvement in health care in the United States as well as current and potential future trends. This knowledge allows consumers and health-care workers to have an understanding of and an informed say (vote) in developing new legislation.

HEALTH-CARE LEGISLATION

In the past, monarchs, the church, or people with specific knowledge or expertise made health-care decisions for the entire population of a locality or a country. These decisions evolved into judgments based on individual case decisions. From repeated judgments, laws were developed that became part of a system of rules. In the United States, as time passed, legislative groups or bodies were added to the lawmaking process, and eventually the congressional system was formed. A system of courts and legislative bodies is organized around three levels of government: the federal, state, and local sectors. Most lawmakers are elected by the people to represent the needs of their communities.

Laws originally revolved around individual rights and property rights, but in the nineteenth century, laws concerning health care were developed based on the fundamental principles of health-care leaders such as Hippocrates, Dorothea Dix, Clara Barton, and Florence Nightingale. The efforts of these and other leaders in the field of health care led to the development of standards of practice (https://www.lawinsider.com/dictionary/generally-accepted-standards-of-medical-practice; standards that are based on credible scientific evidence), which were the foundations of laws related to consumer protection.

The first legal health-care issues concerned the definition of health related to the ability of slaves to work. Early court decisions influenced the methods of health-care delivery systems and the providers within these delivery systems. Patient-care problems included infected wounds, trauma care, and care for specific age-related diseases. Most of the caretakers were self-taught, and the health-care needs of most patients were often attended to by family members. As health-care needs increased, and care became more complex, experts were called in for consultation. In 1750, the first hospital for the poor was established in Philadelphia.

HOSPITALS AND NURSING SCHOOLS

In 1873, the Bellevue Hospital School of Nursing was established in New York as a proponent of the Nightingale principles of nursing care. Clara Barton founded the American Red Cross in 1881, which focused on community health needs. In 1887, the Mayo brothers in Minnesota established the concepts of private-office health-care practice and then group clinics. The formation of the American Medical Association and philanthropic organizations, such as the Rockefeller Foundation and the Carnegie Foundation, advocated professional care, and self-care was devalued. By the end of the nineteenth century, three schools of nursing existed in the United States. A group of nurse leaders formed the American Society of Superintendents of Nurse Training Schools, which adopted a nursing code of ethics based on the Nightingale pledge. The structure was similar to the American Medical Association in elevating professional care.

By 1903, licensure by a state government agency was required to practice nursing, and the original Society for Training Schools evolved into the National League for Nursing (NLN). In 1911, school alumnae formed the American Nurses Association (ANA). Gradually the belief that nurses needed higher education and increased theoretical knowledge led to the opening of a program at Columbia University in New York to train teachers of nursing. The founders of this program for nurse educators, Isabelle Hampton Robb and Mary Adelaide Nutting, advocated the professionalism of nursing.

Hospitals gradually became the centers for health care because they had more resources to provide care compared to a private doctor's office. Health centers developed and specialization increased. Specialty service units appeared in hospitals, including medical, surgical, and obstetrical units. One of the earliest pieces of governmental legislation concerning hospitals was the Hill-Burton Hospital Construction Act of 1946, which provided grants to states for the purpose of building new hospitals.

Although nursing as a career flourished with the establishment of the Army Cadet Nursing Corps to care for military personnel, nursing in civilian life did not receive the respect it deserved until later. Most schools of nursing were managed in hospital settings, but in 1965, the ANA advocated that nursing education take place in a college setting, and a respected profession of nursing was reborn. A standardized national competence examination was determined to be a requirement for nursing licensure, and today almost all registered nurses earn their nursing degrees in college institutions.

The federal government provided funds to train vocational nurses who cared for patients in the community setting. Vocational nursing programs were about 13–18 months in length and focused on skills and theory correlated with clinical practice. Today many licensed practical/vocational nurse programs are based in community-college settings. Bachelor's degree programs and beyond are based in university settings with increasing opportunities for blended and distance learning.

THE MULTIDISCIPLINARY HEALTH-CARE TEAM

Health care soon grew into an industry that depended on multidisciplinary providers, such as doctors, nurses, laboratory technicians, radiology technicians, social workers, and others. The goals of the team are to ensure the optimum physical, social, and mental well-being of the patient, and members work together to provide comprehensive care. Communication among team members and the patient is vital. The plan of care was developed as a tool for this communication and can be an individual patient plan of care, a family plan of care, or a hospital care path that outlines the needs of the patient and the planned approach to meet these needs.

Standards of care provided by nurses and other members of the multidisciplinary team were developed by professional organizations to ensure quality care for patients.

NURSE PRACTICE ACTS

States have government-established nurse practice acts, which define the scope of practice for nurses within that state. The scope of practice is the identification of and legal limitations to the usual and customary skills practiced by a professional. Usual and customary practices are determined by the educational preparation for that profession. Currently each state has its own nurse practice act with some variations in scope of practice, and nurses are responsible for knowing the nurse practice act(s) of the state(s) in which they practice.

The National Council of State Boards of Nursing has designed a broad model Nurse Practice Act that serves as a multistate licensing arrangement (i.e., the Nursing Licensure Compact [NLC]), which enables traveling nurses to function in multiple states (NCSBN, 2020). As of 2020, there were 34 states in which nurses could hold multistate licenses without additional application procedures or fees and nine additional states are pending. The mobility of nurses, the growth of traveling-nurse programs, and the use of Internet services have led to the need for interstate licensing of nurses.

PATIENT'S BILL OF RIGHTS

The President's Advisory Commission on Consumer Protection and Quality in the Health Care Industry adopted a Consumer Bill of Rights and Responsibilities in 2009. This report stressed the importance of the relationship between the health-care provider and the patient and stipulated that the health-care system:

- Is fair and meets patients' needs.
- Gives patients a way to address problems.
- Encourages patients to take active roles in health care.

The key areas in the Consumer Bill of Rights include the rights of the consumer to:

- Have choice of providers.
- Have access to emergency services.
- Take part in treatment decisions.
- Receive respect and nondiscrimination.
- Maintain confidentiality of health-care information.
- Have resources for complaint and appeal.

Minnesota was the first state to establish a Bill of Rights for Patients as a state law in 1973, and the American Hospital Association (AHA) updated *The Patient Care Partnership: Understanding Expectations, Rights, and Responsibilities* in 2003 (Box 2.1). One of the most important rights of patients is the right of informed consent, and the nurse is responsible to sign as a witness that a patient has received information regarding risks, advantages, and alternatives available for a planned procedure in a language that can be understood by the patient.

The U.S. government mandates provision of health-care services to physically handicapped persons, mentally handicapped persons, and pregnant women. These rights must be upheld if the hospital is to remain accredited or approved. Updates to patient's rights under the Affordable Care Act of 2010 ensure insurance coverage for preexisting conditions (CMS, 2010). Accreditation is the process by which an institution is recognized as meeting specific predetermined standards of care. Although the government does not accredit hospitals, a hospital that is not accredited by any group may not be eligible to receive state or federal funding assistance. The Joint Commission adopted criteria for hospitals for the pursuit of accreditation (Box 2.2). Many of these criteria are assessed when the hospital seeks accreditation by various accrediting groups.

BOX 2.1   The Patient Care Partnership: Understanding Expectations, Rights, and Responsibilities

When you need hospital care, your doctor and the nurses and other professionals at our hospital are committed to working with you and your family to meet your health-care needs. Our dedicated doctors and staff serve the community in all its ethnic, religious, and economic diversity. Our goal is for you and your family to have the same care and attention we would want for our families and ourselves.

The sections explain some of the basics about how you can expect to be treated during your hospital stay. They also cover what we will need from you to care for you better. If you have questions at any time, please ask them. Unasked or unanswered questions can add to the stress of being in the hospital. Your comfort and confidence in your care are very important to us.

WHAT TO EXPECT DURING YOUR HOSPITAL STAY

High-Quality Hospital Care

Our first priority is to provide you the care you need, when you need it, with skill, compassion, and respect. Tell your caregivers if you have concerns about your care or if you have pain. You have the right to know the identity of doctors, nurses, and others involved in your care, and you have the right to know when they are students, residents, or other trainees.

A Clean and Safe Environment

Our hospital works hard to keep you safe. We use special policies and procedures to avoid mistakes in your care and keep you free from abuse or neglect. If anything unexpected and significant happens during your hospital stay, you will be told what happened, and any resulting changes in your care will be discussed with you.

Involvement in Your Care

You and your doctor often make decisions about your care before you go to the hospital. Other times, especially in emergencies, those decisions are made during your hospital stay. When decision-making takes place, it should include:

Discussing Your Medical Condition and Information About Medically Appropriate Treatment Choices. To make informed decisions with your doctor, you need to understand:

- The benefits and risks of each treatment
- Whether your treatment is experimental or part of a research study
- What you can reasonably expect from your treatment and any long-term effects it might have on your quality of life
- What you and your family will need to do after you leave the hospital
- The financial consequences of using uncovered services or out-of-network providers
  Please tell your caregivers if you need more information about treatment choices.

Discussing Your Treatment Plan. When you enter the hospital, you sign a general consent to treatment. In some cases, such as surgery or experimental treatment, you may be asked to confirm in writing that you understand what is planned and agree to it. This process protects your right to consent to or refuse a treatment. Your doctor will explain the medical consequences of refusing recommended treatment. It also protects your right to decide if you want to participate in a research study.

Getting Information From You. Your caregivers need complete and correct information about your health and coverage so that they can make good decisions about your care. That includes:

- Past illnesses, surgeries, or hospital stays
- Past allergic reactions
- Any medicines or dietary supplements (such as vitamins and herbs) that you are taking
- Any network or admission requirements under your health plan

Understanding Your Health-Care Goals and Values. You may have health-care goals and values or spiritual beliefs that are important to your well-being. They will be taken into account as much as possible throughout your hospital stay. Make sure your doctor, your family, and your care team know your wishes.

Understanding Who Should Make Decisions When You Cannot. If you have signed a health-care power of attorney stating who should speak for you if you become unable to make health-care decisions for yourself, or a "living will" or "advance directive" that states your wishes about end-of-life care, give copies to your doctor, your family, and your care team. If you or your family need help making difficult decisions, counselors, chaplains, and others are available to help.

Protection of Your Privacy

We respect the confidentiality of your relationship with your doctor and other caregivers, and the sensitive information about your health and health care that are part of that relationship. State and federal laws and hospital operating policies protect the privacy of your medical information. You will receive a Notice of Privacy Practices that describes the ways that we use, disclose, and safeguard patient information and that explains how you can obtain a copy of information from our records about your care.

Help When Leaving the Hospital

Your doctor works with hospital staff and professionals in your community. You and your family also play an important role in your care. The success of your treatment often depends on your efforts to follow medication, diet, and therapy plans. Your family may need to help care for you at home.

You can expect us to help you identify sources of follow-up care and to let you know if our hospital has a financial interest in any referrals. As long as you agree that we can share information about your care with them, we will coordinate our activities with your caregivers outside the hospital. You can also expect to receive information and, when possible, training about the self-care you will need when you go home.

Help With Your Bill and Filing Insurance Claims

Our staff will file claims for you with health-care insurers or other programs such as Medicare and Medicaid. They also will help your doctor with needed documentation. Hospital bills and insurance coverage are often confusing. If you have questions about your bill, contact our business office. If you need help understanding your insurance coverage or health-care plan, start with your insurance company or health benefits manager. If you do not have health-care coverage, we will try to help you and your family find financial help or make other arrangements. We need your help with collecting needed information and other requirements to obtain coverage or assistance.

From the American Hospital Association. (2003). *The patient care partnership. Understanding expectations, rights, and responsibilities.* All rights reserved.

BOX 2.2   Joint Commission Criteria for Hospitals in Pursuit of Accreditation

Infection Prevention and Control – To develop and maintain practices that cover a wide range of infection control situations to reduce health-care associated infections.

Medication Management – Address a well-planned and implemented medication management system including selection and procurement, storage, ordering, preparation and dispensing, administration, and monitoring to reduce medication errors.

Provision of Care, Treatment, and Services – Includes assessment of patient needs, care planning, and providing and coordinating care.

Rights and Responsibilities of the Individual – Includes informing patients of their rights; helping patients understand and exercise their rights; respecting patients' values, beliefs, and preferences; and informing patients of their responsibilities regarding their care, treatment, and services.

Management of the Environment of Care – Promotes a safe, functional, and supportive environment within the hospital so that quality and safety are preserved. Encompasses the building and how its contents are arranged, equipment used to support patients and the people entering the building.

Emergency Management – Includes standards to allow hospitals to plan to respond to the effects of a wide range of potential emergencies.

Human Resources – Standards to verify staff qualifications, orientation, and provision of training.

Management of Information – Address how the hospital obtains, manages, and uses information to provide, coordinate, and integrate services.

Leadership – Address leadership structure, relationships, hospital culture and system performance, and operations.

Life Safety – Address construction and operational conditions to minimize fire hazards and provide systems in case of emergency.

Medical Staff – Structure for self-governing medical staff, licensed independent practitioners, and other medical staff personnel.

Nursing – Address nursing direction, guidelines for delivery of care, and providing nursing services.

Performance Improvement – Standards for measuring performance of care delivery processes and use of data to make improvements.

Record of Care, Treatment, and Services – Comprehensive sets of requirements for medical record contents, policies and procedures that structure the compilations, authentication, retention, and release of records.

Modified from The Joint Commission (2013). *Accreditation guide for hospitals.* Retrieved May 9, 2020, from https://www.jointcommission.org/-/media/deprecated-unorganized/imported-assets/tjc/system-folders/assetmanager/accreditation_guide_hospitals_2011pdf.pdf?db=web&hash=350D19DE3CEF201A9C270B07B7D0FBCD.

THE GOVERNMENT'S ROLE IN HEALTH CARE

The Constitution of the United States, Article 1, section 8, states that a role of the federal government is to provide for the general welfare of the people and provides the spending power to do so. Therefore, the government can act to protect the health, welfare, and safety of the people. For example, to protect the health of the community, state laws require specific immunizations for school children before they are allowed to enter school, although some exemptions are allowed (CDC, 2015).

The involvement of government in health care began gradually. The Children's Bureau, established in 1912, studied the needs of children, established agencies to provide services (e.g., Woman, Infants, and Children program [WIC]), and defined essential community health and nursing responsibilities. The Sheppard-Towner Act of 1921 influenced social welfare policies. President Roosevelt's New Deal, designed to revive the country from the Great Depression, provided government spending for health care. The National Insurance Plan proposed by Mayor Wagner of New York, combined with the passage of the Social Security Act of 1935, were the sparks that ignited expanded government involvement in public health care. In 1937, the Unemployment Compensation and Old Age Benefit laws were passed.

U.S. Department of Health and Human Services

Originally established in 1939 as the Federal Security Agency, the U.S. Department of Health and Human Services (USDHHS) was renamed in 1980. *Healthy People*, published by the USDHHS, is considered by many to be the most important document concerning health in the United States today (see Chapter 1). Under the guidance of this department, the three levels of government (local, state, and federal) provide direct services, financing, information, and setting of policy.

Direct Services

Direct services include providing health care to Native Americans, military personnel and their families, and prisoners. It is also concerned with managing screening clinics for diseases, such as tuberculosis, and managing immunization clinics for children.

Financing

The government funds health education programs and finances health care through Medicare, Medicaid, and Social Security programs (Box 2.3). The government also provides grants for medical and nursing research and education.

Information

Government agencies, such as the National Institutes of Health (NIH) and the Centers for Disease Control and Prevention (CDC), write periodic reports concerning vital statistics, census data, and results of health surveys. Information is published in *Health, United States,* an annual report that provides a snapshot of the health status of U.S. residents.

BOX 2.3   Medicare and Medicaid

Medicare is a type of insurance program in which benefits are received after contributions are made through payroll deductions.

Medicaid is similar to a welfare program in which benefits are provided on a basis of need or poverty.

These programs determine physicians' fees using a complicated formula.

Many services may not be covered or may require a copayment at the time services are rendered.

Policy Setting

Most health-care legislation in the United States is delegated to the USDHHS, although specialties such as environmental health or occupational health may have separate agencies to focus on those specific areas. The Public Health Service sector of the USDHHS, which oversees the health care of U.S. citizens, has a Bureau of Professions responsible for the Division of Nursing, Division of Dentistry, Division of Medicine, and so on.

Federal legislation concerning health care (Table 2.1) is recorded and published in the Federal Register. Revisions of various regulations are based on research findings and public input, and periodic hearings are held. When a law is passed, monitoring of the private sector for compliance occurs.

TABLE 2.1	Examples of Federal Legislation Related to Health Care
1798	The Marine Hospital Service Act provided medical care to merchant marines (eventually became U.S. Public Health Service).
1878	The Port Quarantine Act prevented people with infectious diseases from entering the United States.
1879	A National Health Department was established.
1901	The Pure Food and Drug Act monitored the manufacture, labeling, and sale of food and drugs (later became the Food and Drug Administration [FDA]).
1912	The Children's Health Bureau established and implemented child labor laws. The bureau meets every 10 years to focus on children's needs.
1921	The Sheppard-Towner Maternity-Infant Care Act provided funds for health and welfare of mothers and children.
1935	The Social Security Act passed Title VI to assist states in providing public health services. Enabled development of Medicare and Medicaid programs.
1939	The Federal Security Agency combined health, education, and welfare services.
1940	The Communicable Disease Center (now known as the Centers for Disease Control and Prevention [CDC]) was established in Atlanta, Georgia.
	The Nurse Training Act provided funds to encourage nursing education.
1944	The Public Health Act consolidated public health legislation into one law.
1945	The McCarran-Ferguson Act gave state governments the right to regulate health insurance plans.
1946	The Hill-Burton Act provided for new hospital construction with provisions for care of the uninsured.
1947	The Army Nurse Corps was established.
1948	The National Institutes of Health (NIH) was established.
1954	The Taft Sanitary Engineering Center was established to improve environmental health.
1955	The U.S. Medical Library was formed to provide access to medical literature.
1964	A health amendment provided increased funds for nursing education.

(Continued)

TABLE 2.1   Examples of Federal Legislation Related to Health Care (*Cont.*)

1965	The Title VIII Social Security Amendment created Medicare to care for older adults and the disabled. Title XIX provided access to health care for the poor via Medicaid.
1970	The Occupational Safety and Health Act (OSHA) focused on workplace and environmental health.
1971	The Environmental Protection Agency was formed to monitor all environmental programs.
1972	The National Security Act was amended to encourage health maintenance organizations (HMOs) and preferred provider organizations (PPOs) to manage health care. Provided grants for HMO development.
1973	The Health Maintenance Organization Act required employers to offer federally qualified HMO coverage for employees and mandated state supervision.
1980	Infant Formula Act required standards for the manufacture of infant formulas.
1981	The Omnibus Budget Reconciliation Act provided money for grants for various health promotion projects, such as nursing homes, skilled nursing facilities, and home health agencies.
1982	The Tax Equity Fiscal Responsibility Act (TEFRA) amended the Social Security Act establishing the diagnosis-related group (DRG) system, which changed health care radically by establishing strict rules for reimbursement.
1985	The Consolidated Omnibus Reconciliation Act (COBRA) ensured continuation of health insurance for a time after loss of coverage due to job termination.
1989	Reimbursement of nurse practitioners for care provided was approved.
1990	The Health Objectives Planning Act resulted from the 1979 *Healthy People* report, which identified and monitored the nation's health-care goals. Established *Healthy People 2000* and *Healthy People 2010*.
1996	The Health Insurance Portability and Accountability Act (HIPAA) enabled portability of health insurance, privacy of medical information, and coverage for preexisting conditions.
1997	The Welfare Reform Act regulated restrictions for Aid to Families with Dependent Children (AFDC).
2002	Laws prohibit smoking in some public buildings.
	The use of mercury alloys in dental amalgam for certain patients and the use of mercury in medical devices such as blood pressure machines were prohibited.
	Asbestos abatement programs for school buildings were created.
	Lead and chemical poisoning prevention and screening programs were established.
	The Homeland Security Act addressed the public health and safety of the nation in the event of a terrorist attack.

TABLE 2.1   Examples of Federal Legislation Related to Health Care (*Cont.*)

2003	HIPAA regulations were enforced nationwide.
2005	Public Readiness and Emergency Preparedness Act (PREPA) encouraged rapid production of vaccines to protect Americans in case of a public health emergency threat.
	Patient Safety and Quality Improvement Act (PQIA) encourages reporting to a database to monitor adverse events, near misses, and dangerous conditions.
2006	After a White House conference on aging, the Older American Act of 2006 was passed to provide services to the elderly and was extended in 2020.
2009	Health-Care Recovery and Reinvestment Act. A stimulus package provides for adoption of health information technology, confidentiality of health-care records, and provides new funding for Medicaid and health care for the poor. Promotes prevention and wellness initiatives and provides for medical research.
	Family Smoking Prevention and Tobacco Control Act. Passed in 1990, authorized the FDA to regulate the manufacture, marketing, and distribution of tobacco products, including Bidid, Ktetek, and will include electronic cigarettes, smokeless tobacco, and Hookah. It also prohibits distribution of samples and sponsorship by tobacco companies of school, athletic, or social events. It also prohibits sale of tobacco products in community vending machines (Chen, 2011).
2010	Patient Protection and Affordable Care Act. Extended health-care coverage to 32 million Americans who would otherwise have been uninsured. Medicare payroll taxes were slated to pay for services. Set limits on insurance companies' power to deny coverage to individuals and families.
2017	American Health Care Act repeals and replaces several major items of the Affordable Care Act (AMA, 2017).

Although an individual U.S. citizen has the right to privacy and freedom, a federal law can mandate quarantine if it is deemed necessary to protect the health or welfare of individuals in a community, as was experienced in 2020 with the novel corona virus disease 2019 (COVID-19) pandemic. State laws can also mandate specific health-related actions. For example, some states require all college students to be covered by health insurance, which may be paid for by student fees.

Occupational health is regulated by the federal Occupational Safety and Health Act (OSHA), which requires standards of safety be maintained by employers to protect the health and safety of employees and mandates the reporting of injuries sustained by workers. Workers have the right to know if they are working in a toxic environment. Workers injured on the job also have the right to receive health care and financial compensation for any life-altering injury that occurs while on the job. State laws license and certify home care and hospice facilities and can also regulate, to some extent, insurance companies and labor unions.

Some federal laws can affect the social development of young adults. For example, 18- to 25-year-old men must register with Selective Service. In the event of a crisis requiring a military draft, these men may be called into active service in a sequence based on a random lottery number and the date of birth. Both federal and local laws regulate the age at which one can drink alcohol, drive a car, and work.

The government also defines the age at which senior citizens are eligible for Social Security benefits. Benefits can be accessed as early as age 62, but amounts will be reduced until the full retirement age is reached, which is dependent on the retiree's year of birth (SSA, 2020).

There are also governmental influences on the family, including tough divorce laws in some states and lenient divorce laws in other states. Most states currently have lenient abortion laws and favor the concept of giving custody of children to the biological parent whenever possible in an effort to provide caregivers who will consistently meet the developmental needs of children.

THE RISING COSTS OF HEALTH CARE

Health-Care Delivery Systems

The cost of health care in the United States has steadily increased in recent history and continues to rise. Public health benefits (Medicare and Medicaid) were introduced, but increasing costs threaten their survival. Maintaining quality care while ensuring cost containment is a major challenge in health care today. Cost controls involve addressing issues such as national health goals, entitlements, the right to health care, use of available resources, prescription medication costs, and identification of the changing health-care needs of the people.

The National Committee for Quality Assurance was established to review and accredit managed care organizations (MCOs), which attempt to standardize and control costs of health care. Health maintenance organizations (HMOs) provide care for prepaid members, and preferred provider organizations (PPOs) contract with professionals to provide care to a specific group of patients at an agreed-on fee-for-service rate. Savings realized from government-sponsored health-care programs could be used for other government-sponsored programs or to help reduce the federal budget deficit; therefore, the costs of health care are of interest to all people in the United States.

Private Health Insurance

Increasing health-care costs have also led to higher premiums for membership in private health-care insurance plans. Part of the health insurance costs may be the responsibility of employers who then recoup their costs by increasing the cost of their consumer product, which in turn may raise the cost of living.

 Health Promotion

Prevention and early intervention seem to be the keys to reducing health-care costs and are the core of *Healthy People 2030* (see Chapter 1). The Human Genome Project (see Chapter 6) gives health-care providers the potential to predict, detect, and treat illnesses before they become expensive, chronic problems. The information gained from this project may be used effectively in the future to decrease the occurrence of chronic health-care problems.

Health-Care Reform

Historically, people in the United States oppose the government becoming involved in health-care programs and generally resist "socialized" medicine. Any effort to reform health care must involve managing costs, promoting access, and identifying payors. However, the potential for rationing care and limiting coverage for specific problems are two of consumers' major worries regarding the future of health care. Health-care reform has become a major political issue, and laws and policies passed by one political party may be overturned when another is elected into power.

Resurgence of Self-Care

The focus on illness prevention and early detection and intervention increasingly leads health-care delivery from inpatient to outpatient care settings where education can help to increase healthy behaviors and prevent illness. Self-care is a valuable adjunct to health-care reform, as the focus of health care continues to shift from treatment to prevention of illness and from hospital-centered to community-based care. Self-care is not a new concept. Midwives and lay practitioners were popular in the eighteenth and nineteenth centuries. In the 1830s and 1840s, the interest in self-care peaked, and hydrotherapy (therapy using water) and homeopathy (the use of minute portions of naturally occurring chemicals for their healing powers) flourished.

In 1959, Dorothy Orem developed the self-care model related to nursing practice. In the 1960s, Martha Rogers, a nursing theorist, proposed a holistic view of health care, and in 1989 another theorist, Jean Watson, focused on the value of the nurse-patient relationship in the promotion of health. Today the desire of the individual to have control over their body has resulted in a resurgence of self-care. Many health-care organizations, such as Kaiser Permanente Foundation Health Plan, distribute self-care guides to all members. Self-care, nutrition, and exercise classes are all readily available and are in popular use.

Complementary and alternative medicine (CAM) is practiced by individuals in the community, and many applications have been successfully adopted in traditional care settings (Schiff, 2019). Health-care agencies depend on self-care education to promote health and prevent disease because it is an effective cost-containment technique. Outreach programs target local populations for screening and education based on needs assessments of the community. Providing safe environments in educational institutions and including self-care health concepts in school curricula are essential elements of modern health-care reform. Nursing education programs are increasing students' experiences with healthy individuals in community-based settings. Culturally competent care of a diverse population is being integrated into medical and nursing school programs. Occupational health programs, in the form of supporting employee health, and websites for dissemination of health-care information are also important to the future of health care.

GLOBAL HEALTH

In 1945, the United Nations (UN) was formed by the joining of many nations for the promotion of common goals, including human rights, peace, and the economic and social advancement of all people. The UN headquarters is located in New York City and meets annually with the World Health Organization (WHO), which was created in 1946 to establish worldwide policies and services to promote health and health research (see Chapter 1).

THE FUTURE OF HEALTH CARE

Federal legislation and funding serve to increase the involvement of government in health care. The increasing health-care costs, the increasing need for health care, and the growth of various health-care delivery systems have also resulted in the need for continued federal intervention. Public health programs have the potential for improving health and reducing health-care costs through the early detection of and the intervention in diseases. Government agencies provide vital statistics that aid in identifying areas of need and in developing intervention strategies.

Political influence is promoted by political action committees (PACs). PACs influence legislation by offering monetary contributions to legislators who support their needs and by providing lobbying efforts to create an awareness of needed legislation. The ANA and other medical organizations have PACs to represent the needs of nurses and patients. Many nurses serve as elected public officials, and nurse legislators help in interpreting health-care issues.

Nurses play a key role in the future of health care by supporting and educating patients; providing cost-effective, quality care; and becoming involved in the legislative decisions of local, state, and federal governments. Nurses realize that the role of government related to health care influences the delivery of health care. For that reason, nurses need to be active in the political arena to ensure that the needs of nurses and patients are considered when discussing, creating, and passing laws related to health care.

KEY POINTS

- The role of the government in health care was established in Article 1, section 8, of the U.S. Constitution, which provides spending power to promote the general health, welfare, and safety of the United States. Individual State laws often expand and fund health care of the populace. Standards of health-care practice are the foundation of health-care legislation.
- The Hill-Burton Hospital Construction Act of 1946 provided funding to build new hospitals.
- The Army Cadet Nurse Corps was established to care for military personnel, and nursing as a career began to flourish.
- The multidisciplinary health-care team includes doctors, nurses, lab technicians, radiology technicians, social workers, and others.
- Local governments established guidelines for nursing practice that defined the scope of practice for each level of professional nursing.
- Thirty-four states participate in the NLC multistate nurse licensing partnership.
- Minnesota was the first state to establish the Patient's Bill of Rights as law.
- A hospital that is not accredited may not be eligible to receive state or federal funding assistance.
- The Social Security Act of 1935 expanded government involvement in public health care.
- The Department of Health and Human Services of the federal government

provides direct services, information, and health-care legislation.

- The United Nations meets annually with the World Health Organization to establish worldwide health policies, services, and research.
- Federal legislation that is passed is published in the Federal Register.
- Occupational health is regulated by the Occupational Safety and Health Association (OSHA), which sets standards of health and safety in the workplace.

- The federal government provides legislation and funding to support the goals of *Healthy People 2030*.
- Political influence is promoted by political action committees (PACs), in which nurses can advocate for patient needs and interpret health-care issues.
- The Patient Protection and Affordable Care Act of 2010 addressed the problem of accessibility of health care for all Americans but was revised in 2017 by the administration elected by the people.

Clinical Judgment Case Study

Nurses and other health-care workers may have the opportunity to join political action committees to assist in increasing awareness of the need for health-related legislation. Discuss one topic currently relevant to health-care reform that this committee might promote.

REVIEW QUESTIONS

1. Match the following agencies on the left with their primary functions described on the right:

Agency	Function
Managed Care Organization (MCO)	A. controls the cost of health care.
Health Maintenance Organization (HMO)	B. provides care for prepaid members.
Preferred Provider Organization (PPO)	C. provides care to a specialized group for a fee-for-service-rate.

2. The "Plan of Care" for a multidisciplinary health-care team is: (select all that apply)

A. a tool for communication between health-care providers concerning a patient/client/family.

B. a description of standards of care for a client.

C. identification of health-care providers for a client/patient.

D. a compilation of goals or needs of a client and planned approach to meet those goals.

3. Which of the following is true of the Nurse Practice Act: (select all that apply)

A. defines the scope of practice for a nurse nationwide.

B. defines the scope of practice of a nurse within one state.

C. may include a multistate licensing agreement.

D. defines the functions and limitations of nursing actions.

E. includes patient's bill of rights.

4. The functions of the U.S. Department of Health and Human Services (USDHHS) include: (select all that apply)

A. operating clinics for poor/indigent patients.

B. writing most health-care legislation.

C. overseeing *Health People 2030* document.

D. establishing criteria for hospital excellence.

E. overseeing licensing for most health-care professionals.

5. Political action committees (PACs) influence health care by:

A. writing health-care laws.

B. supporting legislators who vote on health-care policies.

C. studying the needs of local communities.

D. promoting higher salaries for nurses.

Cultural Considerations Across the Lifespan and in Health and Illness

http://evolve.elsevier.com/Leifer/growth

OBJECTIVES

1. Define culture and its expression.
2. Describe the difference between beliefs and values.
3. Identify various beliefs and values in today's adult population.
4. Discuss the relevance of culture and personal values to everyday life and healthy behaviors.
5. Explain the relationship of culture and values to health-promotion teaching.
6. Define complementary and alternative therapies.
7. Discuss the role of the government in promoting culturally competent health care.

KEY TERMS

acculturation
alternative medicine
beliefs
complementary medicine
cultural awareness
cultural care

cultural competence
cultural interventions
cultural sensitivity
cultural stereotyping
culture
ethnicity

ethnocentric
stereotyping
values

Cultural aspects of growth and development for each phase of the life cycle are integrated in the specific chapters later in this text. This chapter is designed to provide some specific illustrations of how being sensitive to the cultural needs of others can improve health-promotion services and outcomes, enhance cost-effectiveness of health care, reduce errors, and increase compliance to healthy behaviors, which will aid in achieving the goals of *Healthy People 2030*.

DEFINITION

Culture is defined as a set of learned values, beliefs, customs, and behaviors that is shared by a common social group and is passed down through generations of family. Culture can influence food choices, parenting styles, and preferences for treatment measures. Health-care workers can demonstrate cultural sensitivity by observing and demonstrating knowledge of culturally appropriate verbal language, body language, use of personal space, and gestures of respect toward family members. Religion is closely related to culture, and religiously appropriate interventions should be integrated sensitively to meet the spiritual needs of patients and their families. An individual person's culture involves dynamic, ever-changing, active or passive elements. An individual's cultural values are unique, developed over time, and guide actions and behaviors that influence self-worth, self-esteem, and life and health decisions. It is increasingly common for younger individuals to identify to various degrees with more than one culture; therefore, cultural sensitivity and awareness is an essential ingredient for effective health care.

Cultural competence is the awareness of, acceptance of, and respect for beliefs, values, traditions, and practice that are different from one's own. The ability to adapt health care so that it does not violate the culture or religion of the patient is at the core of cultural competence.

Cultural competence can assist the health-care worker in devising meaningful interventions to promote optimal health-care practices. The health-care worker must understand that each individual is culturally unique and there is cultural diversity within cultural and racial groups as well as across cultural groups. This chapter provides a suggestion of baseline data relative to specific non-Western cultural groups as a starting point of developing a culturally competent plan of care for an individual patient. Culturally competent care involves assessing six "essential cultural phenomena" (Giger, 2020) that are present in all cultural groups but vary in application across cultures. These six phenomena are outlined in Box 3.1.

The assumption that all people of one culture behave the same way and believe the same thing is called cultural stereotyping, which can be offensive and become a barrier to providing competent care. It is particularly important to be sensitive to individual differences when working with a diverse population.

The United States is a multicultural society. In 2010, approximately 72% of the population was of White/European descent, with 14% African American, 17% Hispanic

---

BOX 3.1 Some Essential Phenomena Present in All Cultural Groups

Communication: such as use of nonverbal/verbal responses.
Touch: such as accepts or stiffens at touch.
Space: such as distance preferred when talking.
Social organization: such as marital status, role in family, work.
Time: such as past, future, or present orientation; importance of timelines.
Environmental control: such as self-control, religion, visitors, room temperature.

Data from Giger, J., & Davidhizar, R. (2002). Transcultural nursing assessment, *International Nursing Review 37(1)*, 199–203.

American, and approximately 5% Asian American, but these statistics are changing (U.S. Department Commerce, Bureau of Census American Community Survey, 2017). It is projected that by the year 2050, the biggest changes will be seen in the White/European population as it decreases to 47%, and Hispanic Americans will increase to 29% (United Nations, 2019). As future generations are born and raised within the Western culture, it will be more difficult to identify a particular race, religion, or culture with pure predictable beliefs. This evolving society will require health-care workers to assess more carefully the response of a patient with a diagnosis such as diabetes mellitus that requires lifestyle changes, and guide those changes in a way that is acceptable to their individual and cultural beliefs.

Beliefs are cultural teachings of practices and values that are handed down for generations and determine how one behaves and responds to daily life and health-care practices. Values are deep feelings about what is right or wrong, good, or bad. Most personal values are learned in childhood and are well established by 10 years of age (Wold, 2008). Values are influenced by culture, and some behaviors that may be valued and encouraged by Western culture may be discouraged by another culture.

Ethnicity is a cultural pattern shared by people with the same cultural heritage. Language, preferred diet, specific customs, family roles, and religious beliefs are often shared among those with the same ethnicity. Cultural awareness involves recognizing the history of patients' ancestry or culture and how their customs influence the handling of problems, issues, or teachings. Health-care workers must be careful not to be ethnocentric, evaluating other peoples and cultures according to the standards of one's own culture, or believing their culture, beliefs, and values to be superior to others. Health-care workers must apply the patients' cultural beliefs, values, and practices to each situation when planning care and health-promotion activities but should avoid stereotyping or making assumptions. Often, acculturation, the adjustment to a new culture, results in differences in practice within the same cultural group. Cultural assessments should be completed on all patients as they enter the health-care system in order to affect a positive outcome.

Cultural care consists of health-promotion activities initiated by a culturally competent health-care worker who enables a patient to modify health behaviors toward beneficial outcomes while respecting the patient's cultural values, beliefs, and practices (Cherry, 2019; Giger, 2020). Cultural interventions are achieved when health-care information is presented in a way that includes specific cultural styles, colors, pictures, symbols, and so forth, which add credibility to the content by reflecting cultural values. Health-care information should be presented in the language of the recipient, using interpreters whenever necessary.

It is important that the patient's traditional practices be incorporated into the care plan as much as possible. For example, a woman who refuses to eat or take oral medication after giving birth may have been offered what she perceived of as an inappropriate beverage or a beverage with an inappropriate temperature with her oral medication. In this example, the care provided conflicted with the woman's cultural practices. However, offering choices such as hot soup or room-temperature water with or without ice with her medications easily solves the problem. A cultural assessment upon admission to the unit should include questions related to these preferences to enable the health-care provider to adapt the plan of care, rather than assuming a specific cultural practice is always preferred. See Table 3.1 for sample questions.

TABLE 3.1   Sample Questions to Ask Related to Cultural Sensitivity

Topic	Sample Questions for Assessment
Diet	*Water:* Do you prefer ice-water or water at room temperature? *Food*: Do you have a personal diet preference or restriction?
Family organization	Who in the family or community would you prefer to participate in discussion of your health problem, plan of care, and recovery options?
Preferred method of communication	Would you prefer a translator to help explain your health problem, and plan of care? What language and dialect do you feel most comfortable with?
Comprehension of information (Gently ask the patient to reconvey the health-care instructions to assure understanding rather than simply asking if they understand your instructions. Depending on a "nod" or "yes" does not always indicate full understanding/agreeing)	Please tell me in your own words what you need to do to continue your healing. Please show me how you will test your blood sugar.

Note: Asking the right questions is the key to providing a culturally sensitive plan of care. Assumptions concerning beliefs or practices are inappropriate.

CULTURE AND PREGNANCY

The cultural background of the family may strongly influence family members' view of the birth experience. An appropriate approach to determine what the pregnant woman considers normal practice is to ask the following questions:

1. Is pregnancy viewed as a healthy time, a vulnerable time, or an illness?
2. Is the birth process viewed as dangerous?
3. Is birth a public or private experience?
4. What type of help is needed/accepted?
5. What is the expected role of the family?

Many non-Western cultures expect the woman to have at least 20 to 40 days of bed rest after giving birth. Some may avoid full washing of the hair or body until vaginal discharge after birth has ceased, and because some cultures consider pregnancy, labor, and delivery to be "cold" conditions, they may prefer to avoid air-conditioned rooms and cold fluids. In some cultures, women discard colostrum (first breast milk) and do not eat vegetables during the first week after delivery, which would be important to include in the individual plan of care. In Western culture, the baby is the focus of gift giving following birth, whereas in many non-Western cultures, the mother is the focus of attention (Giger, 2020).

CULTURE AND THE NEWBORN

The newborn establishes social interactions with parents and is not a "blank slate" at birth. The newborn has the ability to perceive, respond to, and communicate with his or her parents, and the ability of the parents to respond to infant cues is essential for successful relationships to develop. Culture can influence patterns of parent-infant interaction and the developing expression of infant behavior.

CULTURE AND THE CHILD

Cultural practices can influence the timing of developmental stages. For example, the development of initiative may be later for children in families that practice an authoritarian style of parenting, because these families place great value on obedience and conformity in children.

CULTURE AND THE ADOLESCENT

Independence in adolescents is not valued equally by all cultures. Some cultures, for example, do not recognize adolescence as a period of development, so have no word for adolescence in their language. Adolescents understand abstract thinking, and traditional religious practices and symbols can help stabilize the adolescent's developing identity. Many cultures practice specific rituals that recognize passage of the individual from childhood to adulthood. These practices can be symbolic rituals or celebrations, such as a bar mitzvah, or a quinceanera, or can be an actual test that demonstrates mastery of specific survival skills to determine that the adolescent is ready to take on adult responsibilities. Adolescents or young adults often promote unique changes in styles, thoughts, and practices that can collide with their traditional family values and beliefs. Changes in taste for music, clothing styles, and use of social media influence living styles, and often the changes in practices for the younger age group may be quite different from their previous generation's cultural background. These evolving preferences can be either embraced by the family or rejected as a form of rebellion. The changes may be short-lived, or they may persist and affect the following generation's practices and values.

CULTURE AND THE ADULT

In some cultures or religions, women are considered to be in a state of impurity during menstruation and after giving birth. Deeply religious husbands in some religions may not touch their wives during these times. Health-care workers can inquire about and be sensitive to this practice and can provide physical assistance when needed.

In some religions, birth control is discouraged or barred, allowing only natural family planning, using abstinence as the technique of choice. In some cases, health care is performed within a spiritual framework, and adherents may decline preventive medicines, although some required immunizations or personal birth-control drugs may be accepted.

Different cultures place different emphases on women's experiences of menopause. In cultures where age is revered, menopause may be inconsequential. In Western culture where a high value is placed on youth, sex appeal, and physical beauty, menopause and related body changes may challenge feelings of self-worth.

CULTURE AND THE OLDER ADULT

A positive attitude toward life and health is encouraged for older adults in most cultures. Most cultures look to elders as a source of wisdom, and often elders play a major role in raising or disciplining grandchildren. In many cultures, elders are also welcomed as the preferred babysitters and parenting consultants. Many older patients who are confined to wheelchairs or nursing homes may have limited contact with family but may place a high value on any available assistance in accessing family contact.

CULTURE AND HEALTH BELIEFS

Many non-Western cultures believe that balances between hot and cold affect health and illness. This belief is known as the humoral theory in which traditional cold remedies treat hot diseases and hot remedies treat cold diseases. This parallels the idea of the forces of Yang (light, heat, or dryness) and Yin (darkness, cold, or wetness). These forces are believed to influence the balance and harmony of a person's state of health. "Cold illnesses" or conditions include pregnancy, earache, chest pain, paralysis, gastrointestinal diseases, rheumatism, and tuberculosis. These are traditionally treated with hot (Yang) foods such as meat, eggs, hot soup, cantaloupe, and fried foods. "Hot illnesses" include dental problems, sore throat, rashes, and kidney disorders and are traditionally treated with cold (Yin) foods such as fruits, vegetables, cold liquid, and beer. Foods are classified as hot or cold according to their effects on the body when metabolized rather than their thermal temperature. There are also cultural elements that define wellness as harmony in body, mind, and spirit. A holistic approach to healing is valued in these cases.

CULTURE AND ILLNESS

Specific holidays may involve some restriction of activity. Electricity, communication, food, and travel may be restricted during these days. During times of culturally restricted behavior, medical appointments or procedures should be postponed if delay is possible without endangering the patient. Shaving can be done with an electric razor if a beard must be removed, but a razor blade is sometimes not allowed to touch the skin.

In some religions, a sacrament is offered to the seriously ill person. To enable this practice, the health-care worker should notify the religious leader, if possible, before the patient loses consciousness. Abstinence from solid food is generally required for a period of time before clergy offers the consecrated host to people receiving communion. Rosary beads or religious medallions may be pinned to the gown or to the bed of the ill person. Patients may request that a religious text be kept at the bedside and that nothing be placed on top of it. Religious jewelry, prayer strings, or sacred undergarments should not be removed from the body unless medically necessary. Some women may insist on wearing head coverings during hospitalization. Persons of some faiths may decline medications, psychotherapy, blood transfusions, or medications containing blood products, due to religious guidelines. However, today there are some alternatives to blood transfusions such as plasma expanders and autologous transfusions.

Some cultural beliefs suggest that illness is the result of sins committed in a previous life or for the atonement of sins in the present life. Time for concentrated meditation (yoga) may be requested or viewed as required for healing. Social behavior consistent with the "sick persons' role" may vary from being demanding to silent passivity depending on the cultural background and other personal variables of the patient. It is therefore important to ask culturally appropriate questions to assess the cultural needs of the patient when developing a plan of care.

CULTURE AND DEATH

The Self-Determination Act of 1991 granted patients in the United States the legal right to full disclosure of medical information to allow individuals to participate in their own care. In some non-Western cultures, information is released to the patient at the discretion of family members. In most Western cultures, a high value is placed on individual life, and so the patient receives all information and decides what to disclose to family members. In many non-Western cultures, the welfare of the family is primary, and life-and-death decisions are made by group approval.

Some cultures believe that dying persons must have someone with them as their soul leaves the body. Traditionally the body is not left alone until burial, which must occur within 24 hours (or as soon as possible) after death. The body is dressed in a shroud, and no metal objects, including nails, may be in the coffin. No flowers are permitted during the funeral or for the 7 days of mourning immediately following. Mirrors are covered, and immediate family may sit on low, hard benches during the mourning period.

Last rites are obligatory for many cultures. Some prefer cremation to burial, or require the body to be placed in a position facing a spiritual center. According to some cultures, persons do not own their bodies, and so cremation, autopsy, and organ donation are prohibited.

A religious leader may place a thread around the neck or waist of the deceased as a blessing before cremation, which may be preferred over burial. Other cultures teach acceptance of the inevitability of death and believe the person's state of mind at the moment of death influences rebirth. In these cases, suicide, violent death, or the death of a child may require special rituals because the state of mind at death may not have been optimal. Some cultures also consider it to be bad luck for a pregnant woman to attend a funeral.

Some people will prefer that a dying person be surrounded by a positive celebratory atmosphere of family and children. Some believe that dying in the home brings bad luck to the house, and therefore prefer that death occur in a hospital and that professionals prepare the body for burial. In other cultures, death with dignity in the home setting is preferred over a hospital setting, because death is considered a spiritual event.

Some cultures suggest a person must be well dressed at the time of death, therefore it is important the health-care worker assess for this belief so they may inform the family if the patient's death is imminent, allowing them to bring the desired clothing to the hospital. In some cultures, internal metal objects, such as plates, bullets, or medical devices, must be removed from the body before burial, and metal objects such as zippers or buttons are prohibited from touching the body after death.

CULTURE AND TEACHING

In the United States, the myriad of cultures creates an opportunity for misunderstandings and misinterpretations of health-care teachings. People from cultures that place a high value on pleasing others may answer questions with information they think others want to hear to maintain a harmonious relationship. To collect accurate data, questions should be phrased in a neutral fashion. People from some cultures consider direct eye contact impolite and may stare at the floor as a symbol of respect which should not be misinterpreted as inattention. Other patients may view extended eye contact as related to the evil eye, which will bring bad luck. Some people believe the head is sacred and therefore must not be touched or patted. Palpating the fontanel of an infant may be interpreted as a disrespectful action unless the medical procedure is properly explained and is accepted by the parents. Many cultures suggest that silence indicates respect for another person, whereas other cultures may interpret silence as agreement with the speaker. Yet other cultures make every effort to fill silent moments with conversation. These factors should be considered, and interpreters used when appropriate. Whenever possible, family members should not be used as interpreters especially when embarrassing or confidential issues are discussed. Online interpreters are generally available when in-person interpreters are unavailable.

CULTURE AND FOOD

Many cultures and religions include specific foods as an integral part of holiday celebrations and may restrict consumption of specific foods. For example, some do not consume alcohol or hot beverages (The Church of Jesus Christ of Latter-Day Saints, n.d.), while some fast on the first Sunday of each month. A culture may prohibit consumption of all meats, only specific meats such as pork, or provide restrictions regarding the preparation of meats. The health-care worker therefore must be aware that some gelatin preparations and medications with a gelatin base might contain pork products. Mixing dairy and meat products at the same meal, or certain types of fish, may be prohibited in some religions. Nutrition is an important part of the care plan for the individual patient, and questions concerning such practices are important to assure compliance to a special dietary prescription.

COMPLEMENTARY AND ALTERNATIVE THERAPIES AND CULTURE

For many years, Western medicine treated and provided medicines and therapy to the patient in the hospital setting, and the patient had little input regarding the plan of care (which was mostly curative rather than preventive). A growing desire for control of one's own body and health-care decisions, and a desire for consideration of family, cultural beliefs, and values, motivated a self-care movement that is bringing health care out of the hospital and into the community and home (Micozzi, 2018). The focus continues to shift to health promotion and maintenance of wellness, and the health-care provider is more often considered a coordinator of care and facilitator for the consumer to choose options that best meet personal needs and cultural values. The emphasis on self-care, health promotion, and disease prevention is clearly reflected in the *Healthy People 2030* goals.

Complementary and alternative medicine (CAM) has become increasingly popular. Alternative medicines are those therapies that are used *instead* of Western medical care. Complementary medicines are those therapies used *together with* Western therapies. Many CAM practices, such as acupressure during labor and the use of antinausea

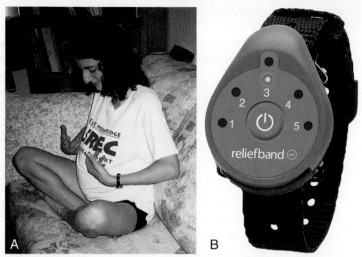

Figure 3.1 (A) Effleurage involves the slow massage of the abdomen in a circular motion using the fingertips to stimulate large-diameter nerve fibers, thus interfering with the transmission of pain sensations. Pressure should be firm enough to avoid a tickling sensation. This form of complementary and alternative medicine (CAM) therapy is used effectively during the active phase of labor. This therapy involves the gate-control theory of pain relief. (B) *Reliefband* is a noninvasive transdermal device cleared by the U.S. Food & Drug Administration (*FDA*) for treatment of pregnancy-induced nausea and vomiting (morning sickness). The device is applied to the ventral side of the wrist where the median nerve is closest to the surface of the skin. It emits a programmed pulse that stimulates the nerve to create electrical signals that travel to the central nervous system to restore normal gastric rhythm. It is a form of CAM therapy involving transcutaneous electrical nerve stimulation. *(Courtesy Reliefband Technologies, www.reliefband,com.)*

bracelets for chemotherapy, have been adopted as valid Western health-care practices (Figure 3.1A and B). Self-care, wellness, and illness prevention are the core aspects of CAM therapy, which considers the whole physiological person as well as social, cultural, and spiritual aspects.

Every patient should be assessed for CAM therapy use because some therapies might interact negatively with medications prescribed during an illness. Some CAM therapies have their roots in "folk medicine" or ancient, time-tested remedies practiced in many countries and passed down through specific cultures. CAM therapies include massage, energy healing, acupuncture and acupressure, reflexology, homeopathy, biofeedback, aromatherapy, guided imagery, herbal remedies, and others.

THE GOVERNMENT'S ROLE IN PROMOTING CULTURALLY COMPETENT CARE

The National Center for Complementary and Integrative Health (NCCIH) is an agency of the National Institutes of Health (NIH) that conducts research on the effectiveness of specific CAM therapies and documents their findings in medical journals. The United States Department of Health and Human Services Office of Minority Health and Cross-Cultural Health Care have a specific Agency for Healthcare Research and Quality (AHRQ) that promotes behaviors and policies related to cultural competence in health care. The U.S.

Office of Minority Health provides information concerning culturally and linguistically (language) appropriate health services (CLAS). One recommended standard of CLAS includes promoting attitudes, behavior, knowledge, and skills necessary to work effectively in a culturally diverse work environment. Culturally competent care can improve communication, enhance education, and aid in achieving the established goals of *Healthy People 2030*. See Appendix A for a multilingual glossary of symptoms for health-care workers to use until an interpreter becomes available.

In 2019, of the 328.2 million residents in the United States, 39.6% of census respondents stated their race was not White alone (U.S. Census Bureau, n.d.). It is predicted that by the year 2055 the United States will not have a single racial or ethnic majority (Pew Research Center, 2016). Culturally diverse (non-White) membership of managed Medicaid programs already has reached 60% (Kaiser Family Foundation, 2013). This trend cannot be ignored, and health-care workers must implement CLAS and provide culturally competent care. Understanding culture as related to health care will:

- Improve services and health-care outcomes.
- Enhance cost-effectiveness of health care.
- Reduce errors caused by misunderstandings.
- Assist in reaching *Healthy People 2030* goals.

Further information concerning cultural practices can be found throughout the text and in the Bibliography.

KEY POINTS

- Culture is defined as patterns of values, beliefs, and practices that are handed down through generations.
- Ethnicity is defined as a cultural pattern shared by a group of families that have a shared cultural heritage.
- Cultural values are established in childhood and are evidenced by 10 years of age.
- Cultural awareness means learning patients' cultural beliefs, practices, and values and understanding how they differ from one's own.
- Cultural competence is the ability to adapt health care so that it does not violate the cultural beliefs or practices of the patient.
- Effective communication and sensitivity to personal space are two important factors in providing culturally competent care.
- The myriad of cultures in the United States provides the opportunity for misunderstanding, misinterpretation, and errors in health care and teaching.
- Alternative medicines are therapies that are used instead of traditional Western medical therapies.
- Complementary medicines are therapies that are used together with traditional Western medical therapies.
- The focus of health care is shifting from the hospital to the home and community with a focus on wellness and prevention of illness.
- The health-care provider is considered a facilitator who empowers the consumer to choose the best available options to meet personal needs and cultural values.
- NCCIH is an agency of the National Institute of Health that researches the effectiveness of CAM therapies.
- The Office of Minority Health provides information concerning culturally and linguistically (language) appropriate services (CLAS).

Clinical Judgment Case Study

A mother who has recently moved from her country of birth to the United States with her children states that she worries she is "losing" her teenage daughter who is dressing and acting differently with her school friends and asks for guidance how to understand and manage this change. What factors would you discuss with this client?

REVIEW QUESTIONS

1. Mark the appropriate box in the table to distinguish between alternative medicine, complementary medicine, and cultural intervention.

	Alternative Medicine	Complementary Medicine	Cultural Intervention
Use of an antinausea bracelet during chemotherapy	☐	☐	☐
Suggesting a plasma expander to a patient who refuses a blood transfusion for religious reasons	☐	☐	☐
Patient chooses to use acupuncture instead of prescribed medication	☐	☐	☐
A patient chooses to undergo chiropractic care instead of prescribed physical therapy	☐	☐	☐
Offering a patient room-temperature water instead of cold, due to a cultural belief	☐	☐	☐
Having a midwife or doula present during childbirth in a hospital setting	☐	☐	☐

2. Which of the following are roles of the government in promoting culturally competent care?
   A. Research and report the effectiveness of CAM therapies.
   B. Enact laws to require that all patients with the same diagnosis receive the same treatments.
   C. Set guidelines for which religious holidays are recognized in the health-care environment.
   D. Promote behaviors and policies related to cultural competence in health care.
   E. Provide information concerning linguistically appropriate health services.
   F. Require health-care workers to speak a minimum of two languages fluently.

3. If a patient refuses to take his vitamin pill because he believes the gelatin base is unhealthy, the nurse should:
   A. challenge his belief.
   B. educate him concerning the need and value of that vitamin pill.
   C. obtain the help of a clergyman to persuade him to take the pill.
   D. respect his belief and find a similar vitamin preparation that does not contain gelatin.

4. When providing health-care information, the health-care worker should (select all that apply):

   A. speak only with the patient.

   B. include the family member who is the decision-maker of the family.

   C. always provide instructions clearly written in English.

   D. include resources to call if there are further questions.

5. Match the terms with the correct definitions.

Term		Definition
Cultural competence	___	A. Evaluating a person's cultural beliefs and values according to standards of one's own practices.
Culture	___	B. Most people of specific cultures believe and practice specific behaviors.
Cultural sensitivity	___	C. Awareness and respect for beliefs and values that may be different from one's own.
Cultural stereotyping	___	D. Use of appropriate verbal and body language and personal space.
Ethnocentric	___	E. Learned values, beliefs, and customs that influence food choices, parenting styles, and treatment preferences.

The Influence of Family on Developing a Lifestyle

http://evolve.elsevier.com/Leifer/growth

OUTLINE

OBJECTIVES

1. Define the various types of family structures.
2. List the developmental stages of a family.
3. Define family systems theory.
4. Give examples of family system stressors.
5. Discuss the effect of the family lifestyle on child development.
6. State three childrearing styles.
7. List three developmental theories.
8. List the effects culture has on personal values, beliefs, and behaviors of family members.
9. Define what makes a family dysfunctional.
10. Discuss one positive and one negative influence of technology and digital media on the family and child development.
11. Understand the effects of a disaster on the family and development.
12. State the effect of the community on the family and child development.

KEY TERMS

blended family	dysfunctional family	posttraumatic stress disorder
cultural assimilation	ethnocentrism	(PTSD)
cultural relativism	Facebook depression	sexting
culture shock	family	sibling rivalry
developmental stage	family systems theory	theory
developmental task		

DEFINITION

The family has been defined as a basic human social system that involves commitment and interaction among its members. This commitment includes a responsibility for the physical and emotional well-being and successful development of the children in that family. For most people, the family is the strongest and most influential group to which a person belongs. A healthy family is not necessarily a family where all members are at the optimum level of health. A healthy family is one that can successfully adapt to crises, challenges, and changes during the life cycle. The role of the nurse or health-care worker is to help the family adapt to these challenges. Health-care workers must understand the many factors that influence family functioning and child development. Comprehensive care involves the patient and the family unit.

Family Structure

Family composition and cultural backgrounds have changed dramatically in the United States during the last 40 years. The traditional nuclear (two-parent) family, where the father works outside the home and the mother remains at home to care for the children, has given way to many other variations. The percentage of married couples with children under the age of 18 in their household has declined from 44% in 1960, to 24% in the year 2000, to 19% in 2020 (PRB, 2020). The daily availability of parents to the children is often decreased because of the demands of the workplace. Working parent(s) may leave the house to travel to work before the child awakens and may return after the child is asleep at night. Flexibility is needed to maintain parental role modeling, mutual respect, and equality of involvement in childrearing.

   Dual-career families, in which both parents work outside the home, have become the norm in modern America and increasing percentages of mothers are the primary or sole earners. In 2019, 64.2% of married-couple families had both husband and wife employed (U.S. Bureau of Labor Statistics, 2020), while in 40% of households, the mother is the primary earner (U.S. Department of Labor, 2017). Conflicting demands among work responsibilities, continuing education for career advancement, and the demands of childrearing often create pressures that require careful scheduling, close communication, flexibility, and mutual support. Children of dual-career families are often expected to be more independent at an earlier age, and parents tend to overestimate the ability of the child to manage without direct supervision. Acute illness, chronic illness, or discipline and behavior problems can create additional stresses in this type of family structure (Box 4.1).

> **BOX 4.1 Ten Potential Challenges in Dual-Career Families**
>
> 1. Need for childcare arrangements.
> 2. Time to participate in children's activities.
> 3. Time to support and encourage academic achievements.
> 4. Time to support and encourage peer interaction.
> 5. Time for child-focused family activities.
> 6. Need for close scheduling and travel away from home on the part of family members.
> 7. Lack of energy for home and childcare activities.
> 8. Difficulty with unexpected illness or injury management.
> 9. Increased need for child to self-manage.
> 10. Maintaining healthy nutrition options at mealtimes.

Same-sex parenting offers wide variation in family structure. Adoption agencies are open to placing children into a same-sex parented family and there is increased social acceptance of this family structure. When measured in self-esteem, personality, peer relationships, behavior problems, and academic success, no major differences have been found between the outcome of children raised in some type of same-sex family or a heterosexual family. Good parenting, regardless of sexual identity, led to positive outcomes, including children of same-sex parenting having more tolerance to diversity and more nurturing attitudes toward other children (Garfield, 2009).

Interracial or interfaith families have increased in recent years and there is increased social acceptance. These couples remain at risk for stigma and separation from their own extended families, which may affect their social support system and influence family stability (Garfield, 2009). However, alliances with other families and institutions with inclusive missions can offer the needed supportive interactions. Children raised in these families often have increased sensitivity toward different ethnicities and religions (Garfield, 2009).

Today, many grandparents serve as head of household and primary caregivers for their grandchildren living with them. Many grandparents accept this responsibility as a "second chance" at parenting and enjoy the close relationship with their grandchildren. Children from these families seem to fare better in behavior and school performance than those dependent on federal aid programs. However, these children often live below the Federal Poverty Level as income of the grandparent is often limited and the grandparent may become isolated from the peer group and be at risk for depression and health problems (Garfield, 2009). Stress may occur if expectations of the grandparent differ from expectations of the parents who remain in contact.

All family variations have some form of influence on childrearing and development. Table 4.1 lists some types of family structures found in the United States. An essential core of parenting within any family structure is commitment to the child. The parenting arrangement may be challenged by divorce, environmental poverty, or illness or death of a parent. Communication between parent and child helps the child adjust to a specific lifestyle that may be different from his or her peers. Children need to have a sense of belonging, support, and consistency in their lives to achieve optimal development (Figure 4.1A).

TABLE 4.1   Various Types of Family Structures

Type of Family*	Description
Nuclear	Traditional – husband, wife, and children (biological or adopted)
Extended	Grandparents, parents, children, and relatives
Single parent	Women or men establishing separate households through individual preferences, divorce, death, or desertion
Foster parent	Parents who care for children who are sent to them via the court system because of dysfunctional families, absent families, or individual family problems
Alternative	Communal family
Dual career	Both parents work because of desire or need
Blended	Mother or father, stepparent, and children
Polygamous	More than one spouse at the same time
Same-sex parents	A single homosexual person or two persons of the same sex who may have children from a previous relationship, who have adopted children, or have children via artificial insemination
Cohabitation	Heterosexual or homosexual couples who live together with their children but remain unmarried (a type of cohabitation may be experienced by college students who live in a dormitory or in off-campus school housing with men and women sharing facilities)

*Not all may be legally sanctioned.
Modified from Leifer, G. (2019). *Introduction to maternity & pediatric nursing* (8th ed.). Elsevier.

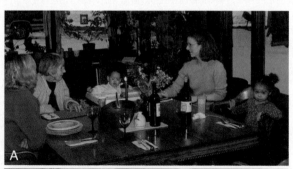
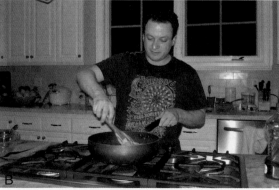

Figure 4.1 (A) Several generations gather around the table for celebrations. Such activities strengthen the family structure. (B) Healthy eating starts with freshly cooked nutritious food.

EFFECT OF FAMILY ON GROWTH AND DEVELOPMENT OF THE CHILD

There are many factors within the family structure, including interactions and lifestyles, that can affect the growth and development of a child. The more common aspects of family variations are discussed in this chapter.

Size of Family

The interpersonal relationship between siblings is unique. The presence of a brother or sister in a family group helps provide support and gives early experience in developing the skills necessary for social interaction. Older children can help younger siblings grasp language skills, but the firstborn or only child may have a longer, more intense verbal interaction with the parent. This one-to-one relationship may result in the development of a wider vocabulary and better conversational skills at an earlier age. Although social experiences may be limited for the single child, the popular use of day care and preschool can provide an opportunity to develop social skills and can decrease the feeling of loneliness for an only child. Extended families who may live nearby may provide opportunities for cousins to interact with the only child of a family to provide opportunities for sharing and the presence of grandparents can offer extra love and attention.

Spacing of Siblings

The age of the older child at the time of the birth of the sibling contributes to the response of the older child. When the new baby arrives, a 1-year-old child may whine and cling, whereas a 2-year-old child may regress in toileting or feeding behaviors, and a 4-year-old may develop temper tantrums. A child older than 5 years may feel protective of the new arrival. Shared experiences among siblings with fewer than 4 years difference in age increase the likelihood of sibling rivalry. Sibling rivalry is a competition or struggle between two or more children in a family. It can contribute positively to child development by offering the opportunity for children to develop interpersonal skills and to handle conflict, but it can also cause stress and chaos in a family.

Divorce

The psychological health and development of the child may be affected by the divorce of his or her parents. The child may be thrust into a single-family home or a newly blended family if remarriage occurs. Children of divorce often have a higher incidence of behavioral or learning difficulties later in life (Kim, 2011). The effect of joint custody on the child is partially determined by the motivation for such an arrangement. The best motivation would be to ensure continuing relationships with both parents, but other reasons often include convenience or lack of commitment by one or both parents. The presence or absence of hostility between the parents is an important factor that influences the psychological adjustment of the child regardless of the type of custody arrangements made.

The child should be prepared for the divorce and assured he or she had no role in the breakup of the marriage. However, self-blame is common despite assurances. Children should be told how the divorce will affect them and their needs, as well as what they can

TABLE 4.2   Responses to Divorce by Age Group

Age Group	Signs and Symptoms	Interventions Needed
Preschool	Regression Returns to thumb sucking Intensified fears Sleep disturbances Fear of abandonment	Maintain household routines Reassure love of child Spend added time with child Establish and maintain bedtime rituals
School age	Shows open grieving Feels rejected Fears being replaced by absent parent Difficulty in concentrating, resulting in poor grades Fears expressing emotions	Allow child to love both parents Help child move from parent to parent Diminish worry about present and future Attend school events Do not use child as confidant or as spouse substitute
Adolescent	Worry about fate of own future marriage Must rethink values and morality of the world May become depressed or suicidal May be expected to assume greater family responsibilities	Avoid delegating too much home responsibility Encourage discussion with neutral party Encourage pursuit of own interests Help in use of support systems
Adult	Increased dependence on eldest child Open expression of fears, anxieties, and anger Inability to focus on needs of children	Counsel to join a single-parent support group Encourage professional counseling Refer to social or financial-aid resources
Geriatric	Depression, loneliness, helplessness, bitterness Increased dependence on children and grandchildren	Encourage joining groups Increase activities that are of personal interest

Data from Tanner, J. L. (2009). Separation, divorce and remarriage. In W. Carey, A. Crocker, W. Coleman, E. Elias, & H. Feldman (Eds.), *Developmental and behavioral pediatrics* (4th ed). Elsevier; Leifer, G. (2019). *Introduction to maternity and pediatric nursing* (8th ed). Elsevier.

expect in terms of living arrangements and continued relationships with both parents. Children need permission to continue to love both parents and to feel free to express these feelings. Table 4.2 shows typical responses to divorce according to age group and developmental level and related guidance or interventions that can be offered by the nurse and the health-care team.

Stepchildren and Foster Children

A blended family is one in which one or both spouses bring children from a previous relationship into a new family unit. The children may have to adjust to a new home and school environment with new rules and new roommates (stepsiblings) who are strangers. This often accompanies a dilution of attention from the biological parent, who must divide attention among a larger family group. Resentment between stepsiblings may occur. A stepparent may be given a name other than "mother" or "father" if the children feel guilty that the stepparent is replacing the biological parent.

Children who enter foster care must face a strange environment without the support of even one biological parent. There is added uncertainty regarding the length of placement, which can result in insecurity and lack of trust in others. In 2017, there were 442,995 children in foster care in the United States (Child Welfare Information Gateway, 2019). Federal legislation in 1980 and 1995 promoted family reunification as the goal for all foster care, so that relatives are now sought first as caregivers for children displaced from biological families before the children are placed in foster care (Child Welfare Information Gateway, 2020).

Chronic Illness

Having a child, parent, or dependent relative with a chronic illness can strain sibling relationships and exact tolls on the emotional, psychological, and economic resources of the family. The healthy child may be expected to be more independent, to carry more responsibilities, or to step into a caregiver role that may keep him or her away from normal activities with peers. Although some healthy children may react with anger at the ill family member, many children develop a greater capacity for empathy because of their experiences with the person who is chronically ill (Table 4.3). Communicating the needs, limitations, and feelings of the ill relative and acknowledging the needs and feelings of caregivers and the impact on the family can make the crucial difference between resentment and attachment for each member of the family. Caregiver group support may be available in local communities.

The death of a child in the family may cause a parent to become overprotective of the surviving children, thus depriving them of normal independence and interaction with their peers. The nurse can explain and discuss terminal illness and its developmental and behavioral consequences by identifying family strengths, coping styles, and strategies. A comprehensive plan for care, continuing education, and promotion of optimal growth and development can then be designed and implemented by the health-care team.

TABLE 4.3 Understanding Chronic Illness at Various Ages

Age	Concept of Illness
Preschool	Magical thoughts
Early school age	Concrete, rigid ideas
Late school age	Little comprehension, although can list symptoms
Adolescent	Child shows greater understanding of cause of illness
Adult	Understands abstract principles and concepts involved in the illness

Data from Thyen, U., & Perrin, J. (2009). Chronic health conditions. In W. Carey, A. Crocker, W. Coleman, E. Elias, & H. Feldman (Eds.), *Developmental and behavioral pediatrics* (4th ed). Elsevier; Kleigman, R., Stanton, B., St. Geme III, J., Schor, N., & Behrman, R. (2016). *Nelson textbook of pediatrics* (20th ed.). Elsevier.

The family that has a newborn child with a chronic illness or deformity goes through a grieving process. This process includes shock, disbelief/denial, anger, depression, withdrawal, adaptation, and adjustment. Any new crises can cause setbacks to previous stages and delay the coping and adjustment of family members. The health-care worker must recognize these stages, determine the resiliency of the family to create a support network, and help them use resources within the family and the community.

Use of Childcare Services

Individual childcare or group day care is a replacement for direct care by a parent and is currently used more often than nannies, extended family members, sibling care, and private babysitters. In 2018, approximately 1.32 million children and 813,200 families per month received childcare assistance (U.S. Department of Health and Human Services, 2019). The terms *day care* and *childcare* do not indicate details about services provided. Childcare services are regulated for health and safety by the American Public Health Association but vary widely in ability to nurture growth and development. High-quality day-care settings can contribute to cognitive development (Chapter 8).

UNDERSTANDING FAMILIES THROUGH THEORIES

A theory is a group of concepts that form the basis for understanding observations. An accepted theory is logical, consistent, and integrates past and current research. Theories provide a way to study family interaction or individual growth and development. The theories are useful because they help us understand why things happen the way they do and help us identify interventions needed for individuals or families that experience problems. Various theories of individual growth and development are discussed in detail in Chapter 5.

Family Systems Theory

Family systems theory is based on the understanding that family functions are interconnected. This means that what happens to one family member affects the entire family. No illness is seen as an isolated, individual event. Everything is viewed in the context of family interactions. For example, when a child has a problem such as anorexia, the entire family is affected. The problem of the child affects the family system, and the family system affects the general maintenance or recovery of the problem that the child is experiencing. Many problems of the individual, such as anorexia, can be manifestations of a dysfunctional family system. Therefore interventions, according to the family systems theory, must involve the whole family, not just the affected individual. Often, stabilizing the family group helps to stabilize the problem of the individual.

Murray Bowen, of Georgetown University, was one of the pioneers of the family systems theory, and Salvador Minuchin, of Argentina, first wrote about the values of family therapy in 1974. They stated that there are interactions among the biological, developmental, psychological, and social factors in the family that determine the individual behaviors of each family member. There is a natural tendency in families to seek a stable state. For example, if one child is overly aggressive and frequently breaks rules, another child in the family will assume the role of the good child to maintain family stability. This process is called *family dynamics*. Child guidance worker John Bowlby (1951) was a pioneer in

---

BOX 4.2   Family Apgar

Adaptation – Sharing of resources and helping of family members.
Partnership – Lines of communication and participation of family members.
Growth – How responsibilities are shared among family members.
Affection – Visible and invisible emotional interactions among family members.
Resolve – How time, money, and space are used for solving or preventing problems among family members.

Modified from Smilkstein, G. (1978). The Family Apgar: a proposal for a family function test and its use by physicians. *Journal of Family Practice (6)*, 1231–1238.

---

describing how a child's distress was a reflection of a family in distress, and treatment of both was essential to a return to optimal health. It is, therefore, important for health-care workers to understand the organization and communication within the family unit. Today, managed health care favors the treatment of the entire family rather than just the affected individual because the results are quicker and longer lasting.

The Family Apgar

In 1978, Gabriel Smilkstein created the Family Apgar as a tool to assess family function (Box 4.2). It was initially used by physicians and psychologists to assess the family's ability to adapt, grow, develop, and resolve issues. The role of the health-care worker on the multidisciplinary health-care team is to observe a family's function and ensure that the needs of each family member are being met. Referral to available community resources, which may include social agencies, school professionals, psychologists, or pediatricians, can help identify problems and initiate appropriate early interventions. Accepting the nontraditional family and helping the adults care for their own physical and psychological needs are the first steps in helping the parents to care for their children and to promote optimal growth and development for the entire family unit (Figure 4.2A and B).

Developmental Theories

There are various theories of growth and development (Chapter 5), and each theory emphasizes specific areas of development, such as motor, cognitive, social, and so on. Piaget offers a developmental theory of cognition, whereas Freud's theories involve behaviors that are motivated by unconscious wishes. Because of the interactions between an individual and the environment, psychosocial theories of development are also important to understand.

Erik Erikson is one of the best-known psychosocial theorists, and his concepts are presented in Chapter 5 and throughout this text. The growth and development of a parent in relation to Erikson's theory of development is described in Table 4.4. A developmental stage is defined as a period in life characterized by the mastery of specific skills or behaviors. Each stage incorporates achievements from the previous stage and contains skills, behaviors, or tasks necessary to enter and successfully master the skills, behaviors, and tasks of the next stage. Handling psychosocial conflicts using coping strategies and support systems or significant relationships has an important effect on the developing personality.

Robert Havighurst was a theorist who described a sequence for learning developmental tasks at each stage of development, including tasks of late adulthood and for the aged. His

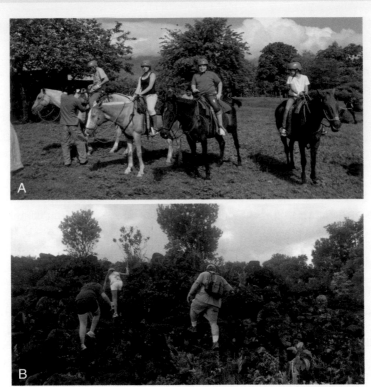

Figure 4.2 (A, B) In accordance with the goals of *Healthy People 2030*, the family that exercises together, or engages in active recreational activities together, promotes positive attitudes about exercise throughout the life cycle. Healthy activity can take place inside or outside of the home setting.

view emphasized that society determines the skills that need to be acquired at each stage of development, but he pointed out that readiness to learn and teachable moments for acquisition of these skills must be utilized, or difficulties in later life can occur.

Betty Neuman, a nursing theorist, believed that nurses and other health-care team members should care for the total patient and family needs, with special efforts directed toward maintaining the interaction of the family within their environment. Specific interventions to reduce stress and to achieve maximal wellness are the basis of the theory.

Evelyn Duvall, a family theorist, proposed specific stages of family development. Each stage of development is unique with new competencies to be mastered. Various stages of physical and psychosocial development occur concurrently, so all processes are integrated.

GROWTH AND DEVELOPMENT OF THE FAMILY

Developmental Tasks of the Family Life Cycle

Parent training programs are available to help parents develop positive parenting styles (Table 4.5). Appropriate discipline management, communication skills, and social support are important.

A developmental task is a competency or skill that helps a person cope with the environment or advance personal development. Tasks occur in sequence, and mastery of

TABLE 4.4 The Growth and Development of a Parent

Child's Tasks (Erikson's Stages)	Parent's Tasks	Nursing Interventions
FIRST PRENATAL TRIMESTER		
Growth	Develop attitude toward newborn: Happy about child? Parent of one disabled child? Unwed mother? These factors and others will affect the developing attitude of the mother.	Develop positive attitude in both parents concerning expected birth of child. Use referrals and agencies as needed.
SECOND PRENATAL TRIMESTER		
Growth	Mother focuses on infant because of fetal movements felt. Parents picture what infant will look like, what future he or she will have, and other ideas.	Parents' focus is on childcare and needs and providing physical environment for expected infant. Therefore, information concerning care of the newborn should be given at this time.
THIRD PRENATAL TRIMESTER		
Growth	Mother feels large. Attention focuses on how fetus is going to get out.	Detailed information should be presented at this time concerning the birth processes, preparation for birth, breastfeeding, and care of siblings at home.
BIRTH		
Adjust to external environment	Elicit positive responses from child and respond by meeting child's need for food and closeness. If parents receive only negative responses (e.g., sleepy infant, crying infant, difficult feeder, congenital anomaly), development of the parent will be inhibited.	Encourage early touch, feeding, and other practices. Explain behavior and appearance of newborn to allay fears. Help parents to identify positive responses. (Use infant's reflexes, such as grasp reflex, to identify a positive response by placing mother's finger into infant's hand.)
INFANT		
Develop trust	Learn "cues" presented by infant to determine individual needs of infant.	Help parents assess and interpret needs of infant (avoid feelings of helplessness or incompetence). Do not let in-laws take over parental tasks. Help parents cope with problems such as colic.

TABLE 4.4   The Growth and Development of a Parent (*Cont.*)

Child's Tasks (Erikson's Stages)	Parent's Tasks	Nursing Interventions
TODDLER		
Autonomy	Try to accept the pattern of growth and development. Accept some loss of control but maintain some limits for safety.	Help parents cope with transient independence of child (e.g., allow child to go on tricycle but do not yell "Don't fall," or anxiety will be radiated).
PRESCHOOL AGE		
Initiative	Learn to separate from child.	Help parents show standards but "let go" so child can develop some independence. A preschool experience may be helpful.
SCHOOL AGE		
Industry	Accept importance of child's peers. Parents must learn to accept some rejection from child at times. Patience is needed to allow children to do for themselves, even if it takes longer. Do not *do* the school project *for* the child. Provide chores for child appropriate to his or her age level.	Help parents to understand that child is developing his or her own limits and self-discipline. Be there to guide child, but do not constantly intrude. Help child get results from his or her own efforts at performance.
ADOLESCENT		
Establishing identity Accepting pubertal changes Developing abstract reasoning Deciding on career Investigating lifestyles Controlling feeling	Parents must learn to let child live his or her own life and not expect total control over the child. Expect, at times, to be discredited by teenager. Expect differences in opinion and respect them. Guide but do not push.	Help parents adjust to changing role and relationship with adolescent (e.g., as child develops his or her own identify, he may become a Democrat if parents are Republican). Expose child to varied career fields and life experiences. Help child to understand emerging emotions and feelings brought about by puberty.

TABLE 4.5   Parent Training Program Components

Component	Activities
Knowledge about child development and behavior	Providing developmentally appropriate environment Learning about child development Promoting positive emotional development
Positive parent-child interactions	Learning the importance of positive, non–discipline-focused interactions Using skills that promote positive interactions Providing positive attention
Responsiveness and warmth	Responding sensitively to the child's emotional needs Providing appropriate physical contact and affection
Emotional communication	Using active listening to foster communication Helping children identify and express emotion
Disciplinary communication	Setting clear, appropriate, and consistent expectations Establishing limits and rules Choosing and following through with appropriate consequences
Discipline and behavior management	Understanding child misbehavior Understanding appropriate discipline strategies Using safe and appropriate monitoring and supervision practices Using reinforcement techniques Using problem solving for challenging behavior Being consistent
Promoting children's social skills and prosocial behavior	Teaching children to share, cooperate, and get along with others Using good manners
Promoting children's cognitive or academic skills	Fostering language and literacy development Promoting school readiness

The nurse can use "teachable moments" to review parenting skills that will enhance the development of positive parent-child interactions and promote optimal developmental and behavioral outcomes. The CDC provides evidence-based resources and content for parent education.
From U.S. Centers for Disease Control and Prevention (2009). *Parent training programs: insight for practitioners*. CDC.

developmental tasks of one stage is usually required to master developmental tasks of the next stage of development. There are physical, cognitive, psychological, motor, and psychosocial developmental tasks. Both the individual and the family have developmental tasks to achieve at specific stages across the lifespan, such as the following:

- *Physical competencies*, which include functional abilities that result from motor and neurological development.
- *Emotional competencies*, which include self-awareness, empathy for others, and using strategies to cope with stress or frustrations.
- *Social competencies*, which include the ability to form positive interpersonal relationships.

The concepts of several theorists are presented in Chapter 5 and in each chapter covering the life cycle. Refer to psychology or anthropology texts for other details concerning individual theorists.

Role of the Health-Care Worker

Understanding the developmental stages and tasks of families and individuals enables the health-care team to provide individualized care. Optimal growth and development results when the person or family masters each task in the various stages of the life cycle. When working with patients or families, health-care team members must consider the developmental stage of the family and the individual, as well as cultural influences, before designing or carrying out a plan of care that will meet comprehensive needs.

Childrearing Styles

Various family styles of functioning can be adopted by a couple in the beginning phases of family development and may be influenced by their cultural backgrounds. Some parents implement an *autocratic style*, where decisions are made without the input of the children. Respect and obedience of authority are expected without discussion. This approach may decrease conflict in the home but can also diminish the child's feelings of self-efficacy and ability to rely on their own instincts. In the *democratic style*, children are encouraged to participate in decision-making, and all members of the family are expected to exhibit mutual respect. This parenting style can contribute to the development of useful collaborative tools but can also lead to debates regarding decisions that affect the family unit. The *laissez-faire style* offers complete freedom for all members, with no rules, minimal discipline (if any), and no effort at impulse control. This parenting strategy can reinforce the concepts of natural consequences and personal responsibility, but it can also create confusion due to lack of structure. Whichever style of childrearing and family development is selected, consistency of that style by both parents is essential for the development of stable family dynamics.

A functional family is a stable unit (firmly established with constant members) with consistent rules whose members are able to deal with conflict, stress, and problems in a way that promotes the physical and psychological well-being of its members. A dysfunctional family is a family unit that does not offer consistency of members or rules, may exhibit poor interpersonal relationships among its members, deals poorly with conflicts and problems, and often cannot reach out to the community for help. Dysfunctional family styles often result in antisocial behaviors of family members, where behavior of individuals may violate the rights of others. Early referral by the health-care team can help family members recapture self-esteem and break the cycle of family dysfunction in future generations.

When a family member has a problem, the health-care worker must determine how the problem is perceived by the family, if coping skills exist, and if support systems are available. This is the core of a family-care plan. The role of the nurse or health-care worker is to help the family manage the problem. Referring the family to available community resources as appropriate and providing follow-up care are important in the plan of care.

Cultural Considerations

Effect of Culture on the Family

Culture is defined as a set of learned values, beliefs, customs, and behaviors that is shared by interacting individuals, such as a family (Chapter 3).

Cultural assimilation is a process by which members of a specific cultural group lose the characteristics of that group and adapt practices of another group. It is often referred to as "Westernization" of a culture when time spent in the United States results in the adoption of an Americanized view of family function and behavior.

Cultural relativism is the concept that normality comes from the standard social practices of a specific culture. What is normal practice in one culture may not be considered normal practice in another culture.

Culture shock is the effect of a sudden, drastic change in the cultural environment of an individual or family.

As people travel around the world with ease and frequency, and families relocate from continent to continent, different cultural groups interact. Cultural backgrounds affect methods of communication and perceptions and response to health and illness. For example, in one culture, the response to a disability may be to hide it, whereas in another culture reentry into society is the treatment goal.

Ethnocentrism is the belief that one's own culture is the standard of behavior and is better than other cultures. Health-care workers need to understand their own cultural beliefs and recognize how they may differ from their patients. It is unrealistic to expect the patient to change his or her cultural beliefs and practices. Health-teaching plans must be designed to avoid conflict with the cultural beliefs and practices of the patient and family. Methods of communication are related to cultural practices. Understanding the culture and knowing who to communicate with in the family is essential in providing effective health care.

Cultural competence involves cultural awareness, acceptance, and respect toward behaviors and practices that are different from one's own. Knowledge of various cultures and the ability to adapt the delivery of health care so that it does not violate the culture or religion of that group are the core of cultural competence. The health-care worker must overcome cultural barriers to communication and behavior to provide effective health care to a culturally diverse society. Some cultural beliefs and practices related to stages within the life cycle were discussed in Chapter 3. Cultural assessment includes values, socioeconomic status, communication patterns, nutrition, language, religious practices, health beliefs, and cultural aspects of the disease and illness. It is important that the health-care worker ask relevant questions to assess how best to handle each individual family culture, rather than making assumptions based on limited information. This is essential to avoid cultural stereotyping. Sample questions for a provider to ask in order to assess an individual's needs are:

- How would you prefer to be addressed?
- Who will participate in decisions affecting your care?
- Tell me what good care means to you.
- Are there personal daily routines you would like to keep the same?
- How do you feel about persons of the opposite gender being involved in your care?

From JAMARDA Resources (2020). *Cultural diversity training and educational products for health care providers.* http://www.jamardaresources.com/

INFLUENCE OF DIGITAL MEDIA AND TECHNOLOGY

Digital media has enabled people to be in immediate contact with the thoughts and actions of others around the world, and the increased exposure of children to digital media can have positive and negative influences on children's development and behavior.

The optimal style of digital media utilization is family viewing where adults select content and share thoughts with the child about what they are watching. Studies have shown, however, that family viewing does not happen routinely (Kaiser Family Foundation, 2010) and with 95% of teens having access to a smartphone, most screen time is independent of parental guidance (Rocha, 2019). Content selected by children may be developmentally inappropriate for their ages.

TV or digital media stream viewing is a passive experience, but the developmental stage of the child influences the ability to understand complex story plots that involve narration, cultural references, or interruptions in the continuity of the story.

Character movements, sound effects, animation, and high-pitched voices capture the attention of young children. Some studies have shown that exposure to violent content can provoke aggressive acts in children who have a tendency for aggression, while others find desensitization (moral disengagement) may occur with repeated viewing of such content (Teng et al., 2019). The Children's Television Act of 1990 defined prime time for family viewing to control program content aired during times children would likely be watching, but with modern streaming devices, prime time is any time. No longer are viewers waiting to watch their favorite shows at a certain airing time. The American Medical Association (AMA) has offered guidance for health-care workers in helping parents monitor their children's viewing habits as part of healthy living counseling (Box 4.3).

Violent video games are of more concern than violent TV programs. The interactive practice, imitation, repetition, reward, and reinforcement involved in the playing of a video game are the same basic elements involved in learning a behavior. Therefore, learning and imitating aggressive behaviors is a definite risk. Physiological changes occur during the interactive playing of video games. Release of a chemical called dopamine in the body increases, and dopamine is known to be related to learning, attention, and motor integration (Pagani et al., 2010). The lesson taught in some violent video games may be that violence is fun and rewarding. Associating violent acts with a pleasant experience may provide the basis for learning violent behavior (Kaiser Permanente, 2019). Many video games can be played real-time over the Internet with strangers around the world which could potentially lead to unhealthy or dangerous relationships among participants. "Cookies" and location tracking can create dangers to children who are unaware of these

---

BOX 4.3   Teaching Parents How to Manage Media

- Monitor TV, video games, and websites that the child views; friend or follow your child's social media accounts.
- Do not use digital content as babysitters (i.e., to keep the child quiet or entertained for long periods).
- Develop family guidelines for movies that are allowed.
- Help the child interpret commercials and other advertising.
- Provide opportunities for active play and socializing in balance with media viewing.
- Ensure privacy settings are turned on to limit personal information access.

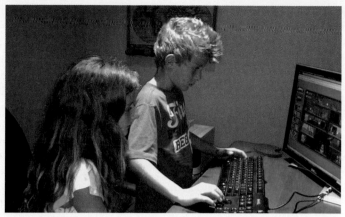

Figure 4.3 Computer games can provide interactive skills, and the Internet can offer a wealth of information to children and adults.

background features. Often parents set limits on screen time but do not restrict the type of application used or game being played. Adults enjoy screen time too, but it is important to be an example by ensuring our children are our priority. Children feel ignored when adults are distracted by their cell phone. Mealtime should be screen-free, and notifications should be silenced during family time.

Video games and applications should not replace other activities such as athletics, chores, outside play, hobbies, reading, music, and homework (Graham & Forstadt, 2010), and parents should avoid using devices to calm kids (Chen & Adler, 2019).

There are many positive outcomes of media use by children. *Sesame Street* is an example of a TV program that provides positive messages and education for young children. Video games can help increase hand-eye coordination, and many games are available without violent content. Digital games and websites can provide interactive stimulation that captures the attention and helps in developing processing skills and problem-solving abilities (Figure 4.3). Drills and repetition with periodic rewards can spark interest, maintain attention, and increase developmental abilities.

Computer-assisted instruction and distance learning is now offered in most schools and community libraries and is accessible at home at minimal or no cost. Distance learning enables an adolescent or adult to obtain college credit for courses without leaving home. Attitude and behavior remediation in the form of online driving schools are also available and are popular.

The Internet is a source of seemingly endless information, but some critical thinking, in the form of evaluating the source of the information to determine validity, is important. Computers and the Internet also allow accessibility to vitally important services and social interactions:
- Banking and other forms of financial activity can be accomplished online.
- Older adults can find information about a health concern, which can increase understanding of their own health problems and augment the teaching of the health-care team.
- Font size on the screen can be adjusted for the visually impaired.
- People for whom English is their second language (ESL) can have information translated into their native language to enhance their pleasure and understanding.

> **BOX 4.4**   Resources for Internet Safety
>
> www.isafe.org – Founded in 1998 and endorsed by the U.S. Congress. The site is dedicated to protecting online experiences of children to make cyberspace a safe and educational place.
> www.getnetwise.org – A public service sponsored by the technology industry to help guide intelligent use of the Internet.
> www.ikeepsafe.org – Founded in 2005 with a mission to provide digital safety for children, schools, and families through data safety certifications, educational resources, and community information.
> www.onguardonline.gov – Offered from the Federal Trade Commission, the website offers free online security tips for educators and parents. Interactive videos and games to teach children about hackers and scammers are also available.

- Disabled persons confined to the home can enjoy personal contacts with the outside world.
- E-mail and programs such as Facetime, Skype, and Zoom enable the elderly to maintain close communication with family and friends.

The Growth of Social Networking Sites

Social media (such as Instagram, Facebook, Twitter, LinkedIn, YouTube, Pinterest, and many others) is accessed by more than 70% of American adults (Pew Research Center, 2019). They allow people to communicate with each other, learn and gain information, share interests, and find support concerning personal illness or problems. Social networking has both positive effects and risks to the healthy growth and development of children.

The American Academy of Child and Adolescent Psychiatry reports that 90% of teens use social media and teens spend an average of 9 hours a day online, not including time for homework (AACAP, 2018). The Children's Online Privacy Protection Act of 1998 states social media platforms set an age limit for use of 13 or older, but younger children easily lie to gain access (FTC, 2013). Facebook depression is a common term used for the teens who overuse social networking to the point of altering sleep and eating habits and isolating themselves from peers and family, eventually succumbing to general depression. Exposure to inappropriate content and dangerous people, being victimized by *cyber bullying*, *body-shaming*, or sexting (sending or receiving of sexually explicit text messages and pictures), sleep alterations, and privacy concerns are all potential risks (AACAP, 2018).

Parents need to learn the technology, monitor their child's activities, and share the journey by discussing networking experiences as they discuss the child's other daily activities. Health-care workers can guide parents toward resources that encourage proper use of technology and media so that they can reap the rewards and avoid the pitfalls (Box 4.4).

EFFECTS OF A DISASTER ON FAMILY AND DEVELOPMENT

Disasters are a part of life and can occur in the form of a natural disaster (e.g., hurricane, earthquake, or flood) or a human-made disaster (e.g., war or catastrophic oil spill). In the past, unless the family was personally involved at the location of the disaster, the event was soon forgotten and the impact thought to be minimal. However, with the current incorporation of media in daily life, disasters in every part of the world can be relayed in explicit detail.

In many homes, the tragic attack on the World Trade Center in New York City on September 11, 2001, was viewed as it was happening and was reviewed on TV for months and years afterward. This event brought terror into private homes and lives as it was occurring and demonstrated that the family does not need to be directly in the area of the disaster to experience such aftereffects. Witnessing the disaster on screen in the privacy of their homes and observing the responses of their parents make children almost as vulnerable as the on-scene victims.

Studies have shown that children can suffer from posttraumatic stress disorder (PTSD) after witnessing parental violence or any event that causes upheaval or disruption of family life (Kleigman et al., 2016). PTSD has been defined as the development of characteristic symptoms following an extreme traumatic stressor (Torres, 2020). Some signs and symptoms of PTSD in children who have experienced a recent traumatic or abusive situation may be social withdrawal; appearing very serious (less playful) than other children of their age; feelings of depression, anxiety, helplessness, or mistrust; giving up rather than displaying self-protective behavior; reacting quickly with fear; or having a dismal view of the future. Adults with PTSD, including adult survivors of childhood trauma, may display similar emotions and behaviors. They may also develop an expectation of abuse or negative experiences and sometimes may unintentionally make choices and have reactions that increase the risk of additional trauma. Symptoms of PTSD can be alleviated or prevented with psychotherapy.

Studies have shown that boys born during wartime had developmental delays that may have been caused by an overattachment to their mothers (Chartrand et al., 2008). This overattachment resulted from an overprotective mother-child relationship that was directly influenced by the stresses of war. Emotional trauma from disasters can affect children and are influenced by parental reactions to the events.

Children respond to personal disaster by exhibiting anxiety, disorganization, confusion, inhibited activity, apathy, withdrawal, and sleeping and eating dysfunctions. These responses can affect school performance and appetite, which impacts growth and development. In response to a disaster event, school-age children may regress to earlier developmental abilities and behavior patterns. Phobias, flashbacks, and reenactments during play are also common. Adolescents may respond with an increase in sexual promiscuity, vandalism, or substance abuse.

These responses are the result of the child's perception of the disaster and the ability of the parents to cope as models of behavior. If a child is intimately involved in the disaster and strangers intrude in his or her life, these responses can intensify. Because children are dependent, they are more vulnerable to further trauma after a disaster occurs. If the community and the parents are personally affected, the child's functioning is disrupted. Symptoms of depression or stress that persist for more than a month after the disaster may warrant referral for a psychiatric evaluation.

Often parents are not aware of the child's responses, or parents tend to minimize the effect of the event on the child. The nurse and health-care worker should look for signs of PTSD when in contact with a child who is going through the aftermath of a disaster.

Children of rescue workers can develop anxiety concerning their parents' risky activities, and professional support may be indicated (as evidenced during the 9/11 disaster).

Nurses, health-care providers, and teachers must advocate preparation and training for disasters and develop an awareness of risks in their own environment. In the COVID-19 pandemic of 2020 families were mandated to be quarantined at home for an extended period in an effort to curb the spread of the virus. This caused major disruptions to routines such as work, school, exercise, sleep, and socializing. New routines had to be established quickly in order to promote resilience and maintain growth. Most professional, educational, and social platforms were moved online while business, schools, and recreation areas were closed. Maintaining social interaction for parents and children was challenging and outlets for energy were few. Lack of appropriate socialization can contribute to anxiety and abnormal development in children (Kleigman et al., 2016). This prolonged stress of the 2020 pandemic was compounded by an economic crisis caused by the closing of businesses and loss of employment income by many families. This also resulted in food shortages and supply insecurities. A "new normal" was formed as a result of that prolonged pandemic that will continue to affect the lives and development of survivors and will be studied for decades to come.

Role of the Health-Care Team

Professionals who care for children have a responsibility to understand and respect the opportunities that the fast-developing electronic media offer for learning and media's role in revolutionizing education. There is also a need to help the child self-regulate choices of what to view and to help parents use media in a positive way to promote a well-balanced lifestyle. Educating the public about quality programming and working with professional groups, industry, and regulating agencies to decrease the violence, pornography, and other negative aspects, and to promote quality programs, are vital.

Nurses and health-care workers must recognize that the response to disasters is influenced not only by a personal threat of injury or being close to the area of the disaster but can be influenced by parental response to the event. Parents should be guided to provide extra emotional support to children, to reassure them that their environment is safe, and to try to maintain a familiar and consistent daily routine. Parents should be urged to discuss the disaster in honest terms at a level appropriate to the child's age. Drawings and play can be used to help children express their feelings. Parents can review how family members can help each other. Coping abilities of the children and the family should be monitored and referral for professional help offered as needed.

EFFECT OF COMMUNITY ON FAMILY AND DEVELOPMENT

In many communities, housing for families with limited income may not be available. The number of children being raised in families without housing has increased dramatically. The psychological well-being and development of social relationships are at risk and family functions are disrupted. Life in homeless shelters is often chaotic and parents feel overwhelmed and powerless. Health-care workers should be aware of these circumstances and try to offer referrals for alternate housing and assistance that may be available.

Initially the family is the center of relationships that influence the development of the child. As the child grows, relationships expand, and outside influences affect the family as well as the child's growth and development. Teachers, coaches, clubs, teams, and peers each place demands on the family unit and have an increased effect on growth and development of its members. Most outside influences aid in learning social rules of behavior, help develop a sense of belonging, and contribute to the development of a positive self-image. The effects of outside influences during the stages of the life cycle are discussed in the following chapters.

HEALTHY LIFESTYLE HABITS

Attitudes toward exercise and food are formed in the home, and the family plays a crucial role in the development of healthy lifestyle habits. Parents are role models for children and have a major part in determining what the child sees as normal. Active parents are more likely to involve their children in regular physical activities, whereas sedentary parents are more likely to create a more inactive environment for their children (Figure 4.2A and B). Replacing 60 minutes of screen time each day with fun family activities (such as taking a walk, playing catch, or bicycling) can foster healthy habits while also improving family relationships. Physically active children are much more likely to become physically active adults who are at decreased risk for disease and disability later in life (Landry, 2016).

Healthy food choices also begin at home. Parents and caregivers must set good examples by consuming mainly fresh foods and water and limiting intake of processed foods and sodas (Figure 4.1B). Children look to parents for the development of lifestyle habits, and adults need to teach by example.

FAMILY-CENTERED HEALTH CARE

In family-centered health care, the family is central to the plan of care for any individual family member. Identifying and valuing the strengths of the family network to cope, support, and assist in the care of a family member are essential. Today the family no longer hands over total responsibility of patients to health-care personnel. Expanded visiting hours in the hospital setting allow family members to participate in care. Home-care services have expanded to allow care of the patient in the home setting, with the family functioning as the experts and the nurse or health-care team functioning as coordinators and consultants in a true partnership experience that empowers the family. To achieve family-centered care, the nurse and health-care worker must first listen to the family's perception of the problem and communicate the perception of the health-care team, identifying similarities and differences. Armed with cultural competence and an understanding of the family as a unit, nurses and health-care workers can provide meaningful, effective, family-centered health care.

KEY POINTS

- The family is a social system that involves interaction with and commitment to its members.
- Family structures include the nuclear two-parent family, the dual-career family, the extended family, the single-parent family, the blended family, and others.
- Traditional family development includes marriage, childbearing, childrearing, child launching, the contracting family, and the aging family.
- A family systems theory is based on understanding that what happens to one member of the family affects the entire family.

- The family lifestyle; size, number, and spacing of siblings; and family health all have an effect on the growth and development of the child.
- Childrearing styles can be classified as autocratic, democratic, or laissez-faire.
- Culture is a set of learned values, beliefs, and customs that are shared by a family.
- Advances in technology and the use of electronic media have allowed for research of information and achievement of educational degrees in the home setting.
- Interactive video games and screen viewing involving violence can have negative effects on the growth and development of children.
- Posttraumatic stress disorder can occur after viewing a disaster scene live, on screen, having a personal experience, or responding to the parents' reaction to the event, can affect growth and development.
- Parents must be guided to monitor the social networking sites used by children to assure positive outcomes.
- The family plays a crucial role in the development of healthy lifestyle habits.
- Community members, such as teachers, coaches, clubs, and peers, influence growth and development and place demands on the family unit.

Clinical Judgment Case Study

A newly divorced mother moves with her teenage daughter and infant son into a new neighborhood. The mother is concerned that she is the only one to guide her daughter who seems sad and has no friends. The daughter is very helpful with her infant brother and with household responsibilities. What interventions could a school nurse or health-care worker use to help the family make a healthy adjustment to their new life?

REVIEW QUESTIONS

1. According to the American Academy of Pediatrics, social networking sites used by children and teens: (select all that apply)
   A. under 13 years of age should be prohibited.
   B. should be monitored by adults.
   C. can cause depression and isolation.
   D. offer opportunities for learning and collaborating with peers.

2. A family is defined as:
   A. a structure consisting of two parents and at least one child.
   B. a social system involving commitment and interaction.
   C. genetically related groups of people.
   D. a group of people living together.

3. Factors within the family that affect the growth and development of the child include: (select all that apply)
   A. size of the family.
   B. spacing of siblings.
   C. divorce.
   D. state in which they live.
   E. political views of the parents.

4. The Children's Television Act of 1990 defined television "prime time" as: (select all that apply)
   A. times during which children are likely to watch TV.

B. times most popular shows should air.

C. times the current newscast should be broadcast.

D. mealtimes when most families are together.

E. times during which families may be able to watch TV together.

5. A developmental task is a competency or skill that: (select all that apply)

A. helps one cope with the environment.

B. occurs in sequence.

C. occurs at a specific age.

D. involves motor skills.

5

Theories of Development

http://evolve.elsevier.com/Leifer/growth

OUTLINE

OBJECTIVES

1. List theories of personality development.
2. Discuss one behavioral theory of development.
3. Discuss one psychosocial theory of development.
4. Discuss one environmental theory of development.
5. Discuss one cognitive theory of development.
6. Discuss the major forces that influence an adult learner.
7. Discuss how understanding developmental theories can enhance the ability to teach an individual who may be in a specific stage of development.
8. List physiological, cognitive, personality, social, and emotional changes that occur over the lifespan.
9. Discuss the uniqueness of individual personality and behavior at each stage of the life cycle.
10. Practice a deeper understanding of self and family.

KEY TERMS

behavioral theories
behaviorist theory
classical conditioning
cognitive theories
Electra anxiety
extrovert

humanist theories
information-processing
  theory
introvert
looking-glass self
moral reasoning

Oedipus complex
operant conditioning
psychodynamic theories
social-learning theory
sociocultural theories

DEFINITION

A theory is a statement based on scientific research that helps to make observations and facts meaningful. Behavioral theories are designed to explain the development of specific behaviors and suggest their relationships to other developing social skills. Psychodynamic theories focus on personality-trait development and psychological challenges at different ages; cognitive theories focus on advancement of the development of thinking; humanist theories describe the influence of human experiences such as love and attachment on behavior and personality development; and sociocultural theories describe how culture influences behavior. There is no single theory of development. Each theory provides important insights into different life stages, and human development is most accurately understood by integrating these theories.

IMPORTANCE OF UNDERSTANDING DEVELOPMENTAL THEORIES

Developmental theories focus on changes in physiology, psychology, and behavior that occur normally at different stages in the lifespan. Behaviors at different stages within the life cycle are influenced by culture, environment, past experiences, family, health status, and the reaction of the individual to all these events.

The study of growth and development starts with conception and extends throughout the lifespan. Understanding what affects growth and development, positively and negatively, helps nurses, health-care workers, and educators predict behaviors and responses at each stage and understand why people behave in certain ways. We now know that adults pass through predictable stages of development just as children do. Therefore studying growth and development in a continuum from birth to the geriatric adult provides a comprehensive understanding of how various life experiences affect growth and development at each stage of the life cycle. This understanding of behavior and personality enables health-care workers and educators to intervene effectively and to foster positive physical and mental health-care practices that will improve the lives of those they serve and teach.

Lifespan Considerations

Specific changes occur in each phase of the life cycle (Figure 5.1). Therefore interventions at the appropriate time within each stage can effectively influence health practices and contribute to the achievement of the goals of *Healthy People 2030*. Anticipation of needs can help in the development of an effective health-teaching plan.

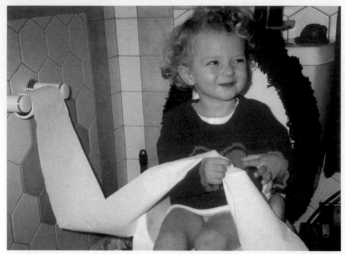

Figure 5.1 Toilet training. Learning self-control of the bowel and bladder is a developmental task of the toddler. There are many child-sized potties available, and eventually the child prefers adult facilities.

THE HISTORY OF DEVELOPMENTAL THEORIES AND BEHAVIORAL PEDIATRICS

Core concepts of development originated in the 1800s when Charles Darwin wrote the *Biographical Sketch of an Infant,* which carefully described how his own son communicated his physical, emotional, and reasoning abilities and is the basis of how we view child development today. In the early 1900s, Frances Galton, Darwin's cousin, studied and designed developmental and intelligence testing, and Alfred Binet and Theodore Simon later developed a scale to identify "norms" or normal behavior versus slow behavior that required intervention. The Binet-Simon test was first published in 1905 and eventually was redesigned to the current Stanford-Binet test of intelligence.

In early 1900 Ivan Pavlov described a "conditioned reflex" (the ability of a neutral stimulus to cause a physiological response) a basis for the concept of phobias (see the following section on Selected Theories of Development).

In 1934, Arnold Gisell published an *Atlas of Infant Behavior,* which identified typical milestones of development. Sigmund Freud is credited with identifying emotions and emotional disorders. He described the five stages of psychosocial development and the concept of conscious and unconscious influences on behavior. Erik Erikson further refined these theories that prevail today. James Baldwin studied the area of sensation and perception and influenced Jean Piaget in the expression of the theory of cognitive development. James Watson, a behaviorist in the United States, wrote of controlling children's behavior through conditioning, and B.F. Skinner further detailed the concept to include "operant conditioning" or use of a reinforcing stimulus to suppress a behavior.

Maria Montessori was an educational theorist who believed children were competent and arranged school levels to reflect competence rather than the age of the child. Her schools remain popular today.

Loris Malaguzzi believed education was a lifelong learning experience that thrives on satisfaction and has creativity, expression, and imagination based on exploring experiences rather than disseminating facts. Studies have shown that even preschoolers left to their own resources are able to solve problems but will not engage in exploring a solution when adults supply them with the answers and solve their problems for them (Gopnik, 2016).

President Theodore Roosevelt convened a "White House conference on children and youth" in 1909 and established the Children's Bureau in 1935 and then included public health and pediatric medical issues to be addressed in future White House conferences that were held every 10 years. After World War II many advocacy organizations focused on the needs of children with disabilities and in 1952, the *Diagnostic and Statistical Manual of Mental Disorders* (DSM) was published to clarify diagnostic criteria of mental and emotional disorders (and revised in 2013). The concept of behavioral pediatrics as a specialty slowly emerged as practicing pediatricians realized special skills were needed to help children with developmental problems. The American Academy of Pediatrics designated the mental health specialty of pediatrics in 1949 and, in 1975, included behavioral pediatrics. The designation was documented in the publication *Pediatric Clinics of North America*, in 1975, with subsequent publications, journals, and training programs, the Pediatric Board certification of behavioral pediatrics as a specialty within pediatrics was born!

SELECTED THEORIES OF DEVELOPMENT

Psychoanalytic Theory (Freud)

Sigmund Freud was a psychoanalytic theorist who identified three interacting parts of a person's psychological functioning. They are as follows:

- *Id* (the unconscious) is present at birth and generates impulses that seek immediate pleasure and satisfaction.
- *Ego* is a view of the self or image a person wants to convey to others.
- *Superego* emerges between 3 and 5 years of age, delays immediate gratification for socially appropriate reasons, and represents recognition of good and bad. It is also known as a moral guide or a conscience.

Freud believed that conflict occurs when society provides mixed messages, causing the unconscious (id) to produce anxiety, which rises to the surface (conscious or ego) and becomes evident to the individual in his or her feelings and behavior. Freud described defense mechanisms that protect the ego by hiding unpleasant feelings from a person's conscious awareness, thus serving as a defense against anxiety (Box 5.1).

Freud believed that personality grows, develops, and changes during the lifespan, but experiences in the early phases of development have a strong impact on the formation of the eventual adult personality. Freud defined sexuality as any expressed bodily stimulation that is perceived to be pleasurable (Gormly & Brodzinsky, 1989). Freud also described specific stages of psychosexual development (Table 5.1).

Freud believed that the Oedipus complex arises during the phallic stage of development (age 3–6 years) and suggested that little boys compete with their fathers for the mother's love and attention. During this stage, the boy prefers attention from the opposite-sex parent. As this stage ends, the boy begins to identify with his father, and attention is desired from both parents again. The Electra anxiety occurs when little girls compete with their mothers for the love and attention of their fathers. At the end of this stage, the little girl stops competing and reidentifies with the mother, again desiring attention from both parents.

BOX 5.1   Defense Mechanisms for Coping

Rationalization – Developing a plausible excuse for unacceptable behavior
Repression – "Forgetting" an unpleasant experience
Projection – Attributing one's thoughts or feelings to another person
Displacement – Expressing feelings (often anger) one has about a person toward another innocent person
Reaction formation – Acting just the opposite of what one feels (e.g., acting sure of oneself when one is really feeling insecure)
Regression – Reverting to immature behavior
Identification – Joining a group so that its positive identity will be reflected on oneself
Sublimation – Rechanneling unacceptable impulses into socially acceptable ones (e.g., channeling aggression into playing football)

TABLE 5.1   Freud's Stages of Psychosexual Development

Stage	Age	Description
Oral	First year of life	Focus is on mouth and the need to suck.
Anal	Toddler age	Focus is on learning self-control of bowels (Figure 5.1).
Phallic	Preschool age	Attention is self-centered during this stage. Some type of masturbation often occurs at this stage. Child identifies with parent of opposite sex. Superego develops at this time.
Latency	School age	Learns to suppress sexual urges and focuses on industry, achievement, and skills.
Genital	Puberty	Deals with sexual urges involving the opposite sex (mature compared with phallic stage). Seeks mutual pleasure with a partner.

Data from Haith, M., & Benson, J. (2008). *Encyclopedia of infant and early childhood development*, Elsevier; Kleigman, R., Stanton, B., Geme, J., Shor, N., & Behrman, R. (2016) *Nelson's textbook of pediatrics* (20th ed.). Elsevier; Carey, W., Crocker, A., Coleman, W., Elias, E., & Feldman, H. (2009). *Developmental-behavioral pediatrics* (4th ed.). W.B. Saunders.

Successful resolution of the Oedipus complex and Electra anxiety were thought to be the basis of the development of a mature sexual role and identity. Freud believed that the experiences of children play a role in forming adult personality, but Freud did not view the adult as a developing being. Thus Freud's theory has no identified stages beyond puberty.

Psychodynamic Theory (Jung)

Carl Jung, a Swiss doctor, studied with Freud but did not believe sexuality was the basis of behavior development. He believed development extended into adulthood and that age 40 was the "noon of life." Jung believed the roots of personality reflected the past culture of the family, which unconsciously molds the way a person perceives experiences as an adult. He was most recognized for describing personality traits, including the introvert (a quiet person who focuses inwardly on self) and the extrovert (an outgoing person who focuses on others in the environment). Jung believed that the personality could be changed in the middle-adulthood phase, when repressed feelings are recognized and coping mechanisms mature. Jung defined the process of recognizing one's own talent and abilities as self-actualization.

Stages of the Life Cycle: A Psychosocial Theory (Erikson)

Erik Erikson's theory describes the parts of personality development that are dependent on the social environment and social interactions. Each stage involves a social crisis or task that must be positively resolved to pass successfully to the next stage. For example, failure to establish trust with caregivers in the infant stage of development may affect intimacy later in life, which is based on the ability to establish trust with another person. Successfully passing through each of these stages is thought to contribute to the overall development of the individual personality and its unique strengths and weaknesses (Table 5.2).

The stage of adulthood also proceeds through phases, which include occupation, marriage and family, friends, culture and religion, and leisure. Each phase has a period of stability, which could last several years, where values are pursued and choices are made. The phases are bridged by a transitional period of change, when reassessment occurs and modifications are made. For example, if a marriage occurred in one phase, divorce can occur in a transitional phase. Choices and changes are discussed in detail in the chapters concerning growth and development during the adult years.

TABLE 5.2 Erikson's Stages of the Life Cycle

Stage	Age	Positive Achievement
Trust vs. mistrust	Infant	Develops trust of others to meet personal needs of self and, as a result, begins to trust others and himself/herself.
Autonomy vs. shame and doubt	Toddler	Ability to act independently is equated with trusting oneself to be good.
Initiative vs. guilt	Preschool	Imitates role models and follows rules. Experiences self-control in social interactions.
Industry vs. inferiority	School age	Develops ability to make friends and independently achieve school tasks.
Identity vs. role confusion	Adolescent	Learns to know oneself and what one believes and develops a career goal.
Intimacy vs. isolation	Young adult	Develops an ability to share all aspects of life with others.
Generativity vs. self absorption	Middle adult	Can contribute to society in a meaningful way.
Integrity vs. despair	Older adult (geriatric)	Maintains a sense of life achievement and absence of deep regret.

Data from Haith, M., & Benson, J. (2008). *Encyclopedia of infant and early childhood development.* Elsevier; Kleigman, R., Stanton, B., Geme, J., Shor, N., & Behrman, R. (2016). *Nelson's textbook of pediatrics* (20th ed.). Elsevier; Carey, W., Crocker, A., Coleman, W., Elias, E., & Feldman, H. (2009). *Developmental-behavioral pediatrics* (4th ed.). W.B. Saunders.

TABLE 5.3   Stages of Parenting Behaviors

Stage	Parenting Behavior
Stage 1: Parental image	Picturing oneself as a parent
Stage 2: Authority	Questioning parental skills as the child becomes autonomous
Stage 3: Integrative	Feeling responsible to motivate child as the child becomes more independent
Stage 4: Independent	Learning how to support teen while maintaining the authority role
Stage 5: Departure	Relating to the child as an adult as child prepares for the future and leaves home

Erikson's theory involves generativity. Erikson believed that parents grow as their children develop and are influenced by parent-child interactions at each stage. He described specific stages of parenting (Table 5.3).

Psychosocial Theory (Levinson)

Daniel J. Levinson was a theorist who elaborated on Erik Erikson's theories. Levinson believed that an interaction among environment, culture, and the individual was the "fabric of life." Levinson believed that each person enters an orderly sequence of events or structures in life. The tasks of each structure are specific and identifiable. For example, Levinson defined the pre-adult as being between 17 and 22 years of age. The pre-adult first leaves the protection of the family, and that period serves as a bridge between adolescence and independent adulthood. He described the early adult (age 22–45 years) as being at the height of vigor and vitality and making important choices such as marriage, career, and lifestyle. He described the middle adult, age 45–65 years, as being in a transition phase with a gradual decrease of mental and physical functioning. He described the late adult, age 65–80 years, as the grandparent generation whose task is to define new goals and levels of involvement with family, friends, and community. The late-late adult (geriatric) stage he described as beginning at 80 years of age and involves the task of facing death, although the individual often continues to be socially interactive. Details of these stages, with more current definitions, are reviewed in later chapters.

Cognitive Theory (Piaget)

Jean Piaget was a Swiss psychologist who emphasized cognitive milestones in development. Piaget described four stages of development related to learning to understand and relate logically to the world (Table 5.4).

Piaget's theory involved sensory and motor interactions with the environment. An infant learns how to grasp a block and learns the relationship it has to the infant's body. The infant then learns when he or she drops the block that it will fall and be out of reach. Gradually the infant learns that he or she can stack the blocks on top of one another, and eventually the infant can use the blocks to build something that represents a house or other object in the environment.

TABLE 5.4 Piaget's Four Stages of Development

Stage	Age	Cognitive Milestones
Sensorimotor	Birth to 2 years	Gains developmental understanding of object permanence. Understands cause and effect. Understands differences in time of day.
Preoperational	2–7 years	Attributes life to inanimate objects. Child believes he or she is the center of world. Sees only the obvious. Understands only one bit of information at a time without seeing abstract relationships. Develops language skills. Uses pretend play. Begins to use logic to understand rules.
Concrete operations	7–11 years	Can understand more than one piece of information simultaneously. Has a realistic understanding of the world. Focuses on the present, not the future.
Formal operations	Adolescent	Can think abstractly and understands symbols. Can think in hypothetical terms. Is future oriented. Understands scientific bases of theories. Cultural practices play a role in helping the adolescent understand "rules" and develop the moral sense of what is right.

Data from Benson, J. (2020). *Encyclopedia of infant and early childhood development*. Elsevier; Kleigman, R., Stanton, B., Geme, J., Shor, N., & Behrman, R. (2016) *Nelson's textbook of pediatrics* (20th ed.). Elsevier; Carey, W., Crocker, A., Coleman, W., Elias, E., & Feldman, H. (2009). *Developmental-behavioral pediatrics* (4th ed.). W.B. Saunders; Piaget, J. (1926). *The language of the child*. Harcourt Brace.

This interaction involves the child's thinking or processing of information at different ages and stages of development. The information-processing theory states that information is input, is processed mentally, and is then followed by an output of judgment and decision-making. This is believed to be the basis of problem-solving and critical-thinking abilities. The basic technique of information processing does not change with age. Only the speed and efficiency of the processing improves with age to adulthood. Piaget's stages involve qualitative, not just quantitative, changes in thought.

Cognitive Theory (Loevinger)

Jane Loevinger extended Piaget's model of development into the stages of adulthood. She believed that the ego adapts to demands and is an important basis for critical thinking. Loevinger believed ego development was progressive, with observable milestones throughout adult life.

Constructive Theory (Kegan)

Robert Kegan expressed a constructive developmental theory similar to Piaget's. Kegan believed that there was a lifelong interaction with the environment, in which the individual

TABLE 5.5   Vygotsky's Language and Development Theory

Age	Verbal Ability	Adult Response
Infant	Cries and coos	Parents respond to cries by cuddling infant and providing toys to stimulate responses.
Toddler	Points to objects	Adults give names and definitions to the objects at which the child is pointing.
Preschool		
3 years old	Speaks to self during play or movement	Parents may or may not listen to all the words.
4 years old	Uses inner speech to guide behavior	Parents praise the child for demonstrating delayed gratification or self-control.
School age	Engages in speech and social interactions	Parents who listen to their child understand the child's interpretation of events and experiences. Parents allow child to discover what he or she can do independently and with the help of others.

Data from Benson, J. (2020). *Encyclopedia of infant and early childhood development.* Elsevier; Kleigman, R., Stanton, B., Geme, J., Shor, N., & Behrman, R. (2016). *Nelson's textbook of pediatrics* (20th ed.). Elsevier; Carey, W., Crocker, A., Coleman, W., Elias, E., & Feldman, H. (2009). *Developmental-behavioral pediatrics* (4th ed.). W.B. Saunders; Vygotsky, L. (1962). *Thoughts and language.* MIT Press.

moved through periods of changes in stability that provided meaning for living. The core of Kegan's theory was the need to be included in reciprocal relationships with others and the need to maintain independence.

Theory of Language and Culture (Vygotsky)

Lev Vygotsky believed that social and cultural experiences were necessary for optimal growth and development. Physiological maturation of the brain enables language development, which influences how a child thinks and behaves. His theory suggested that language was a major force in the growth and development of the personality. Table 5.5 shows how language skills and social interaction affect each other and contribute to learning. People learn what they can achieve for themselves, and, through social interaction, what they can do with the help of others. This has implications for health education.

Social and Economic Influences (Bronfenbrenner)

Urie Bronfenbrenner presented a combination of social and economic factors that influence growth and development (Table 5.6). This theory offers insight into how children may be treated differently in different environments and the effect that those differences may have on a child's understanding of himself or herself.

Hierarchy of Needs (Maslow)

Abraham Maslow described a hierarchy of needs. According to Maslow, if basic needs are met, then the individual can move to higher levels of thought and self-fulfillment. These

TABLE 5.6 Bronfenbrenner's Social Theory of Growth and Development

Social Contacts	Influence on Personality Development
Parents, siblings	Gender of child influences how others treat child, which influences child's behavior. Parental expectations of child influence child's perception of self-worth.
Teachers, babysitters	Teachers' and babysitters' perceptions of the child influence child's sense of self. The active or aggressive child can frustrate teachers and babysitters, and the quiet child is often more appreciated.
School, neighborhood, community	Coach may value an athletically talented child. The academically talented child may not achieve similar recognition.
Political community	Funding for school community centers and programs influences ability of child to experience these social opportunities. Some energy and behaviors, if not appropriately channeled, may become antisocial; poverty can result in poor nutrition that can decrease the ability to learn and develop.

Data from Benson, J. (2020). *Encyclopedia of infant and early childhood development.* Elsevier; Kleigman, R., Stanton, B., Geme, J., Shor, N., & Behrman, R. (2016) *Nelson's textbook of pediatrics* (20th ed.). Elsevier; Carey, W., Crocker, A., Coleman, W., Flias, E., & Feldman, H. (2009). *Developmental-behavioral pediatrics* (4th ed.). W.B. Saunders; Bronfenbrenner, U. (1979). *The ecology of human development.* Harvard University Press.

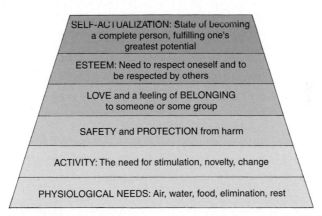

Figure 5.2 Modified version of Maslow's hierarchy of needs. *(From Leifer, G. (2019). Introduction to maternity and pediatric nursing (8th ed.). Elsevier.)*

needs are described using a triangle. The base of the triangle represents the basic physiological needs of survival. As the sides of the triangle narrow, achievement of needs at each level allows movement toward a higher level (Figure 5.2). After basic needs are met, a person can move toward self-actualization. Self-actualization is the realization of one's own talent and abilities and the achievement of satisfaction in life's goals and desires. It is reaching the peak of one's potential. For example, in severe poverty, basic physiological needs for food and shelter may be unmet. The person cannot think beyond meeting these basic needs of survival and so will not proceed to higher goals and ultimate self-actualization. Some characteristics of self-actualization include the accurate understanding of reality, judgments based on evidence, and the acceptance of self as independent and creative.

Environmental Theory (Rogers)

Carl Rogers believed people naturally form their own positive destiny, based on the concept of the self, if obstacles are removed. He theorized that mastery over the environment and positive relationships helped form the self-concept. A person has an idea of the type of person he or she would like to be. Sometimes there are differences between this idealized self and the actual self. If the ideal self shares a lot in common with the actual self, then that person discovers his or her full potential and achieves happiness. According to Rogers, self-actualization happens as a person realizes he or she can do many things to be like the ideal self.

Behaviorist Theory (Watson)

John Watson was known as the father of behaviorism. He believed the environment and experiences molded the personality. Inborn traits or drives are not the basis of his theory. Watson's theories are related to Pavlov's conditioning theory of personality development and Skinner's operant theory.

Behaviorist Theory of Personality (Pavlov and Skinner)

Ivan Pavlov and B.F. Skinner's theories describe learning and interaction with the environment as the center of development. This is known as the behaviorist theory of development. Behaviorists believe that personality and behavior are learned. Therefore they believe that there are no identifiable stages. Each experience helps to mold the adult personality.

These theorists believed that the environment and the way people respond to it influence personality development. Pavlov developed the theory of classical conditioning. Conditioning has to do with associating (pairing) things in the environment. For example, when an individual eats a food that causes the unpleasant symptoms of food poisoning, that individual may develop an aversion to that food. The food poisoning was paired with that food, because they were experienced together. Because of this, that particular food is associated with negative feelings even without food poisoning occurring again.

Skinner attributed learning to operant conditioning, which involves behavioral consequences such as reward or punishment. For example, reinforcing positive behavior with a reward will eventually develop a regular practice of that behavior. Powerful rewards can include praise, recognition, and special attention or can "add up" to be rewards in the form of special privileges, special activities, or occasional material rewards such as toys, money, or favorite foods or desserts, or the removal of a negative stimulus.

These theories are useful in health education, because positive reinforcement of learned information can result in positive health practices. The opposite is also true. If a coach uses exercise as a punishment, by making the student run around a course or do 15 push-ups after bad behavior, then exercise can become perceived as a negative activity and not considered as a pleasurable experience. This can lead to a sedentary lifestyle and obesity later in life. Rewarding healthy behaviors, such as exercise or medical compliance, can increase the occurrence of these behaviors.

Social-Learning Theories of Personality (Bandura and Mischel)

Albert Bandura and Walter Mischel were theorists who believed that social learning formed the basis for personality development (Bandura, 1977). Social-learning theory involves exposure to and imitation of a behavior. Children often imitate what they see. If a father mows the lawn and receives praise for his work, the child witnesses the scenario and receives reinforcement for the positive aspects of that behavior. The child may copy that behavior because of curiosity, a desire to mimic the behavior of people he or she admires, or a desire for the positive reinforcement. In early childhood, these models are usually the parents. In the school-age child, models may be peers or teachers. Therefore, children who receive praise from friends for their illegal or risky behavior can become the behavioral models for the school-age child who is exposed to this type of social environment. The development of aggressive behavior and gender-specific stereotyped behavior may be intensified by the peers the child is exposed to at this age.

Theory of Moral Development (Kohlberg)

Moral reasoning is the development of a set of social rules that enables a person to differentiate right from wrong, and moral behavior is based on perception and integration of these rules. Lawrence Kohlberg's theory of moral development consists of three levels that are closely related to Piaget's views (see Table 5.4). Kohlberg's stages of moral development (Table 5.7) remain a respected theory today, although modification of level three (the postconventional stage) has been suggested as a result of research findings. Carol Gilligan's work challenged the description of postconventional moral thought, and Gilligan also believed that Kohlberg's research excluded women.

TABLE 5.7 Kohlberg's Stages of Moral Development

Stage	Age	Behavior
Preconventional	Toddler	Obeys rules to avoid punishments.
	Early childhood	Seeks to avoid punishment.
Conventional	School age	Conforms to rules to gain recognition or reward.
Postconventional	Adolescent and adult	Follows rules that lead others to perceive person as "good." Develops a sense of responsibility.
	Older adult	Develops own set of principles that may overrule social laws or customs. Is independent.

Data from Benson, J. (2020). *Encyclopedia of infant and early childhood development*, Elsevier; Kleigman, R., Stanton, B., Geme, J., Shor, N., & Behrman, R. (2016) *Nelson's textbook of pediatrics* (20th ed.). Elsevier; Carey, W., Crocker, A., Coleman, W., Elias, E., & Feldman, H. (2009). *Developmental-behavioral pediatrics* (4th ed.). W.B. Saunders; Kohlberg, L (1964). Development of moral character and moral ideology. In H. Hoffman, & L. Hoffman, L. (Eds.), *Review of child development research*. Russell Sage.

Moral behavior is generally considered to be learned. Parents and teachers provide rewards when children demonstrate desired morally sound behaviors. Teaching a child right from wrong in a firm, loving way will result in the development of moral behavior.

Health Promotion

Helping a child understand how someone else feels in reaction to his or her behavior (empathy) is a preferred method for encouraging the development of moral behavior. Punishment often results in resistance and denial and can turn the focus away from learning, and thus punishment may not be an effective tool for teaching moral behavior.

Development of Self-Image (Cooley and Mead)

Charles Horton Cooley created the theory of the looking-glass self, which states that the self-image is formed through three steps: (1) imagining how we portray ourselves to others; (2) imagining how others evaluate us; and (3) combining these impressions to formulate a self-concept or idea of what we are like. For example, if a teacher criticizes a child, the child may think the teacher believes the child is ignorant; therefore, the child's self-image may incorporate the thought that he or she is ignorant.

George Herbert Mead furthered Cooley's theory by presenting three stages in the development of the self. In the first stage, children imitate those around them. The child uses a toy broom to imitate a parent sweeping or a toy lawn mower to imitate an adult mowing the lawn. The child may vicariously feel proud of the clean floor or manicured lawn. When children are ready to experience the world of language, video, and books, they are ready for stage two, which involves the use of language or other symbols during interaction with others, such as making a sad, pouting face; a happy face; and so on. In the third stage, the child pretends to be other people – for instance, a superhero such as Spiderman – and may play the role of the pretend person. In middle childhood, the child understands his or her own role and the way it affects the role of others (Figure 5.3). A child learns about

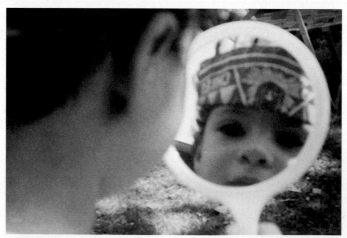

Figure 5.3 A self-image begins to develop with imaginative play during the preschool years.

others' expectations and appreciates that each person assumes multiple roles in life, such as daughter, sister, mother, grandmother, and teacher.

Developmental Tasks of the Older Adult (Peck)

Robert Peck's theory is based on the developmental tasks of the older adult, which include coping with retirement from work, adapting to the normal physiological decline because of aging, and facing the inevitability of death. Peck's theory involved the need to positively meet these challenges to maintain generativity (as described by Erikson) and to avoid despair. Maintaining a positive self-image and feelings of self-worth, despite changing abilities and increasing limitations, is essential to making a healthy transition during this stage.

Developmental Tasks of the Older Adult (Havighurst)

Robert Havighurst (1974) was a theorist who also described the developmental tasks of late adulthood, which involve accepting oneself and maintaining meaning in life. The older adult's developmental tasks include adjusting to a decreasing health status, adjusting to decreased income, adjusting to the death of a spouse, adapting to changing social roles with peer groups, and adapting to changing living arrangements.

Developmental Stages of Retirement (Atchley)

Robert Atchley described five developmental stages in the older adult related to retirement, as described in Table 5.8. See Chapter 13 for further content.

Additional Influences on Growth and Development

In addition to the theories described earlier, there are other influences on growth and development. *Cultural beliefs and practices* (discussed in Chapter 3) and *gender differences* affect development according to how the child is treated by others. Often, beginning at birth a girl is dressed in pink and a boy in blue or brown. Toys selected by parents can also affect gender roles. Increasingly, parents are accepting the importance of gender fluidity, and rejecting the notion of typical gender roles, allowing children to choose their own clothes and toys without judgement (Watkins, 2016).

TABLE 5.8 Atchley's Developmental Stages of Retirement

Stage	Focus
Preretirement	Dreams of retirement
Honeymoon	Enjoys freedom of retirement
Disenchantment	Designs new priorities as a result of boredom
Stability	Begins to feel needed and respected
Terminal	Changes occur because of need for reemployment or decline in health

Poverty can decrease experiences available to the child, and it can also deprive the child of nutrition needed for brain and body development. The homeless child often does not have access to health care, and homeless adolescents may be exposed to drugs, sexual abuse, and other problems that affect growth and development. Parents should be encouraged to partner with educators to enrich the child's experience of learning in the school and in the home.

There are *developmental tasks* to be achieved and challenges to be met in each phase of development through the lifespan. Psychological growth occurs through all stages of the life cycle and can modify a person's personality, behavior, and health.

KEY POINTS

- Personal development is influenced by many factors, including genetics, birth order, gender, and environment.
- A theory is designed to explain the development of specific behaviors and is based on research findings.
- Developmental theories can aid health-care workers, nurses, and educators in understanding needs, learning styles, and behaviors at various stages of the life cycle.
- Understanding needs, learning styles, and behaviors at each stage of development enable the nurse, health-care worker, or educator to plan teaching interventions that will contribute to the goals of *Healthy People 2030*.
- Understanding growth and development can help in the designing of teaching styles that will foster positive health-care practices.
- Freud was a psychoanalyst who identified the id, ego, and superego and described stages of psychosexual development.
- Carl Jung believed that development extended into adulthood, with age 40 as the "noon of life."
- Erik Erikson expressed a psychosocial theory that defined stages of life from infancy through the older-adult phase.
- Jean Piaget developed the cognitive theory of development that centered around understanding and relating to the world environment.

- June Loevinger stretched Piaget's theory of development into adulthood.
- Robert Kegan expressed a constructive developmental theory similar to Piaget's, which involved lifelong periods of change and stability.
- Lev Vygotsky presented a theory of language and culture related to the developmental process.
- Urie Bronfenbrenner believed social and economic pressures influenced growth and development.
- Abraham Maslow described a hierarchy-of-needs theory leading to self-actualization.
- Carl Rogers believed people form their own destinies based on mastery of the environment.
- Ivan Pavlov and B.F. Skinner developed the behaviorist theory of personality development. They described how classical and operant conditioning influence behavior in response to the environment.
- John Watson was known as the father of behaviorism.
- K. Bandura and W. Mischel researched social-learning theory as the basis for personality development.
- Lawrence Kohlberg described personality development based on moral reasoning. He believed moral behavior was a learned behavior.

- Charles Horton Cooley proposed the looking-glass self theory of personality development, and George Herbert Mead expanded the theory by presenting three stages in the development of the self.
- Robert Peck described developmental tasks of the older adult.
- Robert Havighurst described developmental tasks of late adulthood.
- Robert Atchley described developmental stages in the older adult related to the retirement phase of life.
- Maria Montessori was an educational theorist who believed children were competent and designed schools with levels to reflect competence rather than the age of the child.
- Loris Malaguzzi believed that learning should be based on exploration rather than dissemination of facts.

Clinical Judgment Case Study

Using information from established theories of growth and development, explain why the diagnosis listed on the left might have the greatest influence on the development process of the age group listed on the right.

Comparative study:

Diagnosis	Age Group
Fractured jaw	Infant
Fractured leg	Toddler
Fractured arm	School-age child

REVIEW QUESTIONS

1. Mark the box for the appropriate theory of development represented by the description.

	Piaget	Freud	Erikson
Play helps the infant to understand cause and effect in the sensorimotor stage	☐	☐	☐
The infant explores things with his mouth because he is in an oral phase	☐	☐	☐
Playing peek-a-boo helps the infant understand object permanence	☐	☐	☐
Infants who are fed on-demand learn to trust their caregivers	☐	☐	☐

2. Which theorist described a hierarchy of needs that leads to self-actualization?

A. Ivan Pavlov.

B. Abraham Maslow.

C. Lawrence Kohlberg.

D. Robert Peck.

3. Health-care workers need to understand developmental theories because this understanding will help them:

   A. pass the licensing examination.

   B. intervene effectively to promote positive, healthy practices.

   C. design effective discipline for young children.

   D. analyze the goals of *Healthy People 2030.*

4. An understanding of object permanence is part of the stages of development described by:

   A. Jean Piaget.

   B. Abraham Maslow.

   C. Lawrence Kohlberg.

   D. Sigmund Freud.

5. Ivan Pavlov was a behaviorist who believed that personality and behavior develop under the influence of:

   A. conditioning responses.

   B. genetic control.

   C. close parental guidance.

   D. chronological age.

Prenatal Influences on Healthy Development

http://evolve.elsevier.com/Leifer/growth

OUTLINE

OBJECTIVES

1. State the goals of the Human Genome Project.
2. Trace the steps of human fertilization and implantation.
3. Discuss the critical periods of fetal development.
4. Describe how optimal prenatal care can affect the adult health of the newborn and affect the adult health of future generations.
5. Describe the role of exercise during and after pregnancy.
6. Describe the modifications required for exercise during pregnancy.
7. Compare the similarities and differences among two types of twins.
8. Discuss the role of microbiomes in the adult health of the newborn infant.
9. Discuss the emotional changes that occur during transition to motherhood.
10. Discuss the importance of understanding culture as it affects the care of parents and newborns.
11. Discuss bonding and attachment between parents and newborns.
12. Describe the techniques for calming a newborn infant.
13. List the types of toys and activities that foster the growth and development of the neonate.

KEY TERMS

allele	engrossment	monozygotic
Apgar score	fetal alcohol syndrome	multifetal
attachment	fetus	mutated
bonding	gene therapy	neonatal
chromosome	genetic code	sibling rivalry
dizygotic	genetic counseling	syndrome
dominant gene	genome	viable
dysbiosis	gestation	virus vector
ectopic pregnancy	gestational diabetes	
en face	microbiome	

THE HUMAN GENOME PROJECT

Growth and development are influenced by biology and by the environment. Research concerning the maternal-fetal origins of adult disease contributed to the development of the Human Genome Project. The National Institutes of Health (NIH) and the U.S. Department of Energy (DOE) assumed leadership of the many scientists who probed the secrets of human genetic makeup for this project. The Human Genome Project involved gene mapping, which determined the makeup of human genes, and the completion of the project in 2001 resulted in the identification of all human genes. Various grants were awarded to finance the research. The project officially began in 1990, and a draft of the findings was published in 2001. The original goals of the project involved the following:

- Identifying more than 30,000 genes contained in human DNA
- Determining the sequence of the billions of chemicals that are contained in DNA
- Developing tools for analysis of the findings
- Addressing the ethical, legal, and social implications (ELSI) involved
- Transferring the technology for use by the public in the private sector

HEREDITY

Cells are the basic working units of all living systems, and a genome is a complete set of DNA that is contained in all cells. The DNA in the genome is the genetic code of a cell that is carried on the chromosomes. A chromosome is a thread of protein and DNA that is contained in the nucleus of every cell. Each chromosome contains genes, and there are approximately 30,000 genes in a genome. The genes or genetic code within these cells carry information about all the proteins within the cell that will determine the characteristics that will be inherited by the newborn (Figure 6.1).

Heredity is controlled by pairs of genes from both the mother and father. This pairing of genes is called an allele. Genes can be dominant or recessive. A dominant gene will overpower a recessive gene most of the time, so that its characteristic will be inherited in about three of four offspring. One of the four offspring may exhibit characteristics of the recessive trait (Figure 6.2).

INSIDE THE CELL

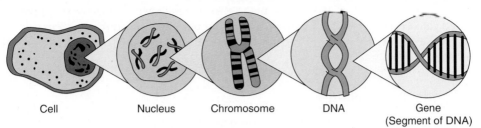

| Cell | Nucleus | Chromosome | DNA | Gene (Segment of DNA) |

Figure 6.1 The cell contains the nucleus, chromosomes, DNA, and genes. (From Leifer, G. (2012). *Maternity nursing, an introductory text* (11th ed.). Saunders.)

Studying the characteristics and roles of mutated (variations that may be abnormal) and normal genes enables genetic therapy to be used to correct mutated genes and to replace missing genes that cause specific syndromes. A syndrome is a group of symptoms or signs of an abnormal condition. It is known that specific genetic syndromes contribute to specific behavior patterns. Behavior patterns can result in a response from

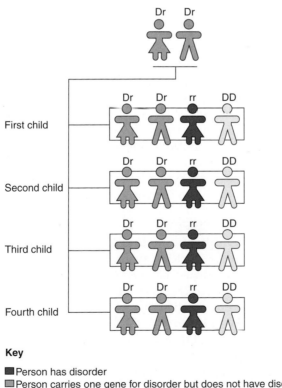

Key

■ Person has disorder
▨ Person carries one gene for disorder but does not have disorder
□ Person has no disorder and does not carry one gene for disorder

Figure 6.2 Transmission of dominant and recessive traits. Each parent has one dominant gene (D) and one recessive gene (r) for a disease. This figure shows the chances of each offspring being affected by the disease. (From Leifer, G. (2012). *Maternity nursing, an introductory text* (11th ed.). Saunders.)

the environment, which can then affect a child's self-image, as well as growth and development. For example, a genetic abnormality that causes Down syndrome, or an uncontrolled glucose (sugar) level in a diabetic mother, or poor nutrition during pregnancy, can each cause cognitive damage in the newborn infant that will impact the child's growth and development.

Genetic Counseling

Genetic counseling is the communication between a geneticist (a specialist in inherited conditions) and the parents to discuss the risk of their infant inheriting genes that could result in an abnormality. It is known that behavior is molded by the influence of genes as well as environmental factors. The success of the Human Genome Project allows more detailed research concerning genetic problems and resulting behaviors. Researchers have developed therapeutic genes that repair defective DNA, suicide genes that can be programmed to destroy defective genes, and pure genes that can replace a missing gene.

Gene Therapy

Gene therapy involves placing a therapeutic gene on the back of a **virus or bacterial vector** (a virus or bacteria that has the ability to enter specific cells in the body). The vector carries the new gene into the cell that has a missing or defective gene and the cell then is able to produce more copies of the inserted gene. The defective cells can also be removed from the body, genetically modified, and returned to the body. Although the majority of gene therapy applications has focused on the treatment of cancer (Lundstrom, 2019), with the discovery of a naturally occurring gene editing system in bacteria, the CRISPR-Cas9 system (short for clustered regularly interspaced short palindromic repeats and CRISPR-associated protein 9) has greatly expanded the approaches and application of genome editing and therapy (National Institutes of Health, 2020). Gene therapy is regulated by the U.S. Food & Drug Administration (FDA) Center for Biological Evaluation and Research (CYBER) and standardized policies have been developed.

Screening Procedures and Therapies

It is possible to screen individual patients for the existence of some specific genetic problems without looking at DNA, such as using hemoglobin electrophoresis for types of anemia or the Guthrie test for phenylketonuria (PKU) (a condition in which phenylalanine accumulates in the body and causes mental retardation). However, DNA-based genetic tests can detect carriers, identify susceptibility, and enable diagnosis before symptoms occur. Carrier testing is possible, and genetic counseling can be initiated for conditions such as sickle cell and thalassemia disease (a genetic trait that causes an abnormal shape or type of red blood cells), Tay-Sachs disease (a destruction of nerve cells that causes mental and motor deterioration and death during early childhood), and cystic fibrosis (a malfunction of the exocrine glands that results in lung and digestive dysfunctions).

Some adult-onset diseases can be diagnosed before symptoms appear, such as Huntington's Chorea and Lou Gehrig's disease (amyotrophic lateral sclerosis). However, genetic specialists are needed to ensure accurate interpretation of test results. This type of testing requires a team of professionals who can determine the psychological impact of this knowledge on the patient and perhaps the impact on the patient's employment or life insurance eligibility, now and in the future. Genetic testing is available but may not always be affordable, appropriate, or relevant to optimal medical management.

ELSI

The **ELSI** program has been developed to study the ethical, legal, and social implications of gene therapy. Techniques of gene therapy still need to be refined to ensure that methods of repairing DNA do not damage the DNA in a way that could potentially cause a new illness. Over the last 15 years research has advanced understanding of the complex societal implications of the study and advance of gene therapy (Bentley et al., 2017).

FETAL DEVELOPMENT

Fertilization occurs when the sperm penetrates the ovum as it enters the upper portion of the woman's fallopian tube. The time in which fertilization can occur is brief. The sperm lives for up to 5 days, but the ovum lives for only 24 hours after ovulation (Chapter 10). The ovum always contributes an X chromosome, and the sperm contributes either an X or a Y chromosome. The combination of XX chromosomes produces a female fetus, whereas an XY combination creates a male fetus. Because it is only the sperm that carries the Y chromosome, the male partner determines the sex of the infant. However, the female has some influence on which sperm fertilizes the ovum because estrogen levels and the pH of the reproductive tract affect the survival rate of the X- or Y-bearing sperm and the speed of their movement to the fallopian tube (Ross & Ervin, 2016).

The *zygote* is the cell formed by the union of the sperm and ovum. The cell rapidly multiplies and develops. Within 1 week it enters the uterus and attaches to the upper posterior portion of the uterine wall. (If the zygote does not move freely through and exit the fallopian tube, its increasing size will rupture the fallopian tube, and this condition is known as an **ectopic pregnancy**.) After implantation into the wall of the uterus, the cells differentiate into layers called the endoderm, mesoderm, and ectoderm. Each layer develops into different organs of the body. After 2 weeks of growth and development, the zygote is called an embryo. From the ninth week of life to birth, the developing baby is called a fetus. Fetal development is shown in Table 6.1.

During the third week after fertilization, the heart begins to beat, and the neural tube (the beginning portion of the central nervous system) forms. For this reason, the mother should take prenatal vitamins to ensure adequate intake of folic acid that is essential for normal neural tube development. It is also prudent to encourage the increased consumption of legumes such as beans, soy, lentils, and peas, and leafy green vegetables such as spinach, which are rich in folate. Conditions such as spina bifida can occur if there is a deficiency of folic acid when the neural tube is forming. The placenta takes control of fetal circulation at the end of the third month of pregnancy. The umbilical cord attaches the fetus to the placenta and a thin membrane separates the maternal and fetal blood because the maternal and fetal blood supplies do not normally mix.

By 20 weeks of gestation (fetal life), the fetus is considered viable (able to survive outside the uterus). However, the lack of a substance called surfactant in the lungs at this stage of fetal development would require that special neonatal intensive care be provided. Some surfactant is produced by 28 weeks' gestation, and another spurt of surfactant is deposited

TABLE 6.1   Embryonic and Fetal Development

Age	Length and Weight	Development
Week 3 Actual size 2.5 mm	1.5–2.5 mm	Single tubular heart is formed. Neural tube forms; primitive spinal cord and brain appear.
Week 4	3.5–4 mm	Heart pumps blood. Esophagus and trachea separate; stomach forms. Neural tube closes; forebrain forms. Upper and lower limb buds appear. Ears and eyes begin to form.
Week 6 Actual size 11.0 mm	11–13 mm	Skull and jaw ossify; hands and elbows differentiate. Auditory canal forms; eye is obvious. Heart has all four chambers. Nasal cavity and upper lip form.

Week 3 figure labels: Neural groove, Cut surface of amnion, Neural groove, Neural fold in region of developing spinal cord, Location of primitive streak, Neural fold in region of developing brain, Yolk sac, First pairs of somites, Connecting stalk, Part of chorionic sac

Week 4 figure labels: Forebrain, Heart, Upper limb bud

Week 6 figure labels: External acoustic meatus, Auricular hillocks forming auricle of external ear, Eyelid, Pigmented eye, Nasolacrimal groove, Nasal pit, Umbilical cord, Heart prominence, Digital rays of hand plate, Foot plate

Age	Length and Weight	Development
Week 8 Scalp vascular plexus, Auricle of external ear, Eyelid, Eye, Shoulder, Nose, Mouth, Lower jaw, Wrist, Umbilical cord, Arm, Toes separated, Elbow, Knee, Sole of foot — Actual size 30.0 mm	30 mm crown-rump 6 g	Embryo has distinct human appearance. Purposeful movements occur. Tail has disappeared. Sex organs form. Beginnings of most external and internal structures are formed. Enters fetal period.
Week 17	150 mm crown-rump 260 g	Genitalia and leg movements are visible on ultrasound; movement may be felt by the mother. Bones are ossified. Eye movements occur. Fetus sucks and swallows amniotic fluid. Ovaries contain ovum. No subcutaneous fat is present. Thin skin allows blood vessels of scalp to be visible.
Week 25	28 cm (11.2 inches) crown-heel 780 g (1 lb, 10 oz)	Wrinkled skin, lean body results from lack of subcutaneous fat. Eyes are open. Fetus is now viable. Mother feels stronger movement (quickening). Fetus has schedule of sleeping and moving. Vernix caseosa is present on skin. Lanugo covers body. Brown fat is formed. Lungs begin to secrete surfactant. Fingernails are present. Respiratory movements begin.

(Continued)

TABLE 6.1   Embryonic and Fetal Development (*Cont.*)

Age	Length and Weight	Development
Week 29	38 cm (15 inches) crown-heel 1260 g (2 lb, 10 oz)	Fetus assumes stable (cephalic) position in utero. Central nervous system is functioning. Skin is less wrinkled because of the presence of subcutaneous fat. Spleen stops forming blood cells, and bone marrow starts to form blood cells. Increased surfactant is present in lungs.
Week 36	48 cm (19 inches) crown-heel 2500 g (5 lb, 12 oz)	Subcutaneous fat is present. Skin is smooth. Grasp reflex is present. Circumferences of head and abdomen are equal. Surge of lung surfactant is produced.

Note: Full term is considered 38–40 weeks. The crown-heel length is 48–52 cm (18–21 inches), and the weight is 3000–3600 g (6 lb, 10 oz to 7 lb, 15 oz). Unnumbered Figures 6.1, 6.2, 6.3, 6.4 from Moore, K.L., & Persaud, T.V.N. (2008). *The developing human: clinically oriented embryology* (8th ed.). Saunders. Unnumbered Figures 6.5, 6.6, 6.7, 6.8 from Jessica Servoss, artist (2020).

into the fetal lungs at 32 weeks' gestation. After 38 weeks of gestation, the fetus is considered to be full term but is normally ready for birth by 40 weeks gestation.

A woman should start prenatal care as early as possible. Adequate nutrition and exercise during pregnancy are beneficial, and monthly visits to the health-care provider enable monitoring of the pregnancy to ensure a healthy outcome for both mother and baby.

Twins

Twins or other multifetal births (e.g., triplets, quadruplets, and so on) can occur. Dizygotic twins, also called fraternal twins, occur when two ova are released at ovulation, and each ovum is fertilized by a separate sperm. The twins may or may not be of the same sex, and they are as alike as any siblings. Monozygotic twins, also called identical twins, occur when one single fertilized ovum separates into two separate embryos. These twins will be of the same sex and will be genetically identical (i.e., they will look very similar to one another). Many twins are born prematurely because the uterus becomes overdistended or the placenta is unable to supply the nourishment required to carry the pregnancy to term.

THE PRENATAL PHASE

Critical Periods

Many of the critical periods during fetal growth occur during the first trimester of pregnancy (first 3 months) when basic structures are developing. Many factors can affect growth and development throughout fetal life. For example, undernutrition can cause a reduction in the number of cells produced, resulting in health problems after birth.

Every system in the body has a critical period in which nutrition, drugs, and other environmental factors influence its development and function. Illness, lack of nutrition, or exposure to toxins during these critical periods can cause a maldevelopment or malfunction of a specific organ or system that may not manifest in the newborn until adult life.

Health Promotion

The well-being of the mother and fetus can influence the life expectancy of the newborn. In accordance with the goals of *Healthy People 2030*, to prevent disease in the next generation we need to improve the nutrition of mothers and babies and reduce exposure to infection in early childhood.

Microbiomes in Pregnancy and Influence on Adult Health of the Newborn

The "Human Microbiome Project" was designed to help understand the relationship of the human microbiome to health and disease (Valentine et al., 2019). Microbiomes, micro (tiny) and biome (organism), are large communities of trillions of tiny organisms that live in our body. Microbiomes play an important role in normal physiology, development, and health.

As the fetus develops in the uterus of the mother, it interacts with microbiomes that are present in her body and influenced by her diet and health practices. Pregnancy-related stress or illness, or medications she consumes, can affect her microbiomes which will then affect the health of the newborn at birth as well as in later life. The exchanges of microbiomes between mother and infant before and after birth are related to the health and disease of the infant in later life (Valentine et al., 2019).

An infant acquires microbiomes during fetal development and at birth as it passes through the birth canal, and during the first hours of life as it interacts with the mother and breastfeeds. These microbiome exchanges have a lasting impact on the health of the newborn as an infant, as a child, and as an adult. Breastfeeding provides different microbiomes to the newborn compared with formula feeding. Events such as fever in the infant can cause shifts in microbiomes that can alter the infant's health and continue its influence even as it progresses to an adult. Antibiotic use can shift microbiomes in a way that allows inflammation or chronic disorders to develop. This shifting or impairment of microbiomes is called *dysbiosis*. Researchers have identified dominant microbiota or microbiomes that are present at different life stages, and, for example, a shift of prominent microbiomes in the elderly stage of life can result in the development of dementia, or dysbiosis of microbiota in early life may result in autism (Wu et al., 2019).

The maintenance of health and the level of immunity to disease are influenced by microbiomes acquired during fetal development and newborn experiences. Proper diet and health practices in stages of early life influence health as an adult.

Toxins

Teratogens (toxins) are harmful influences on fetal growth. Exposure to toxins during fetal development can cause abnormalities, illness, or miscarriage. Maternal ingestion of substances such as alcohol can interfere with cell growth in the developing fetus. For example, fetal alcohol syndrome in the newborn is characterized by mental retardation and abnormal facial features. Recreational drug exposure during pregnancy can cause prematurity, seizure disorders, and learning disabilities in the newborn infant. Maternal cigarette smoking can cause decreased birth weight in the newborn. Mothers are cautioned to avoid contact with cat-litter boxes during pregnancy because of the risk of developing a condition called toxoplasmosis, which can be devastating to the newborn. Careful attention to the prenatal dietary practices of the pregnant woman is essential. For example, excessive ingestion of specific foods during pregnancy (cravings) can impact fetal development and affect the health of the newborn later in life. Glycyrrhizin, a constituent of licorice, can cause an excess of cortisol in the fetus. Some studies have shown that high licorice ingestion during pregnancy resulted in their newborns having deficits in cognitive abilities, memory, and aggression-related problems in adult life (Ross & DeSal, 2017).

Decisions regarding prenatal care and environmental toxins and drugs influence the development of metabolic, developmental, and pathological conditions in the adult life of the fetus with possible influences on multiple generations (Ross & DeSal, 2017). In other words, the health-care practices of grandma during her pregnancy can influence the health of her child, grandchild, and possibly her great-grandchild.

Health Promotion

Maternal illness must be prevented, and certain teratogens should be avoided during pregnancy to prevent untoward effects in the fetus.

Exercise During Pregnancy

While weight loss should not be a goal, exercise is important to maintain levels of health and fitness during pregnancy. Benefits include promoting healthy weight gain, improved energy level, mood, sleep, and muscle tone, as well as decreased risk of gestational diabetes. Diabetes that occurs during pregnancy can negatively affect pregnancy outcome but often disappears after pregnancy. Exercise programs also play a significant role in managing glucose levels in women who have type 2 diabetes mellitus when becoming pregnant (Halvatsiotis et al., 2020). A fitness program can also improve the mother's ability to cope with labor as well as enhance recovery and decrease the risk of postpartum depression (Poyatos-León et al.,

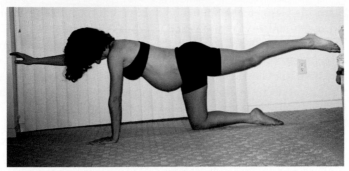

Figure 6.3 Stretch exercises at home are appropriate and healthy for the pregnant woman. Other appropriate activities are step aerobics, swimming, and prenatal yoga, among others.

2017). At least 30 minutes per day, 5 days per week, of moderate exercise also helps prevent excessive weight gain during pregnancy (Vargas-Terrones et al., 2019; Figure 6.3).

A pregnant woman who was previously sedentary can slowly begin a light exercise program that includes walking or swimming. A previously active woman can, in most cases, safely continue her exercise program with a few simple modifications, such as avoiding becoming overheated (since heat is transmitted to the fetus, causing an increase in oxygen needs). There are several safety issues to consider while exercising during pregnancy. Hormones released during pregnancy cause increased joint laxity, which could lead to injury if range of motion is exaggerated. Also, a shift in center of gravity can create balance challenges, thus increasing the risk of falls. The pregnant woman should avoid the supine position during exercises after the first trimester to ensure uninterrupted blood flow to the fetus. Pregnant women should also stay well hydrated and seek guidance from a fitness professional who specializes in exercise during pregnancy.

A pregnant woman should stop exercising if she experiences vaginal bleeding or other discharge, uterine contractions, or decreased fetal movement. Although excessive weight gain should be avoided, food intake must be adequate for appropriate fetal development during pregnancy. An increase of 300 calories per day is a healthy way to achieve the expected 25–30-pound weight gain over the gestational period.

Maternal Adaptations During the Prenatal Phase

The changing patterns of childrearing, the increasing number of dual-career households, and the increasing distances among extended family members influence the social support systems available for parents-to-be. Dependency on physicians is decreased because the large health maintenance organizations (HMOs) or health-care facilities may not guarantee a regular personal physician to follow each pregnant woman throughout her pregnancy.

Health Promotion

Parents need to be well informed to make healthy decisions about pregnancy, delivery, and childcare. Parents need to be involved in developmental issues concerning their parental roles and impending changes in their lifestyles.

If the pregnancy is planned and wanted, attitudes will most likely be positive. If the pregnancy is unintentional, interventions and referrals may be necessary to help the parents develop a positive attitude or to help select alternatives such as adoption or abortion. The timing of the pregnancy in the life of the parents is also an important consideration. Adolescent parents may not have completed the transition to adulthood, may still be in the protective environment of their parents' homes, and so may need a more intensive adjustment period to establish their independence.

The initial phase of establishing a family after marriage (Chapters 4 and 11) involves adjusting to a marital adult affiliation with the establishment of mutual goals, housing, financial responsibilities, educational pursuits, and lifestyle choices. Entering into the role of a parent who is responsible for a dependent child is, according to Erikson, the beginning of the stage of generativity. The mother is motivated to prepare psychologically for the arrival of the infant as she feels the fetus move in her womb (uterus). A state of attachment occurs, and rapport with the fetus develops. The partner may attend parenting classes with the pregnant woman and may be included in the attachment process as the fetus grows and develops (Figure 6.4).

The first period of parental development includes three distinct phases, each with specific tasks. The first phase is the response to discovering that conception has occurred. The parents may be elated or disappointed. Lifestyle changes will be discussed. The second phase occurs in the second trimester (4–6 months of the pregnancy), during which time fetal movement is felt, an ultrasound picture of the fetus is often seen, and the reality of the pregnancy becomes evident. Parents may worry about the health of the infant and

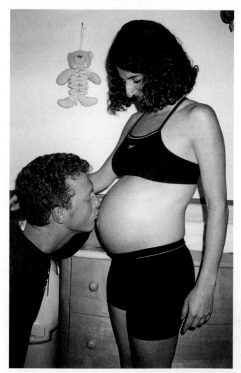

Figure 6.4 The father begins to bond with the fetus as the fetal heart can be heard and fetal movement can be felt.

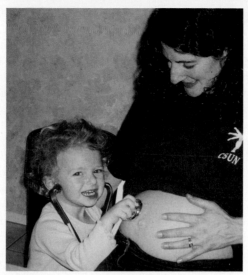

Figure 6.5 A sibling begins to anticipate the birth of her brother.

plan for its place in the home and family (Figure 6.5). The third phase occurs in the third trimester (7–9 months), when plans for the actual birth of the baby become the focus. The partner may worry about competing for attention and may feel left out. Old conflicts may resurface. Parents may feel inadequately prepared for the responsibility of caring for the newborn. Parents can be referred to parenting classes that are available in most communities.

THE BIRTH PROCESS

Childbirth is a normal physiological process that affects the health of the mother and fetus. Labor and delivery are often a family affair with fathers or significant others participating and grandparents actively involved (unless a community is quarantined during an epidemic or pandemic occurrence). Attendance at preparation classes during pregnancy and the cultural background of the parents usually dictate the extent to which the partner or grandparent play supportive roles in the labor and delivery unit. A woman can choose to deliver the baby in a traditional hospital setting, in a freestanding private birthing center, or at home. *Obstetricians* (doctors with special education in women's health), *nurse practitioners* (registered nurses with advanced practice education), or *nurse midwives* (registered nurses with advanced labor and delivery education) may be in attendance to monitor the process. A *doula* is a specially trained labor and delivery coach who may stay with the mother during labor and birth. The birth process occurs in four stages. The first stage is the dilation (opening) and effacement (shortening) of the uterine cervix. The second stage is the descent and birth of the baby, and the third stage is the birth of the placenta (afterbirth). The fetal heart rate and the contractions of the uterus are monitored closely during the birth process. The fourth stage is the recovery stage, when bonding takes place and the family is united and monitored.

THE NEWBORN INFANT

After the infant is born and the umbilical cord is cut, many physiological changes occur in the infant's body to enable it to adjust to life outside of the uterus. The lungs expand and the circulation pattern that allowed bypass of the lungs during fetal life changes so that all blood circulates to the infant's lungs to receive oxygen. The cyanotic (blue) color of the skin quickly changes to its natural color as the infant cries and oxygenation is established. The infant is dried and placed in a prewarmed bed, and the head is covered to minimize heat loss until the infant can stabilize its own body temperature.

The newborn's vital signs are monitored, and an Apgar score is assessed at 1 minute and 5 minutes after birth. The Apgar score is a rating of heart, respiration, muscle tone, color, and reflex irritability (not to be confused with the *family* Apgar described in Chapter 4). A score from 1 to 10 provides an estimate of the condition of the infant and determines the need for further resuscitation efforts. The infant receives vitamin K to aid in blood clotting in the umbilical cord, and an antibiotic ointment is placed in the infant's eyes to prevent ophthalmia neonatorum and chlamydia infection, which if left untreated could lead to blindness in the neonate. An identification band with a special number is placed on the wrist of the infant, mother, and significant other, and the newborn's footprints may be taken.

It is important for the nurse to promote bonding and attachment between parents and newborns as soon as possible after birth (Figure 6.6). Bonding refers to a strong emotional tie between parents and the newborn. Attachment refers to an affectionate tie that occurs over time as a result of parent-infant interaction. Bonding begins during pregnancy, but it is most important that touch and visual interaction occur as soon as possible after birth. The newborn should be placed in the mother's arms, preferably with skin-to-skin contact and put to breast for breastfeeding. (Breastfeeding is discussed in Chapter 7.) The *en face* (face-to-face) position facilitates eye contact between infant and parent (Figure 6.7). The infant can see a short distance at birth and responds to close face-to-face encounters. The

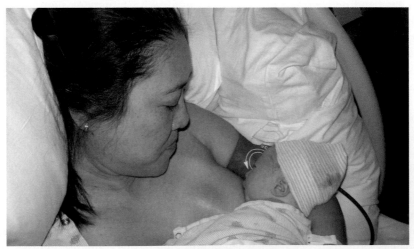

Figure 6.6 A new mother bonds with her newborn infant using skin-to-skin contact during breastfeeding.

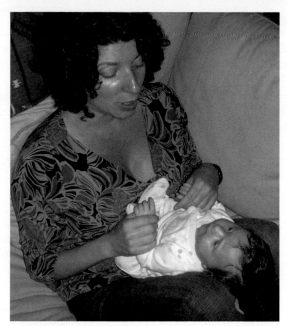

Figure 6.7 The *en face* position between mother and infant. The mother positions her baby to provide close face-to-face interaction to promote bonding. The newborn gazes at the mother and responds to her voice and touch.

infant is most alert in the first hour after birth, and then several hours of sleep and decreased motor activity will follow. Parent-infant bonding should be the focus of care during this first hour of life outside the womb.

THE TRANSITION TO MOTHERHOOD

The transition to motherhood involves hormonal changes, changes in self-image, and reorganization of tasks. The human microbiome plays a major role in maintaining homeostasis and rapid recovery during the postpartum stage. A healthy recovery is best achieved by preventing conditions such as sleep deprivation and inadequate dietary intake, which can alter microbiome gut-brain interaction and contribute to the development of postpartum depression. For example, the new mother should be encouraged to nap while her infant naps and be provided with an adequate nourishing dietary intake to promote a positive outcome in postpartum recovery. Proper instruction concerning breastfeeding techniques, the use of probiotics, and skin-to-skin contact with the newborn are beneficial for a positive postpartum outcome (Dunlop et al., 2015).

Mood swings may occur, with conflicting feelings of joy and depression called *postpartum blues*. The symptoms are typically self-limiting. Discharge teaching concerning self-care and infant care, support, and reassurance should be offered. Rubin's descriptions of the psychological changes that occur after birth have been a framework for the care of new mothers for more than 45 years. The described behavioral changes help health-care workers understand the new mother as she progresses through these stages (Table 6.2).

TABLE 6.2 Rubin's Psychological Changes After Birth

Phase 1	*"Taking in."* The woman is passive, lets others care for her and her infant, and talks about the delivery experience. The mother usually requests food and opportunity to sleep.
Phase 2	*"Taking hold."* The woman begins to initiate care of the infant and assumes responsibility for self-care. The woman is most receptive to teaching at this stage.
Phase 3	*"Letting go."* The parents recognize the reality of the new lifestyle and responsibilities they face and accept the gender and unique appearance of the new child.

Data from Rubin, R. (1967). Attainment of the maternal role: part 1 processes. *Nursing Research, 16*, 237–245; Rubin, R. (1975). Maternal tasks in pregnancy. *Journal of Maternal-Child Nursing, 4*(3), 143; Rubin, R. (1961). Maternal behavior. *Nursing Outlook, 9*, 692; Rubin, R. (1984). *Maternal identity and the maternal experience.* Springer; Rubin, R. (1961). Puerperal change. *Nursing Outlook, 9*(12), 743–755; Rubin, R. (1977). Binding-in in the postpartum period. *American Journal of Maternal Child Nursing, 6*(1), 65–75.

Postnatal Exercise

Exercise can also be an important part of postpartum recovery. In addition to assisting with weight loss, exercise can increase energy levels, restore muscle strength, and decrease the risk of postpartum depression. Exercise in the early postpartum period can include modified sit-ups and *Kegel exercise* (isotonic contraction of the muscles that stop urination) to strengthen abdominal muscles and perineum. Abdominal breathing, head lifts, and modified sit-ups are good beginning exercises.

If there were no complications during labor and delivery, gentle exercises such as walking can begin when the woman feels ready. More vigorous exercises can begin following doctor's approval, usually after about 4–6 weeks of recovery. Caesarean sections and other complicated births may require a longer recovery period before exercise.

FATHERS OR SIGNIFICANT OTHERS

Fathers or significant others often develop an intense focus on the newborn, which is called engrossment (Figure 6.8). A realignment of relationships with parents, past experience with children, and relationship to wife or partner are factors that will affect the bonding experience. When a new infant is added to the family, some of the father's or partner's roles and responsibilities may also change. The partner may be expected to take more time and responsibility for the older sibling or siblings who will need repeated reassurances and validation of continued love. A change in sleep patterns, new financial stresses, and changes in routines can be stressful for some fathers or partners. Fathers may also be prone to postpartum depression that may affect home or workplace functioning and signs should not be overlooked. Plans for childcare for other children, while both parents are focused on the birth of the newborn, need to be in place well before the occasion arises.

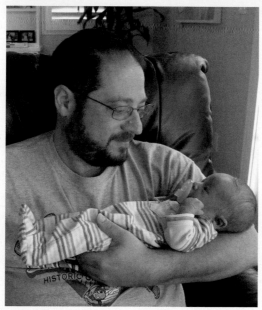

Figure 6.8 The *en face* position between father and infant. The intense fascination that fathers exhibit is called *engrossment*.

SIBLINGS

The influence of the new child's birth on siblings depends on their age and developmental level. Toddlers may regress and be angry. Older children may enjoy helping with the newborn, and adolescents may feel embarrassed about their mother giving birth. A sibling relationship is lifelong and can be characterized by both close friendship and intense rivalry. Sibling rivalry is the competition between siblings, often for parental attention and love.

The initial relationship between a newborn and a sibling is established by the parent's interaction with each child (Figure 6.9). When the newborn is presented to the sibling as being a person with feelings, the sibling is likely to develop positive attitudes and experience good interactions. The birth of a baby is a positive and exciting event for the family, but often a sibling views the event as a loss of the sibling's place in the family. Relationships in the family change, expectations are different, and the parents may become somewhat less accessible, because the parent must focus on the feeding and physical care of the new infant. A 2-year-old may have a low tolerance to change in the relationship with parents, and a 4-year-old may be still struggling to maintain impulse control.

A sibling in the egocentric stage of development cannot be expected to clearly understand the needs of the new baby. Allowing the sibling to participate in the anticipation of the birth may help in the adjustment and transition tasks. Providing an opportunity for the sibling to help with the care of the baby, under the supervision of the parents, can help the sibling feel involved rather than displaced. Major changes in childcare arrangements,

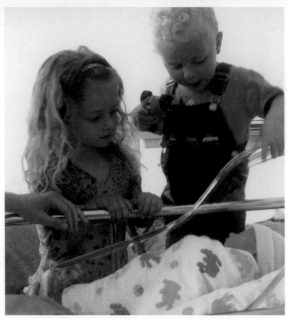

Figure 6.9 Remaining nearby her older children, a mother makes the initial introduction between a newborn and its siblings.

routines, or location of residence should be avoided during the first 6 months after a baby arrives.

Twins often have the opportunity to share experiences early, which can be positive, but when adults compare their achievements with one another, sibling rivalry can intensify. Sibling rivalry may also intensify when a baby is born into a blended family, where a step-child may foster resentment toward the new arrival.

Siblings are often reliable and available playmates in the home and later may become role models and confidants for one another; therefore, sibling relationships generally include long-term benefits.

GRANDPARENTS

Culture and physical distance in living arrangements influence the role of grandparents in the lives of this new family. Some grandparents seek an interactive role, and some grandparents prefer minimal involvement. When parents and grandparents agree on their roles, they can avoid conflict. Because the process of bonding and attachment between parents and the newborn involves learning the cues of newborn behavior, it is essential that parents have the opportunity to spend time with the newborn in the first few weeks or months of life. Grandparents therefore can be most helpful if they assume the role of home manager by preparing meals, shopping, and helping with household tasks. When grandparents take on the care of the newborn, or when a nanny is employed to care for the newborn, the critical time for bonding between parents and the newborn is interrupted and may never be recaptured. This may affect the lifelong relationship between parent and child.

Cultural Considerations

THE INFLUENCE OF CULTURE

The family's cultural background may be different from that of the nurse or health-care worker, but different practices must be understood and respected (Giger, 2016). In some cultures, the husband or partner is expected to be present during the birth process, and in others the presence of the husband or partner is discouraged. In some cases, a male practitioner in attendance at birth may be forbidden. Some parents practice the hot-and-cold theory related to diet, and any diet prescription needs to be carefully designed to ensure compliance. The postpartum phase may last 30 days or longer in some cultures, with the woman forbidden to leave the home. Bathing may be delayed by cultural regulations; cold packs may be refused for perineal comfort. In some cultures, women believe that the colostrum portion of breast milk is unhealthy and therefore do not breastfeed immediately after delivery. Ritual circumcision of the newborn is practiced in some religions, and avoided in others. Some cultures prefer to avoid praise of the newborn to protect the infant from evil influences. This behavior may be misinterpreted as a noncaring attitude or a failure to bond.

Culture may also influence the accuracy of pain assessment. Nurses and health-care workers often use a horizontal illustration of the score of 1–10 to assess the level of pain. Certain cultures read downward rather than left to right and may need a vertical chart for accuracy. In some cultures, women suffer in silence, whereas in others, women chant or moan loudly. Understanding pain and the influence of culture on the expression of pain is essential to providing comprehensive care. Interpreters should be used whenever possible for patients who speak little English. Family members should not serve as the interpreters when sensitive information is discussed, because a family member may interpret selectively (see Chapter 3). For a list of resources for further exploration on cultural competence, access the Health and Human Services Cultural Competence webpage at https://thinkculturalhealth.hhs.gov/

DEVELOPMENTAL TASKS AND RESPONSES OF THE NEONATE

The main task after birth is the establishment of feeding patterns and habits. The infant learns how to latch on to the breast and suck to obtain nourishment, which will last for 2–3 hours. When parents plan to bottle-feed their infants they should be taught about techniques and the types of formulas available. The mother must learn to recognize cues that indicate the infant is hungry even before crying occurs. This is the first *trust* experience. The mother learns to recognize the different cries of the infant and knows whether they mean that feeding, cuddling, or diaper changing is necessary. Various organized behavioral states of the newborn can be observed. They include (1) quiet sleep, (2) active sleep, (3) quiet alert, (4) active alert, and (5) cry.

The neonate sleeps 15–20 hours daily and is most responsive to interaction during the quiet-alert stage of responsiveness. Rocking an infant in a vertical fashion (upright) is likely to maintain alertness, whereas gentle rocking in a horizontal position (lying flat) while wrapped snugly will promote sleep. Each newborn infant has a unique temperament that will influence the intensity of responses to environmental stimuli. The neonatal period (first 30 days of life) serves to solidify parent-infant expectations and relationships. The newborn initiates environmental support by crying or turning away from excess stimulation and learns to self-console and eventually to interact socially by smiling. Nurses and health-care workers can help cement a positive parent-infant relationship by observing parent-infant responses, educating parents concerning the abilities and behaviors of the newborn, and using opportunities to promote bonding and attachment. Newborns who exhibit frequent startles or tremors, gaze away from the face of the caregiver, and appear irritable when stimulated require further professional assessment. Distressed parents who feel inadequate and who believe their infant to be highly vulnerable need special guidance and support to assist the infant to achieve trust and to grow toward autonomy.

Parent Teaching

The alert neonate has predictable responses to environmental stimuli that parents learn to understand and anticipate. This interaction fosters effective parenting and infant growth and development.

During the neonatal period, the infant develops *conditioned responses*, or unconscious responses to external stimuli. For example, the hungry infant who stops crying at the sound of a caregiver's presence, even though food is not yet offered, is exhibiting a conditioned response.

The neonate can hear clearly after the first sneeze clears the eustachian tubes. The newborn's sucking response is increased when stimuli are introduced, and sucking stops when attention is focused elsewhere. The newborn is capable of feeling pain, and pain relief should be offered before any painful procedures are undertaken. Swaddling, cuddling, wrapping, rocking, *nonnutritive sucking* (use of a pacifier), and a quiet environment provide comfort for the neonate. Oral sucrose (a type of sugar) placed on a pacifier often serves as a mild short-acting pain reliever. The behavior and appearance of the newborn are influenced by reflexes that are present at birth and gradually disappear (Table 6.3). These reflexes help the neonate adapt to the environment and gradually disappear as voluntary motor ability develops. Assessment of the neurological system is achieved by testing for the presence of these reflexes.

Development of Intelligence

Intelligence is difficult to define because it includes many aspects and different types of abilities. Intelligence involves the ability to learn from experience and to adapt to the environment and its challenges. It includes the ability to reason, solve problems, and learn. Researchers have classified the study of intelligence to include *psychometric* variables such as reasoning, memory, perception, and abstract thinking; *computational* variables such as the ability to process information; *biological* variables such as neural (brain) functioning; and *complex system* variables that involve language intelligence, spatial intelligence, musical intelligence, interpersonal intelligence, and so on. Each of these areas of intelligence may be studied separately, but they interact to form an individual's intelligence potential.

Both genetics and environment influence the intelligence potential of a newborn infant. Poor nutrition, environmental toxins, or oxygen deprivation can inhibit optimal brain development. Family, schooling, and availability of preschool programs also will influence the infant's ability to reach the full potential of his or her intelligence. Environmental influences affect the potential and rate of development (Chapter 7). The environment can influence

TABLE 6.3 Ages of Appearance and Disappearance of Neurological Reflexes of Infancy

Response	Age at Time of Appearance	Age at Time of Disappearance
REFLEXES OF POSITION AND MOVEMENT		
Moro reflex	Birth	1–3 months

Tonic neck reflex	Birth	5–7 months

Palmar grasp reflex	Birth	4 months

Response	Age at Time of Appearance	Age at Time of Disappearance
Babinski reflex	Birth	Variable*
RESPONSES TO SOUND		
Blinking response	Birth	NA
Turning response	Birth	NA
REFLEXES OF VISION†		
Blinking to threat	6–7 months	NA
Horizontal following	4–6 weeks	NA
Vertical following	2–3 months	NA
Postrotational nystagmus	Birth	NA
FOOD REFLEXES		
Rooting response (awake)	Birth	3–4 months

(Continued)

TABLE 6.3 Ages of Appearance and Disappearance of Neurological Reflexes of Infancy (*Cont.*)

Response	Age at Time of Appearance	Age at Time of Disappearance
Rooting response (asleep)	Birth	7–8 months
Sucking response	Birth	12 months
OTHER SIGNS		
Handedness	2–3 years	NA
Spontaneous stepping	Birth	4–5 months
Straight-line walking	5–6 years	NA

NA, Not applicable.
*Usually of no diagnostic significance until after age 2 years.
†Holding the newborn infant upright under the arms will induce eye opening.
Unnumbered Figure 6.9 from Murray, SS., McKinney, ES., & Gorrie, TM. (2002). *Foundations of newborn nursing* (3rd ed.). Saunders; unnumbered Figures 6.10 and 6.11 from Leifer, G. (2012). *Maternity nursing: An introductory text* (12th ed.). Saunders.

temperament and motivation that then influence the development of intelligence. Intelligence quotient (IQ) scores remain the valid measure of intelligence in research settings. Intelligence testing began with Binet intelligence tests in 1905 and is used for identifying cognitive delays. Intelligence tests can also be used to assess gifted children and those with learning disabilities, or to customize school, vocational, and military placement. Several IQ exams are validated by the American Psychological Association (Chapter 9). Intelligence tests can measure potential, but they may not be a measure of future capabilities (Nio Leon, 2005).

Play Activities and Neonatal Development

Because hearing and vision are present in the newborn, an appropriate toy would include a musical mobile that is placed above the crib within the infant's sight. Music can capture the attention of the newborn. A developmental task of the neonate is to learn how to focus on and follow objects as they move across the field of vision. An overhanging mobile with sharply contrasting colors will foster this development.

The neonate can detect the smell of mother's milk by 6 days of age and prefers sweet tastes. The sense of touch is well developed and stroking the cheek will cause the infant to turn toward the person stroking his or her face. An infant can be quieted, and bonding promoted, by placing the infant in skin-to-skin contact with the parent. A nude infant placed on the nude chest of the parent will quiet and snuggle.

The neonate is in Piaget's sensorimotor stage of cognitive growth (Chapter 5). Infants can learn and repeat behavioral responses. Looking, listening, and touching the environment help the infant master the tasks of this stage. Close contact with the infant will help parents recognize cues to specific needs so that cry time is minimized. The best time to interact with the neonate is during the quiet-alert state of responsiveness. The infant will quickly halt physical activity and become very still when approached and talked to, eyes will focus on the parent's face, and beginning communication will be evident.

KEY POINTS

- A genome is a complete set of DNA contained in all human cells.
- The goal of the Genome Project was to identify the 30,000 or more genes in the DNA; develop tools for analysis; and address the ethical, legal, and social implications of this knowledge and ability.
- The Genome Project enabled gene therapy to correct or replace abnormal genes.
- One of the critical periods during fetal growth occurs during the first 3 months of pregnancy, when basic structures are developing.
- The well-being of the mother and fetus can influence life expectancy of the newborn.
- An expanded goal of prenatal care is to provide optimal maternal-fetal health to prevent or reduce adult-onset diseases in the newborn.
- Exercise during pregnancy contributes to a healthy outcome.
- Improvement in the nutrition and health of mothers and babies may prevent disease in the next generation.
- Microbiomes are large communities of tiny microorganisms that live in our body and play a role in normal physiology, development, and health.
- Microbiomes play a major role during pregnancy and may influence the adult health of the newborn infant.
- Exposure to toxins such as drugs and alcohol during fetal development can cause abnormalities in the newborn.
- According to Erikson, parenting a dependent child is the beginning of the stage of generativity.
- A combination of an XX chromosome from the mother and father will produce a girl, and an XY combination will produce a boy fetus.
- Only the sperm carries the Y chromosome, so the male partner determines the sex of the infant. However, the female has some influence on which sperm may survive to fertilize the ovum.
- An adequate intake of folic acid early in the maternal diet is essential to prevent neural tube defects in the newborn infant.
- Fraternal twins are the result of two ova released at ovulation, each fertilized by a separate sperm. Identical twins are the result of one fertilized ovum separating into two embryos.
- Bonding refers to a strong emotional tie between the parents and the newborn.
- Attachment refers to the affectionate tie that occurs over time because of parent-infant interaction.
- The influence of the new child's birth on siblings depends on their ages and developmental levels.
- Breastfeeding, bonding, and attachment are developmental tasks of parents and the newborn.
- The neonatal period encompasses the first 30 days of life.
- Swaddling, cuddling, rocking, and use of a pacifier calm the newborn infant.
- Newborn reflexes help the neonate adjust to the environment, and reflexes disappear as voluntary motor abilities develop.
- An overhanging mobile with sharply contrasting colors will foster the growth and development of the neonate.

Clinical Judgment Case Study

A woman has just confided with you that she plans to become pregnant and wants to be sure she is doing everything possible to have a healthy baby without completely changing her lifestyle and practices. What guidelines would you discuss with her that are essential for her to know concerning planning a healthy pregnancy experience?

REVIEW QUESTIONS

1. Arrange the following process and developments in proper order.
   A. zygote formation.
   B. implantation.
   C. fertilization.
   D. fetus formation.
   E. viability.
   F. embryo formation.

2. The first period of parental development occurs in three phases, each with specific tasks before birth and after birth. The three columns below indicate which stage of pregnancy is most appropriate to introduce/discuss the specific topic. Place an X in the appropriate column.

Topic	1st trimester	2nd trimester	3rd trimester
Acceptance or denial of pregnancy			
Infant care skills and equipment needed			
Wishes for specific sex of infant			
Concern for parenting skills			
Imagining special features of infant			
Breastfeeding skills			
Fear of birth pain			
Plan for home or hospital delivery			
Hope for future of infant			

3. To promote growth and development in the neonate, which of the following features of an overhead mobile are important to include. Drag and drop (or place an X) next to the essential/appropriate features in column 2.

Possible features of mobile	Most appropriate/important to include
Move across the field of vision	
Offer sound to capture attention	
Be viewed from below the mobile	
Be viewed from side of mobile	
Be home made	
Contain contrasting colors	
Contain bright colors	

Stimulate sense of touch

Be used as distraction during feeding

Include flashing lights to capture attention

Be made of sturdy, washable materials

4. Which of the following information is essential to include when teaching a client about conception? Place an X in column A for essential information and an X in column B for optional/interesting information.

Information	(A) Essential	(B) Optional/Interesting
Sperm lives 5 days after ejaculation		
Ova lives 24 hours after ovulation		
Neural tube development of fetus starts 3 weeks after fertilization		
Prenatal vitamin education		
Implantation of fertilized egg into uterus occurs in 7 days after fertilization		
The sperm contains both X and Y chromosomes		
At 20 weeks' gestation fetus may be viable		

5. Which of the following activities should be encouraged to promote bonding with the neonate? (select all that apply)

A. Use of off-site childcare for older siblings.

B. Holding the infant in an *en face* position.

C. Skin-to-skin contact in the first hour after birth.

D. Immediate removal of the newborn from the mother to allow her to sleep and recover.

E. Maintaining a safe distance between older siblings and the newborn for the first year.

F. Allowing older siblings to assist with caretaking.

G. Allowing the newborn to cry himself to sleep to encourage self-soothing.

H. Breastfeeding.

The Infant

http://evolve.elsevier.com/Leifer/growth

OUTLINE

OBJECTIVES

1. Define the term *infant*.
2. State the developmental tasks of infancy.
3. Describe the physical development of infants from 1 month to 1 year of age.
4. Discuss milestones of motor development.
5. Understand five basic guidelines for physical activity for infants.
6. Discuss the development of language.
7. Describe the theories of Piaget, Freud, and Erikson concerning infant development.
8. Define separation anxiety.
9. Discuss the development of attachment.
10. Describe the basic nutritional needs of infants from 1 month to 1 year of age.
11. List the immunization schedule for infants under 1 year of age.
12. State four safety precautions essential in infant care.

KEY TERMS

autonomy
cephalocaudal
coping skill
defense mechanism
development
expressive language
growth
infant

length
nonverbal language
norms
nursing caries
object permanence
ordinal position
personality

pincer action
preverbal
proximodistal
receptive language
separation anxiety
sudden infant death syndrome
    (SIDS)

DEFINITION

The infant stage of development is the period between ages 4 weeks and 1 year. Growth indicates an increase in size, measured by inches (centimeters) and pounds (kilograms). Development indicates an increase in function and mastery of tasks for the specific phase in the lifespan.

The process of growth and development is orderly and proceeds from simple to complex in an expected pattern but at a variable pace. Growth spurts are common. Norms (averages) are only guidelines concerning the ages at which specific abilities or skills are achieved. Cephalocaudal growth refers to the progression of the growth pattern that proceeds from head to toe. For example, infants are able to lift their heads before they can sit, and they are able to sit before they can stand. Proximodistal growth refers to growth from the center of the body to the periphery. Height refers to a standing measurement, whereas length is measured while the infant is lying down. The average height of a person is generally a result of family traits, although nutrition and other factors may alter the attainment of the specific individual's adult height. Many methods of predicting a child's height have been developed but they are estimates only and not proven to be exact (Hoecker, 2016). One general estimation for infants of potential adult height can be determined by the following formulas:

$$\text{Boys} = \frac{\text{Father's height} + \text{mother's height in inches} + 2.5 \text{ inches}}{2}$$

$$\text{Girls} = \frac{\text{Father's height} + \text{mother's height in inches} - 2.5 \text{ inches}}{2}$$

The length of the newborn is normally about 20 inches (50 cm), and by 1 year of age, the birth length increases by almost 50%. An average newborn weighs approximately 7.5 pounds (3.4 kg). The infant's birth weight doubles by 6 months of age and can be expected to triple within 1 year.

Many factors influence the growth and development of the infant. Development is a process that continues throughout the life cycle, with mastery of specific tasks occurring in each phase. Successful mastery of the tasks in one phase of the life cycle enables the person to proceed more easily to the next phase. Development is an interaction among the child, the parent, and the environment. If there is a problem with the parents or environment, the child responds by developing *defense mechanisms* or *coping skills*. A defense mechanism is a reaction that is protective to the individual or helps conceal conflicts or anxieties. Denial and projection of blame are examples of defense mechanisms. For example, if an infant is hurt, he or she may blame the caregiver for causing the pain and may react by hitting or thrashing (an infant cannot yet understand the concept of an accident).

A coping skill is a behavior that helps an individual adapt to or manage a stressful situation. If a goal is obstructed, the infant may find a way around the obstacle to reach the unachievable goal; modify the goal to an achievable level; or perhaps develop an alternative goal. For example, an infant may learn how to climb over a crib rail to reach a toy.

Infants thrive with parental support and praise. This interaction fosters an attachment between child and parent that provides a sense of security, enabling the infant to try to master developmental tasks. Mutual attachment involves not only a close feeling between the infant and parent but also a responsiveness to needs presented. If the needs of the infant are not met, the development of attachment may not be achieved as easily if at all.

Cultural Considerations

Ethnic and cultural practices influence nutrition and behavior development.

The ordinal position in the family – that is, whether the infant is an only child, an oldest child, a youngest child, or a middle child – may influence the age and rapidity of mastering developmental tasks.

Both the prenatal environment and the home environment influence the growth and development of the infant. The development of personality is an interaction between biological and environmental factors. Personality is most often defined as a unique combination of characteristics that result in the individual's recurrent pattern of behavior. The influences of the family and family interactions on growth and development are discussed in Chapter 4. Theories of behavioral development abound, and a summary of popular theories is presented in Chapter 5. The roles of heredity and prenatal influences are discussed in Chapter 6.

DEVELOPMENTAL TASKS

Trust Versus Mistrust

The functioning of all humans is goal directed and involves the tasks of developing social competence and the mastery of skills necessary for functioning in their environments. Some tasks of infancy include weaning, self-feeding, walking, and acquiring language and communications skills.

Trust versus mistrust is the first psychosocial crisis in infancy that must be resolved (Erikson, 1994) (Chapter 5). In the first year of life, trust develops when infants learn that their basic needs will be met. Crying infants who are left alone cry more at 1 year than infants who are picked up and comforted or who are fed promptly when they evidence hunger. Infants fed on a rigid schedule rather than as a response to hunger signs generally show more spitting up and gastrointestinal disturbances as well as later behavioral problems (Kleigman et al., 2016). By 2 months of age, parents react positively to the infant's responsive smile, and a mutual bond (attachment) is secured.

Intelligence

Understanding Cause and Effect

Infants discover at an early age that there is a relationship between cause and effect, and experiences at each stage of the life cycle build on this discovery. Newborns suck their thumbs to feel secure and will seek out the thumb or pacifier to achieve this feeling of comfort. A cry usually elicits a response from adults, and so the cry becomes a means of communication.

From 1 to 4 months of age, the infant is focused on the parent and, when held, prefers the *en face* (face-to-face) position. After 4 months of age, the infant begins to become more aware of the surroundings and may prefer to be held outwardly or away from the parent, facing the activity happening in the room. By 4 months, infants discover their hands and feet. If a mobile gym is placed above them, infants discover there are predictable sounds and tactile responses that occur when reaching out to touch the mobile. The infant strives to recognize behavior patterns that elicit special responses from the environment. When infants feel secure, they will explore the world around them. Infants who have not developed an attachment to the parental figure do not explore as readily.

At 4 months, the infant drops a toy from the highchair and believes it is gone. By 7 months, the infant will continue to look for it. This is called object permanence, or knowing the object is there even though one cannot see it. Playing peek-a-boo with the infant at this age helps to develop the concept of object permanence.

Memory

Studies have shown that infants can retain memory of a traumatic experience (Czaenabay et al., 2019). General comforting may not be enough to achieve full emotional recovery. Newborns demonstrate a physiological response to pain, and so a stress response can develop and influence later behavior. For example, a choking episode (anoxia) early in breastfeeding may cause an infant to reject further attempts at breastfeeding. One study showed that a 10-week-old infant, repeatedly abused by the father and placed in a foster home, showed an aversion to male caretakers for many months afterward (Gaensbauer, 2002). This evidence has led psychologists to advise parents to talk about stressful events that may have occurred early in the lives of their children, so that the child does not have to deal with those memories alone.

Emotional Development

When placed face-to-face (*en face*) with an adult, an infant will mimic the facial expression of the adult. For example, if the adult's tongue is thrust out, the infant will eventually thrust out his or her tongue also. Smiling, eye widening, and puckering of the lips occur when the infant focuses on the adult or activity that the infant can see. When stimulation reaches a high level, the infant will turn away to rest and then return to the view when ready for further stimulation. If the adult turns away before the infant is ready, the infant will lean forward and attempt to get the adult's attention with sound and movement and will eventually cry with frustration if unsuccessful. When adult stimulation is not available, the infant will eventually lose energy and stop efforts at communication. Interaction between parent and infant is necessary in the first months of life and is important for later social development.

Attachment

The process of attachment begins long before the infant is born, when the mother feels the fetus moving in the womb. The father or partner feels the fetal movement by touching the mother's abdomen and feeling the fetus kick. Both parents can hear the heartbeat with the aid of a stethoscope or a Doppler device. A relationship with an imagined child starts to develop. At birth, the real child emerges, and if he or she is not too different from the imagined child, attachment easily intensifies. However, the infant must respond positively in this mutual interaction. An infant who is sleepy, does not focus on the face of the parent, has difficulty latching on to the breast for breastfeeding, or spits up or vomits during feedings cannot contribute to the attachment process as readily, and the nurse or health-care worker may need to help the process along.

Parents slowly develop an instinctive response to infants' cues. The way infants cry, and the pitch or intensity of the cry, may indicate to the parent whether the infant is expressing a cry of pain, discomfort, hunger, or boredom. If the parent's response is prompt, attachment becomes secure. Providing time for *en face* interactions is important. The infant from birth to age 3 months can respond with varied facial expressions. After age 2 or 3 months, a responsive smile by the infant brings joy to the parent's efforts at interaction. By 5 or 6 months of age, the infant clearly recognizes and prefers the parent to other casual caregivers. The infant also looks to the facial expression and body language of the parent in new situations and responds accordingly. For example, if a relative from out of town visits, and the mother, while holding the infant, smiles and embraces the relative, the infant will likely smile and coo and respond calmly. However, if the person entering the room is a health-care provider for a well-child visit, and the mother is concerned about the pain of the immunizations to be administered, her facial expression and nonverbal behavior or body language (e.g., a stiffened posture) will be communicated to the child, who may then cry as the health-care provider approaches.

Separation anxiety begins at 6 months of age. The infant cries or protests when the parent leaves the room. Stranger anxiety peaks at 9 months of age when the infant is approached by a stranger, babysitter, or substitute caregiver in the absence of the parent. The mastery of object permanence will enable the infant to understand that the parent is still available even though he or she is not visible at the moment.

By 18 months, memory development helps the child remember the parent's image and to trust that the parent will return after an absence. Affectionate, responsive parents who respond to the child's needs help develop a secure attachment and bonding. The process of attachment is a gradual one, but attachment abilities stretch across the lifespan. Mastery of this task is essential for the child to be successful in later attachments to school friends or partners in the adult phase of the life cycle. The infant's temperament can influence the success of the attachment process, because parents usually have expectations concerning temperament of the child. Parents may say, "he is a difficult child," or "she is an easy child." This usually means that the parents' expectations do not exactly fit the infant's temperament, and the health-care worker may need to guide the parent's response (Table 7.1).

Parents who have psychiatric problems or marital stress or who both work long hours may not have the energy to respond to a demanding infant. Infants who receive inconsistent responses to their needs may withdraw from the risks of exploring the world around them, even when the parent is present. These infants or toddlers may become clingy, angry, and rebellious or become nonresponsive to the soothing and care they do receive. Child abuse becomes a risk at this time. The nurse should be alert to signs and symptoms of child abuse (Figure 7.1).

This understanding of attachment behavior is one of the reasons for providing one consistent core teacher in the elementary-school setting, whereas in high school the student usually interacts with multiple teachers in 1 day, because the typical adolescent has achieved independence, trust, and autonomy. It is also the basis of the rooming-in concept,

TABLE 7.1   Temperament

Factors	Characteristics	Interventions
Activity level	Activity level of the infant can be high, medium, or low. It can be assessed by watching activity during feeding, bathing, or playing.	High activity: Provide opportunity for high activity. Low activity: Provide enough time for tasks.
Regularity	Regularity can be assessed by predictability of the infant's sleep-wake cycle, hunger, or elimination schedule.	Make provision for regularity by bringing food and diapers on trips.
Approach/withdrawal	The infant may respond to a stimulus with gusto and exploration or with caution and avoidance. Stimuli include people, foods, and toys.	Use a time-limited trial and praise.
Adaptability	How easily an infant can tolerate and respond to new stimuli.	Provide multiple short exposures to events.
Threshold	The level of stimulation response. Can also indicate hyperreactivity to minor stimuli.	Limit stimuli before bedtime.
Intensity of response	Involves strong focus	Do not yield to the child's will to buy peace.
Distractibility	Easily changes focus of interest.	Calmly redirect wandering attention.
Attention span	Loses interest rapidly.	Plan brief periods of activity; monitor completion of task. Warn if task must be interrupted for meal or sleep.

Modified from Carey, W., Crocker, A., Elias, E., Feldman, H., & Coleman, W. (2016). *Developmental-behavioral pediatrics* (4th ed.). Saunders; Feigelman, S. (2016). Development of behavior: Overview and assessment of variability. In R. Kleigman, B. Stanton, J. St Geme III, N. Schor, & R. Behrman (2016). *Nelson textbook of pediatrics* (20th ed.). Elsevier.

where the parent is encouraged to stay in the room with the infant or child day and night when the child is hospitalized.

Observation of the parents' ability to comfort the infant, distract the infant, and respond to the emotional cues of the infant's behavior can be observed at each well-child visit, and appropriate guidance should be offered as needed. For example, following a clinic immunization, the mother can be encouraged to hold, rock, or breastfeed her infant to calm the infant before leaving the room.

Parents often need help with the separation experience. Sometimes it is not the child who cannot accept separation, but the parent who has the difficulty. Step 1 of separation starts with the placement of infants in their own beds, perhaps in their own rooms. Co-sleeping can prolong this first step in separation. Step 2 involves leaving the infant with a

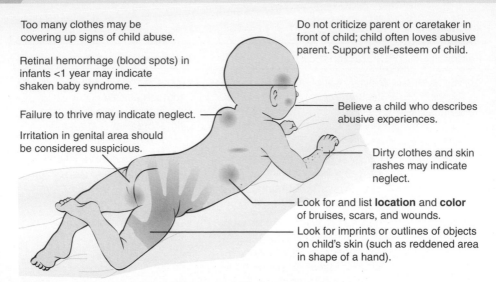

Too many clothes may be covering up signs of child abuse.

Retinal hemorrhage (blood spots) in infants <1 year may indicate shaken baby syndrome.

Failure to thrive may indicate neglect.

Irritation in genital area should be considered suspicious.

Do not criticize parent or caretaker in front of child; child often loves abusive parent. Support self-esteem of child.

Believe a child who describes abusive experiences.

Dirty clothes and skin rashes may indicate neglect.

Look for and list **location** and **color** of bruises, scars, and wounds.

Look for imprints or outlines of objects on child's skin (such as reddened area in shape of a hand).

Divide the body into four planes: front, back, right side, and left side.
Injuries occurring in >1 plane should be considered suspicious.

Figure 7.1 Assessing for child abuse. The nurse should be alert for inconsistent statements about injuries, bruises at various stages of healing, or delay in seeking care. *(From Leifer, G. (2019). Introduction to maternity & pediatric nursing (8th ed.). Elsevier.)*

relative or babysitter. Parents often do not realize that such short separations help infants develop independence and enable them to prepare for the next stage of autonomy. Coping skills are developed, and trust is strengthened when the infant learns from many small experiences with short separations. Protest at the initial separation is to be expected but will diminish as the child learns to trust the caregiver and to trust that the parents will return.

Hospitalization is a unique experience of separation that is filled with strangers, pain, and fear of the unknown. For this separation experience, it is strongly recommended that a parent room-in with the child, and most hospitals have facilities to accommodate parents.

Parents who perceive their child as especially vulnerable and who therefore avoid most separation experiences are exhibiting overprotective parenting, which can stifle the normal process of child development. Crises in separation experiences can recur later in life when the school-age child must leave the home environment to attend elementary school or when the teenage child leaves home to enter college. Leaving home may precipitate a recurrence of the separation anxiety.

Language Development

Language development consists of verbal language that is both expressive (can say it) and receptive (can understand it) and body language that follows a predictable course of development. Body language, also known as nonverbal language, is the language of the motions, postures, and gestures of the body and is learned as part of communication. There appears to be an innate ability to develop language skills.

The first year of life, before the infant can express understandable speech, is called the preverbal stage of language development. In the early months, the infant initially

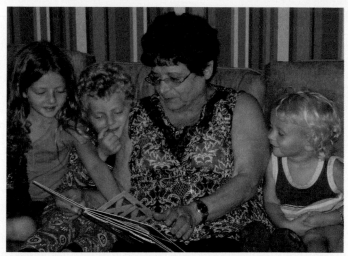

Figure 7.2 Reading to infants and children promotes language development. Infants and young children enjoy books that provide colorful pictures and varied textures.

communicates needs by crying or smiling. The infant will stop all random motor activity when listening to a voice; infants recognize mother's or caregiver's voice; and learn the rhythms and speech patterns of what will be his or her native or primary language. At 3 or 4 months of age, the infant will search for the source of sounds and utter repetitive sounds, which develops into babbling, using combinations of vowels with some consonants. By 7–8 months, syllables using the D, P, and B sounds appear, and parents are gleeful when they hear "ma" or "da." By 9 or 10 months of age, specific sounds are used consistently to refer to objects or events and the infant recognizes his name and simple words like "no." At this age, infants share their emotions by showing a favorite toy to an adult, because they are sure it will bring joy to the adult also.

The first words may occur between 10 and 13 months of age. Body language, such as pointing, leaning, or staring, assists the infant to make desires or needs understood. The first single words used often have multiple meanings. For example, "ball" can mean "that is a ball" or "give me the ball." Nonverbal behavior often assists the parent to understand what the infant means.

By the time infants are 1 year old, their brain is committed to the language that is used regularly in the environment around them and can follow a simple command. Infants soon learn combinations of syllables that separate words by hearing them often and separating them according to the frequency heard. For example, in the phrase "pretty girl," babies learn that "ty" goes with "pret," not "girl." It is not "pret-tygirl," it is "pretty-girl." This is a learned skill and is an important reason parents should talk to their infants in a natural language and should not use slang or baby talk (Figure 7.2).

Motor Development

The development of motor skills is closely related to the development of perception, emotion, and cognition. Reaching out and touching what they see enable infants to establish visual-motor skills. Many motor skills are dependent on the disappearance of newborn reflexes (Chapter 6). With the disappearance of the tonic neck reflex (the arm extends when the head turns to the side), the infant is able to bring both hands to the midline of the body into prayer position. At 3 months, the infant attempts to grasp whatever he or she touches. At 6 months, the infant shapes the hand to prepare to touch and grasp an observed object. By 9 months, the pincer action enables the infant to grasp with the thumb and forefinger. By 2 years, wrist action enables the use of spoons during feeding.

As posture and balance develop, infants first learn to lift their heads, then to sit and stand, and then to take their first steps around 1 year of age. Infants start to walk about 4–5 months after they are able to pull themselves up to a standing position (Table 7.2).

Physical Activity

The acquisition of motor skills in infancy lays the foundation for a lifetime of physical activity. In order to develop fine and gross motor skills, an infant must be provided with a safe and stimulating environment to move and explore. Early motor competence and confidence can contribute to the enjoyment of physical activity throughout childhood and beyond (Figure 7.3). The National Association for Sport and Physical Education (NASPE, 2009) recommends five basic guidelines for physical activity during infancy (Box 7.1).

Autonomy

Autonomy refers to independence. Striving for independence starts early in infancy. Self-consoling behavior is an early form of independence. Infants learn to bring their hands to their mouths and to suck their fingers to bring comfort or to relieve boredom. At 6–10 months of age, body rocking is used to achieve self-comforting. Nine-month-old babies with newly developed pincer ability will insist on self–finger feeding and will resist the attempts of parents to feed them with a spoon at mealtime.

Sleep Patterns

A maturing central nervous system combined with parental responses aids in the development of sleep patterns. By 3 months, most infants develop a pattern of sustained sleep between midnight and 5:00 a.m., but a few do not develop this pattern before 1 year of age. In the first year, waking at night is considered normal. Supplemental foods, such as rice cereal, should not be added to the infant's bottle in an effort to promote sleep. The goal is to help infants develop self-regulatory skills so that they return to sleep without prompting. This can occur more quickly if parents wait until there is evidence that infants are fully awake before picking them up. In a semi-wakened state, gentle body patting or use of a pacifier should be enough consolation to help the infant return to sleep. The establishment of a pre-bedtime routine of quiet activity (e.g., rocking or reading to the infant) helps with the acceptance of bedtime during the first years of life.

Health Promotion

The establishment of an appropriate sleep pattern is important, because adequate sleep is related to memory, attention, learning, and general behavior.

TABLE 7.2   The Development of Locomotion, Prehension, and Perception

Age	Locomotion	Prehension	Perception
1 month	Chin up.	Hand held closed. Fingers move without coordination from mind.	Able to focus on sharply contrasted, angled mobile above.
2 months	Chest up. Elevates self with arms.	Hand held open most of the time.	Selectively responds to patterns, colors. Imitates expressions. Is self-centered. Prefers to look at familiar sights.
4 months	Rolls over at will.	Reaches for overhead objects with fingers, with hit-and-miss action.	Perceives differences in facial expressions.
5 months	Sits alone momentarily.	Picks up toy with squeeze action.	

(Continued)

TABLE 7.2   The Development of Locomotion, Prehension, and Perception (*Cont.*)

Age	Locomotion	Prehension	Perception
6 months	Sits alone steadily with hands forward for support.	Grasps with thumb on one side and three fingers on other.	Can distinguish between familiar and unfamiliar sights. Separation anxiety begins. Sees self and parent as one.
8 months	Sits with support. Pulls to standing position.	Thumb and index finger can hold object without pressing it into palm. Can transfer from one hand to the other.	Can distinguish happy from fearful face.
9 months	Creeps.	Uses finger to explore what eye sees. Has hand-mouth coordination.	Fears strangers. Recognizes self as separate from parent.

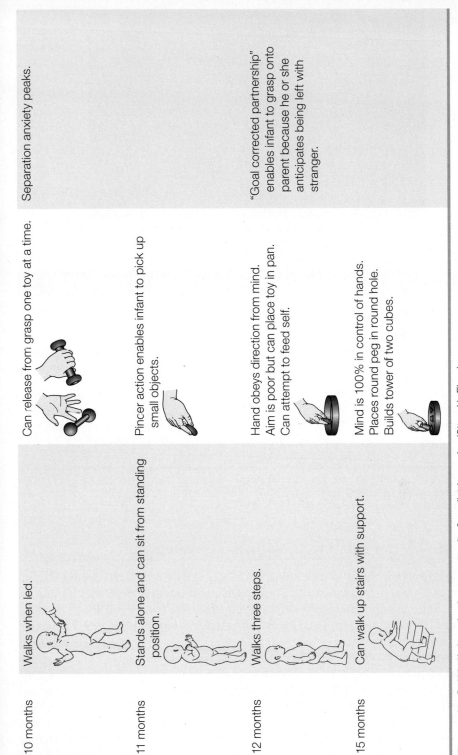

10 months	Walks when led.	Can release from grasp one toy at a time.	Separation anxiety peaks.
11 months	Stands alone and can sit from standing position.	Pincer action enables infant to pick up small objects.	
12 months	Walks three steps.	Hand obeys direction from mind. Aim is poor but can place toy in pan. Can attempt to feed self.	
15 months	Can walk up stairs with support.	Mind is 100% in control of hands. Places round peg in round hole. Builds tower of two cubes.	"Goal corrected partnership" enables infant to grasp onto parent because he or she anticipates being left with stranger.

From Leifer, G. (2019). *Introduction to maternity & pediatric nursing* (8th ed.). Elsevier.

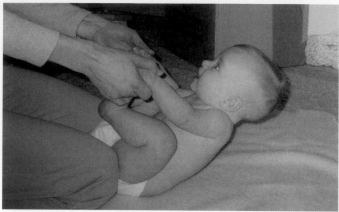

Figure 7.3 Age-appropriate exercise for the infant. The infant learns head control by gentle lifting. The infant will soon assist in pulling up by using her arm muscles.

BOX 7.1   Physical Activity Guidelines for Infants

Guideline 1: Infants should interact with caregivers in daily physical activities that are dedicated to exploring movement and the environment.

Guideline 2: Caregivers should place infants in settings that encourage and stimulate movement experiences and active play for short periods of time, several times each day.

Guideline 3: Infants' physical activity should promote the development of movement and skills.

Guideline 4: Whenever possible, caregivers should ensure an environment for infants that meets or exceeds recommended safety standards for performing large muscle activities.

Guideline 5: Those responsible for infants' well-being are responsible for understanding the importance of physical activity and promoting movement skills by providing opportunities for structured and unstructured physical activity.

Modified from Society of Health and Physical Educators: Virgilio, S., Clements, R. (2020) *Active start: A statement of physical activity guidelines for children birth to age 5* (3rd ed.). www.ShapeAmerica. org/standards/guidelines/activestart.aspx

---

Role of Play in Fostering Growth and Development

Piaget's sensorimotor theory of development (Chapter 5) is evident in the infant's play activities, which are activated by sensations and relate to the infant directly. Play is the work of a child, and age-appropriate play activities can effectively foster growth and development. For example, a newborn must learn to focus and follow with the eyes. Hanging a bright mobile with contrasting colors (such as black and white) above the crib within sight of the infant can promote the development of this skill. At 3 months, an interactive mobile that is activated by kicking helps develop the cause-effect understanding. At 6–7 months of age, playing peek-a-boo helps solidify the object permanence concept. Dropping food from the highchair when someone is there to pick it up is also part of the learning process, although the messiness involved often tries the patience of parents. In the young infant, all toys are explored for taste and touch, but by 1 year, the infant typically understands the function of the toy. A car will be pushed; a telephone will be put to the ear. All toys and activities are related to the child's body. Egocentric behavior is evident in 1-year-olds who drink from a toy cup or place a toy telephone to their ear, but a toddler at 18 months of age will offer the drink to a doll. The 1-year-old enjoys push toys that foster the newly mastered walking abilities.

According to Freud's theory of development, the infant is in an oral phase, which involves exploring with the mouth (Chapter 5). Oral sucking, biting, and chewing toys are appropriate activities for this stage of development.

By applying learned skills to environmental experiences, children learn about the world around them. Often the health-care worker must reassure parents that a child picking up everything from the floor and placing it in the mouth, or a child intentionally dropping food from the highchair tray onto the floor, are developmentally normal behaviors and are definitely not signs of a child who is behaving badly.

HEALTH MAINTENANCE
Nutrition

In the first year of life, the brain and the body grow and develop rapidly. Proper nutritional intake is essential to support optimum development. The newborn has a rooting reflex that seeks out the nipple and a sucking reflex that is elicited when the nipple touches the lips. A tongue extrusion reflex prevents ingestion of solid foods in the first few months of life.

Health Promotion

The best nutrition for the newborn is breast milk, which contains antibodies and easy-to-digest fats. For mothers who cannot breastfeed, most commercial formulas provide adequate nutrition, although they do not have the extra benefits of the antibodies and other protective ingredients in breastmilk. Breastfeeding should not be considered a lifestyle choice, but a choice to provide documented health benefits for the infant (Parks et al., 2016).

Cultural Considerations

Breastfeeding

Cultural factors influence breastfeeding choices. Some mothers from North American or European backgrounds are uncomfortable with the body contact and exposure required for breastfeeding. In American cultures, returning to the workplace soon after delivery may influence the mother's choice to bottle-feed her newborn, although many workplace environments provide accommodations for breastfeeding mothers. User-friendly breast pumps and milk storage containers are available and inexpensive. In some cultures, breast pumping is discouraged as a relief for engorgement or as a convenience for working mothers.

In some cultures colostrum is discarded, and sterile water may be provided for the newborn to drink until maternal milk flow is well established. Contraindications to breastfeeding are rare and include women with active human immunodeficiency virus/acquired immunodeficiency syndrome (HIV/AIDS); active tuberculosis; active herpes lesions on the breast; and in women receiving chemotherapy or medications that may pass into the breast milk and cause adverse effects in the newborn (Parks et al., 2016).

Newborns are usually fed on demand at 2- to 3-hour intervals, and by 4–6 months of age infants may skip a nighttime feeding. If the newborn is lethargic, efforts to maintain a state of alertness will aid nutritional intake. Supplemental feedings of fluids should not be given to breastfeeding newborns. Pacifiers can be offered no earlier than 4 weeks of age after breastfeeding is well established to avoid nipple confusion (Parks et al., 2016). Infants should be fed breast milk (or formula) for at least 1 full year. At 1 year of age, the infant can be placed on cow's milk or a plant-based alternative. Low-fat milk should not be given to children under age 2, because the fats are necessary for development of the nervous system. At 4–6 months of age, the tongue extrusion reflex has disappeared. The infant will no longer spit out solid foods and is ready for strained rice cereal. Gradually, vegetables and fruits are added to the diet, but only one at a time to allow identification of foods that may upset the infant's stomach or result in a food allergy response. By 11 months of age, meat and eggs can be added to the diet. By 1 year, the infant typically eats table food three times a day and can join the family meal schedule.

Introduction of foods before 4–6 months of age is not recommended, because the infant does not have the digestive enzymes necessary for complete digestion and utilization of the nutrients. Foods such as nuts, jellied candy, and large pieces of solid foods should not be offered to the infant, because these items present a choking hazard. Honey should not be given to children under 2 years of age because of the risk of botulism poisoning. Home-made foods for the baby can be simple to make and economically beneficial. This also allows for simplification and control of ingredients to avoid unhealthy and hidden additives. Commercially prepared foods such as beets, turnips, celery, and collard greens are high in nitrates and should be used sparingly for infants under 1 year of age. Commercially prepared baby food in jars are vacuum packed, and parents should check the safety seals and expiration dates before purchase. When a jar is first opened, a pop should be heard as the vacuum is broken. Foods should not be fed directly from the jar, and leftovers should not be returned to the jar, because saliva contamination can alter the foods. Parents should avoid tasting the food from the same spoon used to feed the infant, because organisms from their mouth will be passed to the baby.

The development of autonomy dictates the need for finger foods by 9 or 10 months, when the infant can be expected to prefer self-feeding. The temperament of the infant will influence the development of mealtime challenges. For example, infants with a high activity level should not be expected to sit for a long period at the family meal table. Infants who are highly distractible may not even finish a meal. Infants who are slow to adapt may not easily try new foods.

Health Promotion

The health-care worker can help the parent develop strategies to accommodate temperament as it relates to feeding, so that conflicts will not arise. The prevention of obesity is a *Healthy People 2030* goal and overfeeding during infancy is thought to be a contributing factor to obesity later in life. The health-care worker can provide parents with information regarding feeding concerns during the first years.

Teeth

The eruption of the first 20 deciduous teeth, which are also known as *primary* or *baby teeth*, usually begins at 5–7 months of age (Box 7.2). The upper and lower central incisors

BOX 7.2 Estimating the Number of Erupted Primary Teeth

The number of primary teeth that should be present in an infant or toddler can be anticipated using the following formula: Age in months − 6

are usually the first to emerge. At this time, the infant enjoys holding toys that can be chewed. The primary teeth serve the purpose of helping the intake of nutrition by allowing the chewing of foods, and they also help in the formation of the jaw. If an infant or child loses a primary tooth because of an accident, a spacer is usually inserted by the dentist to preserve the space for the later eruption of the permanent tooth, thus avoiding expensive orthodontic care. Nursing caries (cavities) occur when the infant is put to bed while sucking on milk or juice from a bottle. The sugars in the milk or juice coat the teeth and promote tooth decay. If the infant insists on a bottle at bedtime, it should be a bottle of water to prevent the development of nursing caries.

Immunizations

Well-child visits should be scheduled after birth before the newborn is discharged from the hospital. Community resources should be assessed, and the parents informed about available help for breastfeeding problems, such as the La Leche League or Healthy Starts programs offered by some health-insurance companies. Home visits are often available through the Visiting Nurse Association, the local health department, or through the home-health services of a hospital for new mothers of high-risk newborns. The growth, development, health, and nutrition of the infant should be checked every 2 months and appropriate immunizations scheduled. Recommended immunization schedules are updated each year. Current immunization schedules can be accessed at www.CDC.gov/vaccines/index.HTML.

Parent Teaching

Well-child checkups are the best time to answer questions the parents may have and to provide anticipatory guidance concerning the developmental stages and needs of the growing infant.

www.Zerotothree.org is a resource for parents concerning information about ages and stages, health and nutrition, and general developmental assessments.

Accident Prevention

Accidents are a major cause of morbidity (illness) and mortality (death). The first injury prevention activity for the newborn, now required by law in most states, is the use of car seats. When held in the lap of a parent instead of in a car seat, the infant becomes a high-speed missile in the event of a motor vehicle accident. Also, front-seat airbags in cars can be lifesaving for adults but can be lethal to infants or young children during accidents (Chapter 8).

Safety Alert

A safe or "childproof" home is essential for the prevention of accidents. There are private agencies in many communities that will come to the home to evaluate safety and offer childproofing suggestions for parents. Local police stations or highway patrol stations offer assistance in assessing car-seat installations. Falls are common causes of injury to infants younger than 1 year.

Following are some guidelines to help prevent common accidents:

- Keep the crib's mattress height set at the appropriate height for the child's age to prevent rolling out of the crib.
- Use safety straps when infants are placed in highchairs or strollers to prevent falls.
- Install gates at the top and bottom of stairs to prevent the infant from falling.
- Place the infant supine, to sleep on their back, and avoid using pillows or blankets in the crib to prevent accidental suffocation or **sudden infant death syndrome (SIDS)**.
- Keep small objects out of an infant's reach to avoid choking, especially after the development of the pincer action.
- Do not leave infants unattended in a bathtub. Infants can drown quickly, even in shallow water.
- Avoid burns by moving electrical cords and pot handles out of reach, and by keeping electrical outlets covered.

KEY POINTS

- Infancy includes the period between 4 weeks and 1 year of age.
- Developmental tasks involve the goals of developing social competence and mastery of skills necessary for functioning in an environment.
- Some developmental tasks of infancy include weaning, locomotion, self-feeding, and acquiring language.
- The development of a sense of trust begins in infancy.
- The infant's birth weight doubles by 6 months and triples by 1 year of age.
- The infant is in Piaget's sensorimotor stage of development.
- Object permanence involves knowing an object is there even though it is not in sight.
- The infant is in Freud's oral stage of development. Sucking and exploring textures with the mouth are normal behaviors.
- Separation anxiety begins at 6 months of age, when the infant protests if the parent leaves the room.

- Language development involves both verbal language and body language.
- Verbal language involves expression and receiving (understanding) communication from others.
- Egocentric behavior is evidenced by the 1-year-old, who relates all toys to his or her own body.
- Overfeeding during infancy is thought to be a contributing factor to obesity later in life.
- Infants should be placed in environments that stimulate movements and exercise.
- A natural pattern of intermittent play is age-appropriate physical activity for infants.
- Breast milk is the best food for infants under 6 months of age, and mothers should be encouraged to continue to provide breast milk until 1 year of age.
- To prevent SIDS, infants should be placed on their backs to sleep.
- By 1 year of age, the infant eats table food three times a day.

- At 1 year of age, whole milk can be introduced, but low-fat milk should not be provided to children under 2 years of age.
- The most common type of dental caries in infants is nursing caries, which are preventable.

- By 9 months of age, the pincer action enables the infant to grasp small objects with the thumb and forefinger.
- A childproof home is essential for preventing accidents.

Clinical Judgment Case Study

A mother discusses her 8-month-old infants' behavior with you and states that she and her husband have not been out of the house alone together since the infant was born. She states the infant picks up the tiniest objects from the floor and puts it into his mouth and when in the highchair, he throws everything from the tray onto the floor. The infant gets very upset if they leave him and she hesitates to leave her "problem child" with a babysitter. What suggestions would you give the mother on how to prepare the infant for a babysitter and how to handle the "behavior problems"?

REVIEW QUESTIONS

1. The nutritional needs of the infant develop markedly in the first year of life. Place an X in the appropriate column to designate the following statements as true or false.

	True	False
Breastmilk contains antibodies not found in formula		
Supplemental formula should be offered to breastfeeding infants		
Children should be placed on low-fat milk at 1 year of age		
The tongue extrusion reflex disappears between 4 and 6 months of age		
At 1 year, the infant typically eats table food three times per day		
3-month-old infants do not have the enzymes to properly digest food		
Baby foods should not be fed directly from a jar		
Honey is not safe for children under the age of 2		
Parents should taste baby food from the same spoon to check temperature		
An infant under 1 year of age should not be allowed to self-feed finger foods		

2. Arrange the following developmental milestones in the order they typically occur.
   A. Separation anxiety.
   B. First responsive smile.
   C. Pincer action.
   D. First steps.
   E. Recognize and prefer parent.
   F. First repetitive syllables.

(Continued)

3. When observing a 9-month-old infant, which of the following developmental tasks would be expected to have been achieved? Place an X next to the achieved developmental tasks and those that require safety precautions that should be discussed with the parent.

Developmental task	Achieved	Safety precautions required
Weaning	☐	☐
Walks independently	☐	☐
Hand-mouth coordination	☐	☐
Crawls	☐	☐
Speaks meaningful words	☐	☐
Rolls over	☐	☐
Birth weight tripled	☐	☐
Birth weight quadrupled	☐	☐
Pincer action	☐	☐
Fed breastmilk	☐	☐
Fed low-fat milk	☐	☐
Has two teeth	☐	☐

4. A 3-month-old infant is observed during a clinic visit. Highlight the observations in the following report that would suggest a follow-up would be indicated.

"The infant appears well-developed and weighs 16 pounds today. The mother initially placed the infant on his abdomen. The infant made no effort to lift his head or roll over. The mother then places the infant on his back and engages in animated speech with him. The infant reaches out toward the mother's face with an open hand but does not smile responsively. The infant sucks energetically while breastfeeding and accepts strained baby food offered by the mother."

5. Which of the following interactions would promote a healthy attachment with an infant?

A. Consistent use of the *en face* position.

B. Speaking in a quiet, monotone voice to avoid startling the infant.

C. Recognizing and responding to hunger cues before crying begins.

D. Promoting independence in the infant by allowing self-soothing in the 1-month-old.

E. Making eye contact while breastfeeding.

F. Keeping the newborn in the same room as the mother in the hospital.

G. Leaving the 9-month-old with a new caregiver every weekend.

H. Labeling the infant as "difficult."

Early Childhood

http://evolve.elsevier.com/Leifer/growth

OUTLINE

OBJECTIVES

1. Define early childhood.
2. Describe characteristics common to toddlers.
3. Describe characteristics common to preschool children.
4. Discuss the developmental tasks of early childhood.
5. Review healthy food choices for growing children.
6. List three factors that aid in the development of language skills.
7. List at least three guidelines for selecting a preschool or day care center.
8. Describe the role of physical activity in maintaining health.
9. Describe the characteristic play and appropriate toys for a toddler and preschool child.
10. List three safety risks common to the early childhood years.
11. Discuss the principles of guidance and discipline for children during the early childhood years.

KEY TERMS

age-appropriate toys
cooperative play
corporal punishment
dental caries
discipline

early childhood
immunity
oropharynx
parallel play

pincer grasp
preschool phase
time-out
toddler phase

DEFINITION

The early childhood period includes children from 1 to 6 years of age. Early childhood is typically separated into two phases; 1–2 years of age is the toddler phase, and 2–6 years is the preschool phase. During early childhood, physical growth slows and stabilizes.

DEVELOPMENTAL TASKS

Tasks to be mastered include acquiring *receptive language* and *expressive language* (understanding and speaking words); developing social interaction skills; mastering self-control in such areas as toilet training; and beginning to develop a self-image and sense of autonomy. The toddler, between 1 and 4 years of age, is in Erikson's stage of autonomy versus shame or doubt. The preschooler, between 4 and 6 years of age, is in Erikson's stage of initiative versus guilt.

Increased motor ability allows expanded exploration in the family and within the community. The willingness to separate from the mother and to explore enhances the development of autonomy and communication skills.

PHYSIOLOGICAL CHANGES

Most children learn to walk steadily between 12 and 15 months of age. By age 2, an exaggerated lumbar curve of the spine causes the abdomen to protrude. By age 3, the posture is more erect. The legs appear bowed between 12 and 18 months of age, and the feet strike the floor flat when walking. A knock-knee appearance develops between 18 months and 2 years. The gait gradually becomes steadier, and by age 2 the knees and toes appear more in alignment. At age 2, the child can run. By age 2½ the child can climb stairs gracefully; by age 3 the child can alternate feet when climbing stairs and can ride a tricycle. By age 4 the child can hop and by age 5 can skip.

The anterior fontanel of the skull closes at 18 months. By age 2, 20 primary teeth have erupted. Continued myelinization of neurons within the brain increases brain function. Although complete myelinization of the brain does not occur before 6–7 years of age, the rate of brain and body development during the preschool years influences behavior and motor coordination. The neocortex of the brain is responsible for thought, emotion, and higher-level brain functions. The frontal lobes are responsible for memory, attention, behavior, and emotions. For example, the skill of bike riding involves vision, hearing, sensation, balance, and using the thalamus and neocortex brain functions (Figure 8.1). A school-age child can ride a two-wheel bicycle, whereas a toddler struggles to learn skills involved in controlling a tricycle. The left hemisphere of the brain has been implicated in language disorders, cerebral palsy, and deafness (Shaywitz & Shaywitz, 2016). Language-rich interactive play helps to enhance language development. Children who have difficulty in one area of brain development may be predisposed to other areas of developmental delay. Developmental screening should be part of every well-child visit.

The preschooler on average gains 4–5 pounds (2 kg) and grows 2–3 inches (7–8 cm) per year. Approximately half of the adult height is achieved by age 2, and the birth weight is quadrupled by 2½ years of age (Feigelman, 2016). Growth charts can be accessed on the Centers for Disease Control and Prevention website (http://www.cdc.gov/growth charts/).

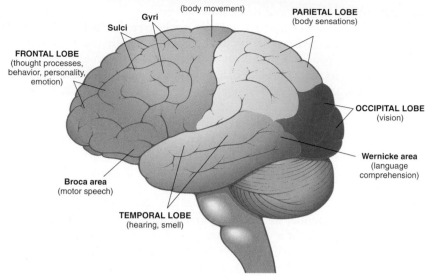

Figure 8.1 Anatomy of brain function.

The toddler has a well-developed pincer grasp (the ability to pick up small objects with the thumb and forefinger) by age 1 and can touch the thumb to each finger sequentially by age 5. A 2-year-old can copy a straight line on paper; a 3-year-old can copy a circle and can use safe scissors. A 4-year-old can draw a person with three body parts, and most 5-year-olds can print their names. Between 18 months and 5 years, the child shows a preference for using one hand or the other and so becomes left-handed or right-handed. Attempts to change hand preference are often met with frustration and are rarely successful. The eye muscles strengthen, depth perception increases during the preschool period, and 20/20 vision is usually achieved by age 4. When asked to find a specific picture on a page while reading a book, the toddler will examine the page in a random pattern to find the specific picture. However, in the same situation with a preschool-age child, the child will examine the page in an organized fashion (up and down or side to side), indicating reading readiness has occurred. Successful reading requires examining the page in an organized pattern.

Hearing is fully developed in the toddler and is necessary for speech development to occur. The eustachian tube connects the middle ear to the oropharynx (back of the throat). The eustachian tube is short and straight allowing bacteria to easily travel from the throat to the middle ear causing an ear infection. A child who is put to bed while drinking milk or juice from a bottle may have a pooling of the sugary fluid in the back of the throat that enables bacteria to grow. These bacteria then have easy access to the ear through the eustachian tube and can cause a middle-ear infection. If a child must be put to bed with a bottle, only water should be in the bottle to prevent development of frequent ear infections, as well as dental caries (cavities).

During early childhood, fine motor skills develop, which include self-feeding, dressing, and undressing. Toddlers are able to eat with a fork and spoon but often prefer finger foods. At age 2, the appetite decreases.

Toilet (potty) training occurs as sphincter control develops and the child masters some form of communication to indicate the need to use the toilet. Modeling behavior, using specially equipped dolls and celebrating successes, aids in achieving toilet training, but the process cannot be hurried and may not be complete before 3½–4½ years of age (Feigelman, 2016). Bowel control occurs before full-bladder control, and nighttime or stress accidents are common. Accidents should not result in scolding or punishment because mastering sphincter control is related to the development of the self-concept. The child may appreciate the power of flushing the toilet after successful use, as he produced the contents.

During toilet training, a child's refusal to sit on a toilet may stem from the fear of falling in or being flushed away. The child's fear is real, and the parents cannot dismiss it and expect to gain cooperation.

Nutrition

Adequate nutrition is essential for optimal physical and mental development in young children. The U.S. Department of Agriculture (USDA) recommends the consumption of nutrient-dense foods during early childhood to ensure nutritional and caloric needs are met. Macronutrients (carbohydrates, fats, and proteins) are required in various amounts and can be consumed from a variety of sources. A varied diet is more likely to provide adequate amounts of the necessary micronutrients (such as vitamins and minerals) than a restricted one. While total caloric requirements can vary widely by age, the recommended proportions of macronutrients remain consistent across the lifespan. The USDA recommends approximately 52% of total calories be consumed in the form of carbohydrates, with most of those being complex. *Complex carbohydrates* include whole grains, vegetables, starches, beans, and whole fruits. Refined sugars and fruit juices are *simple carbohydrates*, and their consumption should be limited. Caloric intake of about 30% should be from fat, and the remaining 18% from protein (USDA, 2020). During the early childhood years, the dependent child is fed by adults whose eating habits may be based on ethnic, cultural, folklore, or fad concepts. Some families are economically disadvantaged, some need guidance on how to select nutritious foods, and many need support on how to cook foods to preserve the nutritious qualities. The USDA MyPlate food guide is a guideline for an optimal diet for children and adults (http://www.choosemyplate.gov) and is based upon Dietary Guidelines for Americans (see Figure 11.3 in Chapter 11). The choices adults make when buying groceries are affected by marketing and coupons. When food is marketed to children, purchases can be influenced by the inclusion of toys or "surprises," shelf placement, and even videogames (Parks et al., 2016). Using food as a reward or withholding a food as punishment is discouraged.

High-fiber diets are not advised for children because the foods are filling but do not provide all of the essential nutrients for growth and development. Children 1–6 years old are susceptible to nutritional deficiencies because growth is rapid and energy output is high. The vegetarian diet is a diet that excludes animal flesh foods and is often referred to as a "plant-based diet." Variations in the vegetarian diet include:

- Veganism: excludes animal flesh and products produced from animals such as dairy products.
- Ovo-vegetarianism: includes eggs but excludes dairy products.
- Lacto-vegetarianism: includes dairy products but excludes eggs.
- Lacto-ovo-vegetarianism: includes eggs and dairy products.
- Flexitarian: a vegetarian who will occasionally eat meat.

There are other variations of plant-based diets that are more restrictive and have not been studied in children. Vegetarianism is considered a healthful diet by the Academy of Nutrition and Dietetics and can satisfy the goals of nutrition in all stages of life, with many health advantages compared with the nonvegetarian diet. Specific nutrients that need special attention for growing children who are vegetarian include vitamin B12, iron, and zinc because their absorption is limited due to the phylates in high-fiber foods (Greenbaum, 2016). Trace elements are important for the growing child and supplementation is advised.

There are no known advantages in consuming excess nutrients or vitamins, only disadvantages. Obesity should be prevented and support for growth and development should be provided through a varied and nutritious diet. Eating habits are developed during the early childhood years, and children may carry these healthy (or unhealthy) habits with them into adulthood. The effect of childhood nutrition on adult health and illness has been well established.

Healthy People 2030

Worldwide nutritional goals for *Healthy People 2030* include a 30% reduction in low birth weight, a 50% reduction in women of reproductive age who have unintended pregnancies, and access to a stable food supply for all.

PSYCHOSOCIAL DEVELOPMENT

Language Development and Communication Skills

The Toddler

Children develop *receptive* language before *expressive* language. That is, they are able to understand words before they can express them. Communication is evidenced in the neonatal period by the cry, coo, or smile. The initial purpose is to communicate needs, to regulate another's behavior, to attract attention, and to interact socially.

By 1 year of age, the toddler usually says the first clear word and responds to simple, single demands or statements such as "bye-bye" or "no!" By 15 months, the toddler may speak four to six words and typically uses one finger to point to various parts of the body. By 18 months the toddler speaks about 15 words and by 19 months may speak in two-word sentences. By age 2, the child has a vocabulary exceeding 100 words and can follow two-step commands such as "pick up the toy and put it away." When learning to speak, the toddler can learn more than one language if both languages are used at home. When one language is used at home and a different language is used at school, difficulties tend to arise. By age 5, most children achieve competence in their native language.

The Preschooler

Language development occurs rapidly during the preschool years. A typical 2-year-old has a vocabulary of just over 100 words, whereas a typical 5-year-old has a vocabulary exceeding 2000 words. In a preschool child, the number of words in a typical sentence is equal to the child's age (Feigelman, 2016). By age 2½ the child expresses possession, as in "my doll." By age 4, the past tense is expressed, and by age 5 the child can express the future tense. Although speech development is directly influenced by the experiences of others talking to the child and encouraging the child to verbalize, speech development follows a predictable sequence and occurs even without the benefit of encouragement or imitating

TABLE 8.1   Literacy Milestones

Age	Motor	Cognitive/Language	Interaction
6–12 months	Reaches for book Puts book to mouth	Looks at pictures Vocalizes, pats picture	Face-to-face gaze Parents follow baby's cues for "more" and "stop"
12–18 months	Holds book with help Turns several pages at a time	Points at pictures with one finger Labels pictures with same sound	May bring book to read Child becomes upset if parent does not let child "control" reading
18–36 months	Turns one page at a time Carries book around house	Names familiar pictures Attention highly variable Demands story over and over	Parent asks, "what's happening?" questions Parent shows pleasure when child supplies word

Modified from Feldman, H., & Messick, C. (2009). Language and speech disorders. In W. Carey, A. Crocker, W. Coleman, E. Elias, & H. Feldman (2009). *Developmental-behavioral pediatrics* (4th ed.). Elsevier; Simms, M. (2016). Language development and communication disorders. In R. Kleigman, B. Stanton, J. St. Geme III, N. Schor, & R. Behrman (2016). *Nelson pediatrics* (20th ed.). Elsevier.

the words of others, albeit at a much slower pace. Speech development reflects mental and emotional development, and often delays can be detected by age 2, when speech delay is obvious. However, speech can also be delayed under conditions of abuse and neglect.

By age 2, a child can be heard to repeat the commands of others. When tempted to touch a forbidden object, the child can be heard to state, "don't touch." From this observation it is apparent that the child's own internal language plays a part in the child's behavior. When the child's skill at language allows him or her to express basic fears, the need for acting out on the fears or frustrations decreases. For this reason, language-delayed children are apt to experience more frequent behavioral outbursts or temper tantrums.

The language skills acquired during the preschool years set the stage for success for the school-age child in the task of achieving literacy at school. A school-age child is expected to enter the classroom with competency in his or her native language. Literacy milestones can be used to aid in the assessment of the child's development (Table 8.1).

For example, a child may use only single words at 18 months, few vocabulary words by age 2, or words that are not clearly understood by age 3. In these cases, a referral for speech and hearing evaluations should be offered (Table 8.2).

Cognitive Development

The sensorimotor stage of cognition ends and the beginning of symbolic thought begins when the toddler begins to use words to express ideas and to solve problems. By age 1, the toddler can push aside an obstacle to gain access to a toy. By 18 months, the toddler learns that dropping a ball, block, or stuffed toy down a flight of stairs results in different rates of descent and heights of bounce. By age 2, the toddler remembers past experiences and adjusts behavior accordingly. A 1-year-old child may exhibit stranger anxiety when the

TABLE 8.2 When a Child With a Communication Disorder Needs Help

Age	Behavior Indicating Help Is Needed
0–11 months	Before 6 months the child does not startle, blink, or change immediate activity in response to sudden loud sounds. Before 6 months the child does not attend to the human voice and is not soothed by the mother's voice. By 6 months the child does not babble strings of consonant + vowel syllables or imitate gurgling or cooing sounds. By 10 months the child does not respond to his or her name. At 10 months the child's sound making is limited to shrieks, grunts, or sustained vowel production.
12–23 months	At 12 months the child's babbling or speech is limited to vowel sounds. By 15 months the child does not respond to "no," "bye-bye," or "bottle." By 15 months the child will not imitate sounds or words. By 18 months the child is not consistently using at least six words with appropriate meaning. By 21 months the child does not respond correctly to "give me …," "sit down," or "come here" when spoken without gestural cues. By 23 months two-word phrases have not emerged that are spoken as single units (e.g., "whatzit," "thank you," or "all gone").
24–36 months	By 24 months at least 50% of the child's speech is not understood by familiar listeners. By 24 months the child does not point to body parts without gestural cues. By 24 months the child is not combining words into phrases ("Go bye-bye," "Go car," "Want cookie"). By 30 months the child does not demonstrate understanding of the words "on," "in," "under," "front," or "back." By 30 months the child is not using short sentences ("Daddy went bye-bye"). By 30 months the child has not begun to ask questions using "where," "what," and "why." By 36 months the child's speech is not understood by unfamiliar listeners.
All ages	At any age, the child is consistently dysfluent, exhibiting repetitions and hesitations. Child evidences blocks or struggles in saying words. Struggle may be accompanied by grimaces, eye blinks, or hand gestures.

Data from Mac Dante, K., & Kleigman, R. (2019). *Nelson's essentials of pediatrics.* Elsevier; originally modified from Weiss, C.E., & Lillywhite, H.E. (1976). *Communication disorders: a handbook for prevention and early detection.* Mosby.

parent leaves the room. By age 2, the child can anticipate a temporary absence (e.g., a parent going to work) in an accepting manner knowing the person will return.

Preschool thinking involves Piaget's preoperational or prelogical characteristics, such as magical thinking and egocentrism (Chapter 5). Two-year-old's attribute life qualities to inanimate dolls or toys and typically feel their wishes caused things to happen. They feel

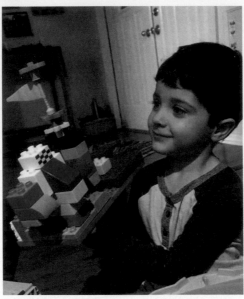

Figure 8.2 This boy proudly examines the unique toy he created.

their point of view must be the same as everyone else's. Although preschoolers are empathetic, they believe that whatever comforts them will also serve to comfort others.

Through experience, preschoolers gradually learn about cause and effect and how to solve problems. Having one object represent another, such as a box representing a train, evidences symbolism and fantasy play. Pretend play is common at age 2. By age 3, children can understand the motivations of others that may differ from their own, and by age 5 they can role-play scenarios with elaborate plots and characters and create toys with building blocks that represent a unique character or castle (Figure 8.2). During the preschool years, while the child is trying to understand the differing opinions of others, fears and other forces in life may be represented by monsters, bad people, or invisible friends.

One of the major tasks of the child during preschool years is to develop impulse control for behaviors such as biting, kicking, and throwing toys. Impulse control is typically achieved by age 4, with minor relapses in times of stress. By 18 months, the toddler develops a sense of self and by age 3 is able to express complex feelings and ideas through pretend play. At age 4, the child can understand the wishes and emotions of others and how they differ from the child's own. Whatever the preschooler cannot understand or express is often acted out in the form of negativism or tantrums. The natural temperament of the child influences the intensity of the emotional responses of joy, anger, or frustration. Many parents need guidance in helping their toddlers manage these challenges in a positive way. Parents can access resources for understanding ages and stages of early childhood by accessing http://www.zerotothree.org.

Moral Development

According to Kohlberg, learning self-control and learning to share with others are moral tasks of early childhood (Chapter 5). Preschoolers look carefully at parents as models of

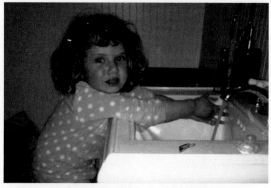

Figure 8.3 Children can learn to wash their hands at an early age. Regular handwashing can prevent the spread of infection and can assist in meeting some of the goals of *Healthy People 2030*.

moral behavior, and this is often acted out in their play. Preschoolers must organize and synthesize what they view at home, in the community, and on television. They constantly test limits either to confirm that a behavior is unacceptable or just to gain attention. A child of 3 becomes ritualistic and aware of rules that he or she feels must be obeyed, and the child will feel guilty if scolded (Figure 8.3). A 2-year-old cannot differentiate between intentional acts and accidents and readily assigns blame. A 3-year-old can understand the difference between intentional acts and accidents but still may extend blame to another. By age 5, the child extends blame for only the intentional act and easily excuses the accident.

Some parents complain that their preschool child lies. Preschoolers do not have the abstract reasoning to lie for the purpose of deceiving others. They tell the truth as they interpret it or wish it to be true. Stealing is a behavior that a preschooler does not feel is wrong because ownership is not completely understood. Respecting the property of others is a learned behavior. A child will learn socially acceptable behavior through consistent, positive reinforcement, and discipline.

Discipline

Discipline must have as its basic purpose the guiding, teaching, or correcting of behavior, not punishment. Preschoolers are naturally egocentric and may not understand the rights and needs of others. The preschooler may hit the mother in anger yet expect to be loved, hugged, and comforted by the mother in his or her frustration.

The purpose of discipline for toddlers should be to help them develop self-control while maintaining positive self-esteem. Setting limits should include praise for good behavior. A time-out response to unacceptable behavior is effective for children between the ages of 1 and 6 years. This response places the child in a safe place with time for self-regulation. The child is removed from the situation, is placed in time-out with just a very brief explanation of why it is happening, and is reminded of the cause at the end of time-out (Figure 8.4). Time-outs usually are limited to 1 minute per year of age. With consistent use, the child will learn to anticipate this disciplinary response to certain behaviors and will learn to control those behaviors.

Corporal punishment (spanking) focuses on the pain of the punishment, can model aggression, and rarely accomplishes the true goal of discipline. Young children may model the behavior of the parent and may hit the parent. Children can also become accustomed

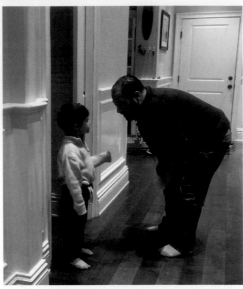

Figure 8.4 By 4 years of age the child understands the rules of behavior. An important teaching approach of the parent is to discuss the behavior of the child and use "time-out" when appropriate.

to the spanking, so that the parent must hit harder, and child abuse can become a risk. Severe physical punishment may affect the psychological health of the child and result in more aggressive behavior of the child.

Rewarding good behavior is the positive and most effective technique of discipline. A hug, smile, praise, or material reward for good behavior is effective. Consistency in parental response is the key to successful discipline. It is effective to ignore the behavior of a child who whines, nags, or has a tantrum and to express frequent praise when the behavior is good. If any behavior receives attention, it will be used again with more intensity to attract attention. Operant conditioning, as described by B.F. Skinner, occurs when the learner repeats behaviors that result in the positive outcome of reaching his or her goals, and the learner stops behaviors that have negative outcomes. The operant theory of discipline is described in Table 8.3. An example of the operant theory during play is the use of an interactive mobile that is activated when the infant kicks or touches a footpad. The infant's kicking will increase if the infant enjoys the resulting sound and movement of the mobile.

When discussing disciplinary techniques for children, the health-care worker should be nonjudgmental and should help parents develop a mutually acceptable plan that will be consistent and safe. Support groups, parenting classes, and counseling should be available for referral as needed.

Sexuality

In the past, toddlers and preschool-age children were thought to be free of sexuality or in a period of sexual dormancy (see Chapter 10 for definitions of sexuality). Today it is recognized that children in early childhood do have the capacity for sexual pleasure and response including penile erection, pelvic thrusting, rhythmic movements, and masturbation. Kinsey et al. (1948) and other researchers have shown that children between the

TABLE 8.3 The Operant Theory of Effective Discipline Techniques

Type of Discipline	Example	Effect
Positive reinforcement	Child receives a treat or toy for helping mommy	Increases the "helping mommy" behavior
Negative reinforcement	Restrict privileges for bad behavior Remove restrictions for good behavior	Increases likelihood of desired behavior occurring again (useful in older children)
Negative punishment	Take away fun and interaction with others Ignore behavior	Excessive limits can undermine a child's sense of initiative Tantrums between 2 and 4 years of age should not result in a reward of positive attention

Effective discipline helps the child internalize behavior control. Discipline should be immediate, specific, and time limited.

TABLE 8.4 Sexual Behavior in Early Childhood

Normal	Requires Referral
When diapers are changed, child may touch own genitals	Prefers touching genitals instead of playing with toys
Plays with feces	Repeatedly uses feces as a toy
Touches genitals, breasts of family and peers	Asks to be touched in genital area
Removes clothes, likes to play nude	Removes clothes in public repeatedly even after correction
Shows interest in watching bathroom functions	Often insists on watching bathroom functions of others
Plays "doctor" to inspect body of others	Forces peers to remove clothes
Places objects against genital area	Insists on placing objects against genital area of self or peers
Plays house, with mommy and daddy roles assigned to peers	Simulates sexual intercourse activities; draws genitals on figures

Data from Hillman, J., & Spigarelli, M. (2009). Sexuality: Its development and direction. In W. Carey, A. Crocker, W. Coleman, E. Elias, & H. Feldman (2009). *Developmental-behavioral pediatrics* (4th ed.). Elsevier.

ages of 4 and 7 years' experience play activities that involve viewing or touching the genitals which results from normal curiosity (Table 8.4).

Parents have an impact on the molding of sexuality in their infants and children. The parents' response to the child's urinary and fecal elimination is an early influence related to sexuality. A negative response to a dirty diaper, the label of "stinky" to the soiled underpants of a toddler, or forced toilet training all influence the development of sexuality. Treating the natural process of bodily functions as secret or as dirty promotes embarrassment or discomfort related to the genital area. The acceptance or rejection of hugging and kissing as an expression of emotion by parents can influence sexuality and the ability of the child to establish intimate relationships in later life (Hillman & Spigarelli, 2016). Modesty appears gradually between 5 and 6 years of age. Preschool day care centers typically do not separate boys' and girls' bathrooms, and viewing the body is treated as normal and natural. Masturbation or sexual curiosity that interferes with normal play activities, or acting out sexual intercourse with dolls or playmates, however, may be indications of sexual abuse, and the child should be referred for counseling.

Physical Activity

National health guidelines recommend at least 60 minutes of daily physical activity for children to increase aerobic capacity, functional ability, fitness, and quality of life. Preschool and school recess, physical education programs, organized sports, and community recreational programs support activity greater than the minimum recommendation. A combination of nutrition and physical activity during childhood is the key ingredient for weight control and prevention of some adult-onset illnesses such as heart disease, high blood pressure, and diabetes, as well as establish a foundation of healthy habits for adolescence and adulthood (Turk, 2016).

Age-appropriate activities should range from moderate to vigorous, often following a natural pattern of intermittent play. Running, jumping, hopping, and climbing are all age-appropriate physical activities for young children. Organized sports can also be good sources of regular physical activity. Caregivers should limit sedentary activities such as television, computers, and video games and should ensure that young children have access to safe, active play.

Caregivers can keep children safe during physical activity by providing appropriate footwear and protective gear for each activity. Shoes should be cushioned and supportive with a good fit. Protective gear may include helmets, pads, mouthguards, and shin guards, among others. Equipment and play surfaces should be well maintained to avoid injuries. Children should be kept hydrated by offering water before, during, and after exercise. For details on protective gear for specific physical activities see https://www.medic8.com/healthguide/sports-medicine/prevention/equipment.html.

Play

In the toddler period, play reflects the child's experiences. Age-appropriate toys are those that are safe and promote the cognitive and motor development of the specific age group. The toddler may pretend to put a baby to bed or to shop at a store. The 2-year-old exhibits parallel play, in which he or she plays next to a friend but does not interact with the friend. The 3- to 4-year-old exhibits cooperative play, in which a group of children can cooperate by acting out a scene together or by building a tower of blocks together. By age 5, there is organized group play with assigned roles, such as playing house with one child assigned the mother role, one the father role, and so on.

Play allows the child to imitate adult roles, be the aggressor, assume superpowers, and solve problems. The child's drawings often reflect his or her inner emotional issues or conflicts. According to the preschool child, rules of play are absolute, and fairness means

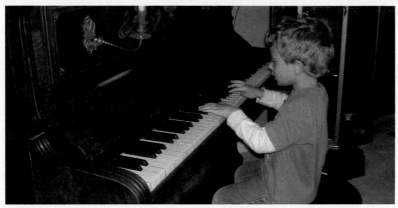

Figure 8.5 Preschoolers share a love of music. This child enjoys playing the piano.

equal treatment regardless of circumstances. Group songs and music are enjoyed by both the toddler and the preschool child who respond with unique dancing and random movements (Figure 8.5). Many 2-year-olds enjoy singing along with recorded songs.

Day Care

The experience of spending time in day care or preschool is a big step toward developing independence. The child must accept that the parent will leave and must trust that the parent will return. There are several types of day care settings that may be available in communities for parents who work outside the home.

Parents may also choose a private babysitter or nannies to come into their home to offer personal attention to their child. Family care centers provide childcare for small groups of children, and often parents take turns providing childcare in this type of setting. *Day care centers* offer structured play and rest activities for groups of children who are supervised by professional staff. Some employers offer day care within the workplace as a service to their employees. *Preschool centers* offer structured activities that foster growth and development and teach coping skills. A good preschool program can help a child gain self-confidence and positive self-esteem. Parents may be offered the following suggestions to help them select a facility that will best meet the needs of their child:

- State licensing agencies offer lists of local day care centers and preschools.
- The school or center should meet accreditation standards set by the National Association for Education of Young Children.
- Staff should have school preparation in early childhood education.
- Student-to-staff ratios should be established with clear limits.
- Techniques of discipline, philosophy of care or education, safety, and sanitary conditions of the environment should be reviewed.
- Facilities for snacks and rest should be reviewed.
- Health history requirements for children should be reviewed.
- Toys and facilities for indoor and outdoor play should be reviewed.
- Parents should visit the school and should observe staff-child interactions.
- Parents can speak to parents of other children in the school to evaluate their input and opinions.

TEACHING TECHNIQUES

When parents respond to the words of a toddler appropriately, they stimulate the development of positive communication. The use of picture books at regular interactive reading sessions with the toddler also aids in language development. Parents should not demand correct speech of a 2-year-old, and accurate pronunciation should not be a major focus. If speech difficulties are associated with other oral problems, such as the inability to blow a kiss or to eat, medical evaluation should be sought.

Parents can be taught methods for helping the preschooler to express feelings through words such as "You feel angry now, and I understand." Teaching the preschooler how to express feelings verbally rather than by acting out is a key to positive social development. Preschool children who are learning to be autonomous often rapidly shift between dependence and independence, joy and rage, and this changing behavior can cause parents to feel frustrated and inadequate. Parents need to be counseled concerning the normal development and behavior of the toddler and preschool child.

The child should be introduced to the dentist by age 1 and have the first dental exam by age 2 followed by visits every 6 months. Dental X-rays may be done between 4 and 6 years of age. The infant's gums can be wiped with a soft damp cloth, and a toothbrush initiated when the first tooth erupts. Regular toothbrushing twice daily with a soft toothbrush and age-appropriate toothpaste should be routine by age 2 to maintain oral health (Douglass & Clark, 2015). Parents can often model behavior that they wish their child to imitate (Figure 8.6).

The behaviors of the child and the responses of the parent should be discussed at well-child visits. When a parent does not offer any positive statements about his or her child, and the child misbehaves in preschool and at home, more detailed assessment may be necessary.

Safety and Accident Prevention

Accidents are a major threat during the early childhood years. Young children play hard and have little understanding of the potential dangers around them.

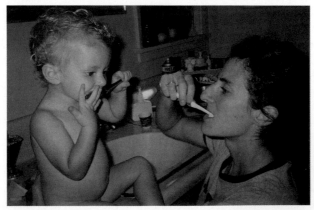

Figure 8.6 The child imitates the mother and brushes her own teeth. The child also "helps" brush the mother's teeth in this nightly ritual.

Safety Alert

- Parents may need guidance concerning the need to childproof the house, to keep stairways safe, and to avoid clutter.
- Toys should be sturdy and age appropriate without sharp edges.
- Preschoolers should not be allowed to carry breakable items or sharp objects.
- The appropriate use of car seats is essential (Figure 8.7).
- A child should not sit in the front seat of a car until older than 13 years of age as inflating airbags can be lethal.
- Children should not be left inside cars alone.
- Pot handles should not overhang the edge of stovetops, because accidental burns are common dangers in the home.
- Medicines should have childproof bottle caps and should not be left within the sight or reach of a young child.
- Preschool children can be taught the dangers of talking with strangers and should know where to go if a parent or sitter is not in sight.
- Accident prevention techniques should be discussed at every well-child visit (Table 8.5).
- The use of dishes that have a high lead content should be avoided as lead can seep into the food and cause lead toxicity that can impair growth and development.

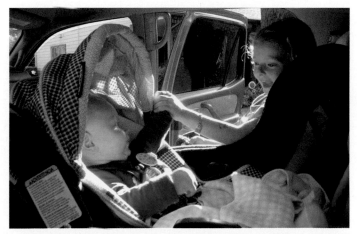

Figure 8.7 An older child, in a front-facing car seat, entertains the infant in a rear-facing car seat. The infant who is less than 2 years of age or weighs less than 35 pounds is secured in a rear-facing car seat behind the driver in the car's back seat to prevent the large and heavy head from falling forward and obstructing the airway when the car stops suddenly or in case of an accident. The driver can look through the car's rearview mirror toward a mirror mounted on the rear window to see the face of the infant. A child of more than 35–40 pounds is secured in a front-facing car seat in the center of the car's back seat. An older child should use a booster seat until (1) the vehicle safety belt fits properly flat across the chest, (2) the lap belt fits low and snug across the thighs, and (3) the child can sit firmly against the seatback with the legs bent at the knees over the seat edge. A child should not sit in the front seat of a car until over 13 years of age. Information concerning safe car seat use can be accessed at https://www.nhtsa.gov/equipment/car-seats-and-booster-seats.

TABLE 8.5 How to Prevent Hazards Caused by the Behavioral Characteristics of Toddlers

Behavioral Characteristics	Hazard and Prevention Strategies*
AUTOMOBILE	
Impulsive, unable to delay gratification, increased mobility, egocentric	Teach child safety rules of the street. Teach child the meaning of red, yellow, and green traffic lights. Caution child not to run from behind parked cars or snowbanks. Use car-seat restraints appropriately. Hold toddler's hand when crossing street. Supervise tricycle riding. Do not allow child to play in car alone. Driver must look carefully in front and behind vehicles before accelerating. Teach child safe areas around house. Supervise young toddlers and preschoolers at all times.
BURNS	
Fascination with fire Toddler can reach articles by climbing, pokes fingers in holes and openings; can open doors and drawers; is unaware of cause and effect	Teach child the meaning of "hot" (e.g., allow child to touch sun-warmed beach sand). Put matches, cigarettes, candles, and incense out of reach and sight. Turn handles of cooking pots toward back of stove. Beware of hot coffee; avoid overhanging tablecloths. Keep appliances such as coffee pots, electric frying pans, and food warmers and their cords out of reach. Test food and fluids heated in microwave ovens to ensure that center is not too hot. Beware of hot charcoal in grills. Use snug fireplace screens. Mark children's room locations to alert firefighters in emergency. Keep a pressure-type fire extinguisher available and teach all family members who are old enough how to use it. Practice what to do in case of home fire. Install smoke detectors. Check bathwater temperature before placing child in water. Do not allow child to handle hot water faucets. Protect child from sun with sunscreen and clothing.
FALLS	
Exploring different parts of house; can open doors and lean out open windows; toddlers' depth perception immature Capabilities change quickly; may seem grown up at times, but still requires constant supervision at home and on playground	Teach children how to go up and down stairs when they show readiness for these tasks. Use side rails on large beds when child graduates from crib. Lock basement doors or use gates at top and bottom of stairs. Mop spilled liquids from floor immediately. Use window guards. Use car-seat restraints appropriately. Keep scissors and other sharp objects away from toddler's reach. Use childproof doorknobs and drawer closures. Secure child in shopping cart at store. Supervise when child is climbing in playground. Clothing and shoelaces should be appropriate to prevent tripping.

TABLE 8.5   How to Prevent Hazards Caused by the Behavioral Characteristics of Toddlers (*Cont.*)

Behavioral Characteristics	Hazard and Prevention Strategies*
SUFFOCATION AND CHOKING	
Explores with senses, likes to bite on and taste things Eats on the run	Do not allow small children to play with deflating balloons, which can be sucked into windpipe. Inspect toys for small or loose parts. Remove small objects such as coins, buttons, and pins from reach. Avoid popcorn, nuts, small hard candies, chewing gum, or large chunks of meat. Child should not jump and run with food in the mouth. De-bone fish and chicken. Learn Heimlich maneuver and CPR. Inspect width of crib and playpen slats. Keep plastic bags away from small children. If child is vomiting, turn him or her on side. Avoid nightclothes with drawstring necks. Discard old refrigerators and appliances or remove doors.
POISONING	
Ingenuity increases, can open most containers Increased mobility provides access to cupboards, medicine cabinets, bedside stands, interiors of closets Looks at and touches everything Learns by trial and error Puts objects in mouth	Store household detergents and cleaning supplies out of reach in a locked cabinet. Do not put chemicals or other potentially harmful substances into food or beverage containers. Keep medicines in locked cabinets; put them away immediately after use. Use child-resistant caps and packaging. Discard unused/expired medicine appropriately. Follow physician's directions when administering medication. Do not refer to pills as "candy." Explain poison symbols to child and to parents. Keep telephone number of poison-control center available. When painting, use paint marked "for indoor use" or one that conforms to standards for use on surfaces that may be chewed by children. Wash fruits and vegetables before eating. Obtain and record name of any new plant purchased. Alert family of location and appearance of poisonous plants on or around property or commonly encountered when camping. Use childproof locks on cabinets. Use dishes that do not have high lead content.
DROWNING	
Lacks depth perception Does not realize danger Loves water play	Watch child continuously while at beach or near a pool or water-filled bathtub. Empty wading pools when child has finished playing. Cover wells securely. Wear recommended life jackets in boats. Begin teaching water safety and swimming skills early. Lock fences surrounding swimming pools. Supervise tub baths; be aware that a young child can drown in a small amount of water.

(Continued)

TABLE 8.5 How to Prevent Hazards Caused by the Behavioral Characteristics of Toddlers (*Cont.*)

Behavioral Characteristics	Hazard and Prevention Strategies*
ELECTRIC SHOCK Pokes and probes with fingers	Cover electrical outlets. Cap unused sockets with safety plugs. Water conducts electricity; teach child not to touch electrical appliances when wet; keep appliances out of reach. Keep electrical appliances away from tub and sink areas.
ANIMAL BITES Immature judgment	Teach child to avoid stray animals. Do not allow toddler to abuse household pets. Supervise closely.
SAFETY Easily distracted Trusting of others Falls frequently	Teach toddler safety related to strangers. Do not personalize clothes. Do not allow toddler to eat or suck lollipops while running or playing. Keep sharp-edged objects out of reach. Keep sharp-edged furniture out of play areas.

CPR, Cardiopulmonary resuscitation.
*In every situation, keep first-aid chart and emergency numbers handy. Know location of and how to get to nearest emergency facility.
Modified from Leifer, G. (2019). *Introduction to maternity & pediatric nursing* (8th ed.). Elsevier.

Immunizations

Immunity is defined as the body's resistance to disease-causing organisms. Newborns have immunity protection transferred via the placenta from the mother, but this immunity lasts for only a few months. In infants and young children, the immune system is immature, and the child is vulnerable to life-threatening infections. After the newborn is discharged from the hospital, an active immunization program starts at 2 months when the child is capable of producing his or her own antibodies; well-child checkups and immunizations are scheduled at 2-month intervals.

 Health Promotion

The current recommended American Academy of Pediatrics (AAP) immunization schedule for infants and children can be accessed at http://www.CDC.gov/vaccines.

Sometimes teaching a preschooler about health issues requires the child's participation, interaction, or cooperation. A preschool child knows that a pin or needle stuck into a balloon will pop the balloon. Therefore, it is no surprise that children fear that a pin (or needle) stuck into their arm or leg will cause their body to pop or explode too. One possible approach to relieve this fear is to allow the child to handle the syringe (without the needle) and to administer pretend injections to a doll. The immediate presence of a calm, reassuring parent who is holding the child in a firm hug will assuage fear and anxiety better than any verbal explanation or reassurance.

When teaching parents, it is important to develop a partnership with them and to understand their values so that anticipatory guidance can be provided. The nurse can offer tools to the parents to help them manage their child's behavior, including an explanation of the ongoing developmental process.

Information concerning preventative health care for infants, children, and adolescents can be accessed at http://www.AAP.org/periodicityschedule.

KEY POINTS

- The early childhood period is between 1 and 6 years of age and is separated into the toddler phase and the preschool phase.
- Tasks to be mastered during early childhood include understanding and speaking words, social interaction, mastery of self-control in feeding and toileting, and beginning to develop a self-concept and a sense of autonomy.
- Toilet training occurs as sphincter control develops and the child masters basic communication skills to indicate the need to use the toilet. Complete bowel and bladder control is typically achieved by age 3½–4½ years.
- Adequate nutrition is essential for optimum physical and mental development.
- A 2-year-old child exhibits negativistic behavior and tantrums because of frustrations and struggles for independence.
- Preschool thinking involves Piaget's preoperational or prelogical characteristics.
- A 2-year-old cannot distinguish between intentional acts and mistakes.
- Impulse control is typically achieved by age 4.
- A 3-year-old is ritualistic and feels all rules must be obeyed.
- According to Kohlberg, the preconventional stage of moral development begins during the preschool age.

- Discipline should have as its purpose the guiding, teaching, or correcting of behavior rather than punishment.
- Toddlers and preschoolers do not completely understand the rights of others.
- According to Freud, a conscience begins to develop in the preschool phase, and children begin then to understand how their behavior affects others.
- Age-appropriate, daily, moderate, and vigorous physical activities are important to maintain the health of children.
- Children should be kept well hydrated by offering water before, during, and after exercise.
- Sports-appropriate protective equipment should be worn by children to prevent injuries.
- Play is an important part of a child's life. Appropriate toys can promote growth and development.
- Twenty primary teeth erupt by age 2 and the birth weight quadruples.
- The preschool child can easily learn more than one language when the different languages are used in the home.
- Language milestones can be used to assess the child's development.
- In a preschool child, the number or words in a typical sentence is equal to the child's age in years.

(Continued)

- A preschool child learns socially acceptable behavior by positive reinforcement.
- Time-outs should last 1 minute per year of age.
- A 2-year-old exhibits parallel play, whereas a 3-year-old engages in cooperative play with groups using a high level of imagination.
- Parents who hold, hug, and rock their children can influence the ability of the child to establish intimate relationships later in life.
- Accident prevention techniques should be discussed with parents.
- An active immunization program schedule starts at 2 months and continues through the preschool years. Many communicable diseases in childhood can be prevented through immunization.

Clinical Judgment Case Study

When discussing disciplinary techniques for children, the health-care worker can help parents develop a plan that is mutually agreeable. Discuss three appropriate types of disciplinary techniques that can be used consistently and safely for the early childhood years. List examples of how these techniques can be implemented.

REVIEW QUESTIONS

1. A parent brings an 18-month-old child to the clinic. The parent discusses the behavior of the child and the following assessments are written. **Highlight the assessments that are not age appropriate and should be recorded and reported for follow-up by a professional.**

   "The child is standing next to the mother. It is noted that his knees and toes are not in alignment and he is wearing a diaper. As the mother reads a book to him, he smiles, pats the pictures with his open hand, and speaks mostly using vowel sounds and occasional D and B sounds. He appears to throw his toys on impulse and the mother states he sometimes has temper tantrums. He sits down and plays with a toy car next to a friend who is also playing with a toy car, but he does not make an attempt to play with that friend or initiate contact."

2. Helping a parent set guidelines for discipline for a preschool child is often a challenge. Review the situation described below and drag the words to fill in the blanks in the following sentences that best describe the most appropriate response.

   "To aid the preschooler in making safe decisions, the parent should----------1----------- for poor behavior and when a breach of behavior occurs, the best response is-----2-----------------, and action initiated such as--------3-------------------. After the punishment is administered the parent should------------4-------------."

Choices:

1. A. set limits; or B. verbally admonish
2. A. immediate; or B. scheduled
3. A. gentle spanking; or B. time-out
4. A. explain why the punishment occurred; or B. offer time-out in his room

3. Which of the following statements are true regarding early childhood nutrition? (select all that apply)

   A. A 6-year-old child needs a higher percentage of protein than the average adult.
   B. 52% of total calories should be from carbohydrates.
   C. A young child's diet should be high in fiber to promote satiety.
   D. The consumption of fruit juices should be limited because the carbohydrates are simple instead of complex.
   E. A vegetarian diet can be healthy for a young child.
   F. A young child's eating habits are influenced by those of their family.
   G. Using food as a reward is discouraged.

4. Mark the box in the table indicating which behaviors are typical for a toddler or a preschooler.

Behavior	Toddler	Preschooler
Has a vocabulary of about 100 words	☐	☐
Uses future tense	☐	☐
Develops impulse control	☐	☐
Exhibits stranger anxiety	☐	☐
Speaks in sentences	☐	☐
Exhibits modesty	☐	☐
Prefers to eat with fingers rather than spoon	☐	☐
Enjoys organized group play	☐	☐

5. Choose the correct answers to fill in the blanks in the following paragraph.

   Physical activity during early childhood should be a minimum of -----1----- minutes per day. Most of this activity should be -----2-----, and -----3-----. Regular physical activity, in combination with good nutrition, can prevent -----4-----. Caregivers should provide -----5-----. The best hydration for a young child is -----6-----.

   1. A. 30 minutes, or B. 60 minutes
   2. A. intermittent, or B. continuous
   3. A. light/moderate, or B. moderate/vigorous
   4. A. heart disease, or B. dental caries
   5. A. gym membership, or B. protective equipment
   6. A. water, or B. sports drinks

Middle Childhood

http://evolve.elsevier.com/Leifer/growth

OUTLINE

OBJECTIVES

1. Define middle childhood.
2. Describe the physiological changes and developmental tasks that occur in middle childhood.
3. Describe the role of daily physical activity and play activities in nurturing growth and development and in preventing illness in later life.
4. Discuss advantages and disadvantages in the use of electronic media by children.
5. Describe the cognitive development that occurs in middle childhood and its effect on the development of learning styles.
6. List at least three ways in which Erikson's task of industry can be fostered in middle childhood.
7. Trace the development of moral behavior in the school-age child.
8. Discuss the discipline techniques that are effective in middle childhood.
9. Discuss the use of intelligence testing for school-age children.
10. Discuss the psychosocial development that occurs in middle childhood.
11. Discuss the role of peer groups in the growth and development during middle childhood.
12. Discuss the sexual development of and education appropriate for school-age children.
13. List the major health-teaching needs of school-age children.

KEY TERMS

cognitive style
corporal punishment
discipline
exercise
gamification

gingivitis
latchkey children
middle childhood
mnemonic technique
moral behaviors

moral reasoning
physical activity
plaque
social cognition

DEFINITION

Middle childhood encompasses the ages of 6 and 12 years. These school-age children differ from preschoolers because they focus more on fact rather than fantasy. School-age children interact more with teachers and others outside the family who will have a significant impact on their growth, development, and education. One of the major developmental tasks of this age group is forming positive self-esteem from internal sources rather than depending solely on feedback from elders for self-esteem. The ability to develop close peer relationships will affect the development of new ideas, skills, and tools that will enhance the child's advancement toward maturity. Other developmental tasks include changing from concrete thinking to abstract thinking, developing secondary sex characteristics, and accepting more responsibility.

PHYSIOLOGICAL CHANGES

Myelinization of the brain slows during middle childhood but continues through adolescence. The bones continue to ossify and grow, and the body develops a lower center of gravity than in preschool years due in part to a shift in posture and an increase in leg length. Physical growth is slow until a growth spurt occurs just before puberty. The average weight gain is 5.5–7 pounds (2.5–3.2 kg) per year, and average height increase per year is about 2 inches (5 cm). Children who are taller than their peers may face an extra challenge because they are likely to be treated as if they are older or more mature. The self-concept may suffer if the tall child does not live up to these inflated expectations.

The loss of primary teeth begins at about age 6; the lower central incisor is normally the first tooth to be lost (Figure 9.1). Parents often treat the loss of primary teeth as a sign that the child is growing up and many parents reward the child whenever a tooth falls out. About four permanent teeth erupt each year in the same order as deciduous (primary)

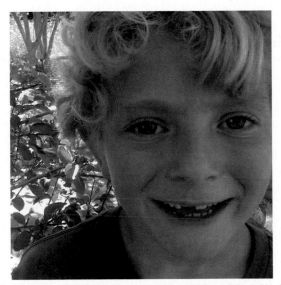

Figure 9.1 One of the most obvious physical changes of middle childhood is the loss of the primary teeth. The loss of primary teeth begins at age 6, and about four permanent teeth erupt each year.

teeth (Chapter 7). Premolars usually erupt about 11 years of age. Regular dental check-ups should be a part of routine health care to screen for dental problems and to have the teeth cleaned. Prevention of dental caries includes fluoridated water, daily brushing with fluoridated toothpaste, and routine application of a topical fluoride by a health professional (American Academy of Pediatric Dentistry, 2019). Limiting intake of sticky sweets and chocolates, and instead encouraging snacks such as apples, raw carrots, and sugarless gum, can reduce plaque formation. Plaque is a sticky, colorless, or pale-yellow mass of bacteria that grows on the surfaces of teeth and spreads to the roots. Plaque buildup can harden into white or yellow tartar, which contributes to gum irritation or infection (gingivitis). Plaque can be prevented by regular tooth brushing and flossing. Flossing between teeth can be modeled by parents and can be quickly learned by the school-age child.

The gastrointestinal tract of the school-age child is more mature than that of the preschooler, and stomach capacity increases but the rate of stomach emptying also increases, which may affect absorption of medications (Rappley & Kallman, 2009). The school-age child requires less caloric intake than the preschooler, and the older child usually snacks less. Preferences for specific foods develop. Sensory organs mature and sharpen the senses of taste, smell, and touch. Large-print books are no longer necessary because visual maturity (20/30 to 20/20 acuity) is achieved sometime between preschool age and age 6 (Olitsky et al., 2016).

Newly developed fine and gross motor skills, increased muscle strength, coordination, and interest increase enjoyment of physical activities. School-age children master coordination and control, allowing them to enjoy activities that require more skill such as team sports, playing a musical instrument, or dance, but high stress or impact sports such as tackle football or power lifting are not recommended as skeletal immaturity increases the risk of injury.

Exercise and Play

Physical activity is bodily movement produced by contraction of skeletal muscle that increases energy expenditure above a basal level. Exercise is a subcategory of physical activity that is planned, structured, repetitive, purposeful, and maintains one or more components of physical fitness as an objective (World Health Organization, 2018).

Children between the ages of 5 and 7 achieve their activity engaging in vigorous play. After age 7, children are able to participate in competitive play and use coping strategies to manage team cooperation, conflict, losing, and winning. Participation in organized sports can develop teamwork, physical fitness, and foster emerging social skills. While competition can be a welcome challenge, the development of these physical, emotional, and social skills is the priority in middle childhood. For this reason, all children should be encouraged to participate in team sports without excluding those who are less physically talented. High stress and excessive pressure to win are not helpful and should be avoided. Understanding the competitive nature of sports occurs around 9 years of age, while mastery occurs around 12 years of age. The ability to wait for a delayed reward is important. Repeated failure impacts self-esteem and may prevent the child from taking future risks (Feigelman, 2016).

School-age children need daily physical activity for the same reasons that younger children do: to build strength, endurance, and coordination; to slow the development of coronary risk factors; and to build a foundation of healthy lifestyle habits. Exercise in childhood also promotes a healthy body composition and bone mass, and there is ample evidence to show that active children are more likely to become active adults. School-age children should continue to engage in 60 minutes of moderate to vigorous levels of physical activity daily. Organized team sports can contribute to meeting the guidelines as well as contribute to the psychosocial development of the child through increased confidence, focus, and respect for authority. Moderate intensity exercises appropriate for children include hiking, skateboarding, rollerblading, and bicycle riding. Vigorous activities can include running games (such as tag), jumping rope, soccer, basketball, and swimming. Tug-of-war, tree climbing, push-ups, swinging on monkey bars, hopscotch, and trampoline are all examples of appropriate muscle and bone strengthening exercises for children. A summary of growth and development, nutrition, play, and safety is reviewed in Table 9.1.

Asthma is a common childhood health problem and some types of asthma are exercise induced, but exercise should not be abandoned but rather managed in a way that enables the asthmatic child to achieve the benefits of healthy exercise and activities that are important for all children.

The best tolerated exercises for children with asthma include those with intermittent activity such as volleyball, baseball, gymnastics, and swimming. Warm-up and cool-down activities before and after exercise are helpful.

Health Promotion

The American Academy of Pediatrics Committee on Sports Medicine and School Health recommends teaching motor skills and fitness exercises in the school setting to develop skills and to promote positive attitudes toward exercise, which may lead to a positive lifelong health and fitness philosophy. The focus should be on mastery and enjoyment rather than on winning. The assignment of the extra running of laps or extra exercise as punishment promotes negative attitudes toward exercise. Protective accessories appropriate to the sport should be worn to prevent injury to the immature skeletal system.

Activities, such as collecting things or playing board games, are often enjoyed by the school-age child. Internet or video games can help develop hand-eye coordination and can challenge intellect. These games are healthy outlets as long as they do not replace daily physical activity and should not be used in excess of 2 hours per day (Felt & Robb, 2016). Creativity should be encouraged because it helps to develop general thinking and problem-solving skills. Art and music lessons, appropriately encouraged, can help to develop lifelong interests, appreciation, and talents in the child.

Health Promotion

Many schools have physical-fitness programs that promote healthy lifestyles consistent with the goals of *Healthy People 2030*.

Eight-year-olds take pride in mastering skills and in showing off their accomplishments. By age 9 or 10, physical strength is greatly increased and interest in specific sports or other activities develops. Increased understanding of rules and teamwork enables these children to participate in competitive games. School-age children often compare themselves with one another according to their ability to master academics or to excel at sports. This tendency to compare affects the development of self-esteem. Maintaining optimum nutrition and preventing injury are two additional health challenges that exist during the school-age years.

TABLE 9.1   Summary of Growth and Development and Health Maintenance of School-Age Children

Age (Years)	Physiological Growth	Intellectual Competency	Emotional-Social Competency	Nutrition	Play	Safety
General: 6–12 years	Gains an average of 2.5–3.2 kg/yr (5.0–7.0 lb/yr). Has overall height gains of 5.0 cm/yr (2 in/yr); growth occurs in spurts and mainly in the trunk and extremities. Loses deciduous teeth; most permanent teeth erupt. Progressively more coordinated in both gross and fine motor skills. Caloric needs increase during growth spurts.	Masters concrete operations. Moves from egocentrism; learns that he/she is not always right. Learns grammar and expression of emotions and thoughts. Vocabulary increases to 3000 words or more. Handles complex sentences.	Central crisis; industry vs. inferiority; wants to do and make things. Progressive sex education needed. Wants to be like friends; competition is important. Fears body mutilation, alterations in body image; earlier phobias may recur; nightmares; fear of death. Nervous habits are common.	Fluctuations in appetite because of uneven growth pattern and tendency to become more involved in activities. Tendency to neglect breakfast in rush to get to school. Although lunch is provided in most schools, child does not always eat it.	Plays in groups, mostly of same sex; gang activities predominate. Enjoys reading age-appropriate books. Bicycles important. Sports equipment, cards, board and table games. Most play is active games requiring little or no equipment.	Enforce continued use of seat belts during car travel. Bicycle safety must be taught and enforced. Teach safety related to hobbies, handicrafts, mechanical equipment.

| 6–7 years | Gross motor skills exceed fine motor coordination. Has good balance and rhythm – runs, skips, jumps, climbs, gallops. Throws and catches ball. Dresses self with little or no help. | Has vocabulary of 2500 words. Learns to read and print. Begins concrete concepts of numbers, general classifications of items. Knows concepts of right and left; morning, afternoon, and evening; coinage. Has intuitive thought process. Is verbally aggressive, bossy, opinionated, argumentative. Likes simple games with basic rules. | Boisterous, outgoing, and a know-it-all. Whiny; parents should sidestep power struggles, offer choices. Becomes quiet and reflective during seventh year; very sensitive. Can use telephone. Likes to make things; starts many projects, finishes few. Adults should give some responsibility for household duties. | Persistence of preschool food dislikes. Tendency for deficiencies in iron, vitamin A, and riboflavin. 100 mL/kg of water per day, 3 g/kg protein daily needed. | Still enjoys dolls, cars, and trucks. Plays well alone but enjoys small groups of both sexes; begins to prefer same-sex peers during seventh year. Ready to learn how to ride a bicycle. Prefers imaginary, dramatic play with real costumes. Begins collecting items for quantity, not quality. Enjoys active games such as hide-and-seek, tag, jumping rope, in-line skating, soccer. | Teach and reinforce traffic safety. Child needs adult supervision of play. Teach child to avoid strangers and never to take anything from strangers. Teach illness prevention and reinforce continued practice of other health habits. Restrict bicycle use to home ground and no traffic areas; teach bicycle safety. Child should wear helmet. Teach and set examples about harmful use of drugs, alcohol, and smoking. |

(Continued)

TABLE 9.1 Summary of Growth and Development and Health Maintenance of School-Age Children *(Cont.)*

Age (Years)	Physiological Growth	Intellectual Competency	Emotional-Social Competency	Nutrition	Play	Safety
8–10 years	Myopia may appear. Secondary sex characteristics begin in girls. Hand-eye coordination and fine motor skills are well established. Movements are graceful, coordinated. Cares for own physical needs completely; is constantly on the move; plays and works hard.	Learning correct grammar and expression of feelings in words. Likes books he/she can read alone; will read funny papers and scan newspaper. Enjoys making detailed drawings. Mastering, classification, serialization, spatial, temporal, and numerical concepts. Uses language as an effective communication tool; likes riddles, jokes, word games. Rules are a guiding force in life now. Very interested in what things are and how they work, such as weather, seasons, and the like.	Strong preference for same-sex peers. Antagonizes opposite-sex peers. Self-assured and pragmatic at home; questions parental values and ideas. Has a strong sense of humor. Enjoys clubs, group projects, outings, large groups, camp. Modesty about own body increases over time; sex conscious. Works diligently to perfect the skills he/she does best. Happy, cooperative, relaxed, and casual in relationships. Increasingly courteous and well mannered with adults. Gang-group stage at a peak; secret codes and rituals prevail. Responds better to suggestion than to dictatorial approach.	Needs about 2100 calories/day; nutritious snacks. Tends to be too busy to bother to eat. Tendency for deficiencies in calcium, iron, and thiamine. Problem of obesity may begin now. Has good table manners. Able to help with food preparation.	Ready for lessons in dancing, gymnastics, music. Restrict screen time to 1–2 hours daily. Enjoys hiking, sports. Enjoys cooking, woodworking, crafts. Enjoys cards and table games. Likes radio and music. Begins qualitative collecting.	Stress safety with firearms. Keep them out of reach and allow their use only with adult supervision. Know who the child's friends are; parents should still have some control over friend selection. Teach water safety; swimming should be supervised by an adult. Enforce balance in rest and activity.

11–12 years	Vital signs approximate adult norms. Growth spurt for girls. Differences between sexes increasingly noticeable, with boys having greater physical strength. Eruption of permanent teeth complete except for third molars. Secondary sex characteristics begin in boys. Menstruation may begin.	Able to think about social problems and prejudices; sees others' points of view. Enjoys reading mysteries or love stories. Begins considering abstract ideas. Interested in the reasons for health measures and understands human reproduction. Very moralistic; religious commitment often made during this time.	Intense team loyalty; boys begin teasing girls, and girls flirt with boys. Wants unreasonable independence; is rebellious about routines; has wide mood swings; needs some time daily for privacy. Very critical of own work. Hero worship prevails. Facts-of-life chats with friends prevail. Masturbation increases. Appears under constant tension.	Male needs 2500 calories/day; female needs 2250 (70 calories/kg/day); both need 75 mL/kg of water/day and 2 g/kg protein daily.	Enjoys projects and working with hands. Likes to do errands and jobs to earn money. Very involved in sports, dancing, talking/texting on phone. Enjoys all aspects of acting and drama.	Continue monitoring friends. Stress bicycle and in-line skate safety on streets and in traffic and the use of helmets and other protective gear.

Modified from Betz, C., Hunsberger, M., & Wright, S. (1994). *Family centered nursing care of children* (2nd ed.). Saunders; Carey, W., Crocker, A., Coleman, W., Elias, E., & Feldman, H. (2009). *Developmental-behavioral medicine* (4th ed.). Elsevier.

Electronic Media

Traditional media such as radio, passive TV, and magazines have been replaced by interactive media devices on various devices connected to the Internet. This allows access to a multitude of videos, shows, and interactive multiplayer videogames where players can create virtual worlds. Communication via texting a written message or symbol (emoji) and direct messaging through media sites has become popular (Kabali et al., 2016).

Gamification applies gaming elements to real-world activity. Cutting edge graphics and rewards for reaching specific levels of play are offered and valued, adding game-like elements to a task in order to encourage participation (Kim, 2015).

Social media offers many benefits including exposure to new ideas and knowledge, increased social contact and support, streamlined collaboration on projects, and easier access to health promotion information. With this access there is also the danger of encountering content inappropriate for the school-age child who is unsupervised. Inappropriate and unsafe social contact can compromise confidentiality, and some sites offer violent or sexual content inappropriate for the school-aged child. Use of screens for entertainment should not exceed 2 hours a day and should not replace valued physical activity and personal interaction (Rodesky et al., 2016). Physical fitness suffers from sedentary habits fostered by an increased preference for social media and Internet (Figure 9.2). Studies have shown that 96% of school-aged children have used mobile devices and more than 75% own their own device. Elementary schools require some assignments be accessed on computer sites and uploaded to another site to be graded by the teacher (Guernsey & Levine, 2015). Some schools require reading assignments of downloaded books to offer a wide range of material, and character-focused media may help children understand people who are different from themselves (Bus et al., 2015). Many school-aged children have preferred media sites and may have a "media portfolio" including Facebook, Instagram, Twitter, Snapchat, TikTok, and others. Often school-aged children focus on features of digital media such as animation and sound that they can tap/swipe and modify.

Parents offer an important role in modeling behaviors for children. Adult use of media can interrupt parent-child interaction causing conflicts. Interruptions between child and

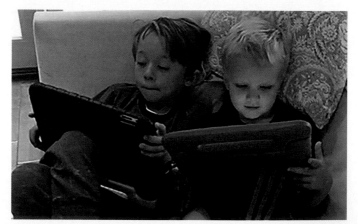

Figure 9.2 Children may be sitting next to each other but are not communicating or interacting when they are using iPads or electronic devices. The American Academy of Pediatrics recommends no more than 2 hours a day of non-educational screen time for school-aged children. *(From Leifer, G. (2019). Introduction to maternity and pediatric nursing (8th ed.). Elsevier.)*

parent communication due to mobile phone or Internet use can result in decreased development of language, social skills, and emotional regulation. There should be "unplugged zones" in the house, such as while seated at the dinner table, where parents and children can communicate without distraction (Reed et al., 2017).

COGNITIVE DEVELOPMENT

According to Piaget, school-age children are concrete thinkers. They think logically and understand rules, although they learn best when they can see and handle objects. Hands-on learning is the most effective educational method for school-age children. Table 9.2 lists mastery of tasks and behaviors necessary for success in school and also lists the related

TABLE 9.2   Mastery of Tasks Necessary for School Success

Child's Tasks	Parent's Tasks	Interventions
Adapt to differences in expectations of various teachers. Compete with 30 or more peers for adult attention.	Communicate with teacher to maintain consistency in expectations and discipline. Praise child's accomplishments. Avoid comparisons to other children.	School nurse can be contacted to facilitate parent-teacher-child interaction. Observe parent-teacher interactions and provide guidance and positive support.
Learn to accept criticism from peers and teachers without losing self-esteem.	Supervise peer activities. Facilitate constructive communication.	Provide teacher-parent guidance. Teach constructive and positive feedback.
Assimilate peer values with family values.	Maintain open communication. Encourage peer activity. Introduce and accept other cultures in community.	Provide anticipatory guidance in handling behavior problems. Observe and address signs of prejudice.
Find satisfaction in school achievements.	Help children to achieve. Do not complete tasks for them.	Provide suggestions for identifying strengths and weaknesses. Build on strengths.
Participate in group activities.	Encourage child to join a group or club and actively participate as a member.	Refer to community agencies such as churches, organizations, and club activities as needed.
Learn behavioral self-control. Cope with negative treatment from others in a constructive way.	Encourage participation in activities away from home and with peers. Help build faith in child's problem-solving skills. Discuss coping with prejudices.	Encourage parents to let go and to provide guidance while encouraging independence.

Modified from Leifer, G. (2019). *Introduction to maternity & pediatric nursing* (8th ed.). Elsevier Saunders.

TABLE 9.3   Cognitive Deficits and Their Effect on School Performance

Deficit	Related School Problem
Inability to understand spatial relationships by visual examination.	Repeatedly confuse letters b, d, and g. Difficulty with basic reading and writing.
Difficulty in sensing body position and in programming movements.	Poor handwriting; tight grasp of pencil.
Inability to decipher similar sounding words.	Difficulty following directions, leading to short attention span and behavior problems.
Difficulty with long-term memory and recall.	Delayed mastery of counting and alphabet recital.
Easily distracted.	Difficulty following complex instructions.
Difficulty remembering items in order.	Difficulty in organizing assignments and planning completion.
Difficulty in receptive language.	Difficulty in following directions; attention cannot remain focused.
Impaired expressive language.	Difficulty with recall memory. Difficulty expressing feelings or talking spontaneously in a group setting.

Modified from Kleigman, R., Stanton, B., St. Geme, J., Schor, N., & Behrmann, R. (2016). *Nelson's textbook of pediatrics* (20th ed.). Elsevier.

parental guidance that can be offered. Cognitive deficits must be assessed and addressed early so that the child can be successful in school (Table 9.3).

Erikson refers to the school age as the stage of industry. In this stage, the child develops a thirst for knowledge and a desire to master skills and to emulate role models or heroes. If a parent intrudes on children's efforts at achieving a skill – perhaps by helping too much or by doing the task for the child – a sense of inferiority can develop in the child's mind. Even if children receive an excellent grade for a project, they may not attain a sense of industry if they know the work was not really the result of their own efforts.

School-age children can group similar items together and can understand that words have more than one meaning. Children may delight in telling jokes to one another, and they may tell jokes to entertain friends or to tease adults.

By age 7, egocentrism decreases. Children realize others may have valid opinions that differ from their own, and they may seek another person's opinion concerning an issue. With a decrease in egocentrism, children become more cooperative and begin to understand how their actions may affect other people. This understanding, called social cognition, enables children to interact better with peers and can enhance their self-concept.

The development of moral reasoning happens as the child learns to understand rules and to determine if an action is right or wrong. Moral behaviors are actions based on moral reasoning. In early childhood, rules are important. A 5-year-old child may show intense frustration if a peer breaks a rule. In later childhood, the 10-year-old may enjoy making his or her own rules for a game or bartering to change the rules.

Culture or an environment such as poverty or war can influence moral behavior. Knowing what is culturally or morally right does not guarantee acting in accordance with

BOX 9.1   Moral Behavior Includes Three Phases

1. **Knowledge (logic)** – Knowing what is right
2. **Emotion** – Feeling good or bad about what is right
3. **Action (behavior)** – Behaving according to the rule of what is right

that knowledge. Lying, stealing, and cheating behaviors are common in school-age children even as they learn moral behavior. Therefore, adult modeling of honesty and fairness is essential as the child is learning moral behavior (Box 9.1).

Lawrence Kohlberg was a theorist who suggested that moral reasoning develops as cognitive function matures (Chapter 5), so the ability to think logically is related to moral behavior. Other theorists emphasize that moral behavior is learned through positive reinforcement. Parents teach by rewarding desired behavior. Punishment for undesirable behavior is less effective. Punished children may feel less motivated, less capable, or confused, or may focus on the punishment and its emotional consequences rather than the behavior. In addition to using reward or punishment in guiding children's learning, modeling how a child's actions may affect others is also helpful in developing moral behavior.

Cognitive Styles

A school-age child must have an attention span of 45 minutes to process information, encode it into memory, and retrieve or remember it later. Children approach learning and problem solving in various ways. A cognitive style refers to a pattern of thought and reasoning. Some children take a cluster of knowledge and group it in a certain way to better remember the information. Some use mnemonic techniques, such as the rhyme for remembering the number of days in each month of the year.

The elementary-school curriculum is designed to increase cognitive demands gradually for students. The first 2 years of elementary school focus on learning to read, write, and do basic math. By the fourth grade, the volume and complexity of the work increases. If basic skills were not mastered, the child might not progress smoothly. Other factors that affect success in school include the child's desire to please teachers and parents, to compete with other children, to work for delayed rewards, and to take risks by trying new things. Feelings of success encourage the child to continue making efforts. Feelings of failure may lead to avoidance of risks or low self-confidence.

Communication Skills

Grammatical rules are recognized and used by 7–8 years of age, and children often use language as an effective communication tool in their relationships with others. They can tell jokes and express sarcasm and use fill-in-the-blank words. At 8–11 years of age, children enter the phase of concrete operations (Chapter 5) and have the ability to problem solve. Rehearsing memorization is important at this age for cognitive development and is part of school curricula. Emerging skills of verbal counting rather than finger counting are essential for success in later grades. Math skills are related to the development of reading skills. The goal of reading in middle childhood is to understand the content rather than just understanding the words and the goal of writing is composition and no longer just spelling and penmanship (Feigelman, 2016). A child who has a language or other communication problem is at risk for social isolation and underachievement in school.

Cultural Considerations

Bilingual education programs are offered to school-age children who speak English as their second language. However, if the teachers are not proficient in the child's primary language, the child may have to learn English by a total immersion technique, which means the child learns the language by hearing it used every day in the classroom. This may add stress socially, academically, and emotionally. It is important that schools offer support programs for bilingual or language-impaired children to reduce stress and associated behavior problems such as frustration, anger, and rebellion.

Intelligence Tests

The original version of the Stanford-Binet intelligence quotient (IQ) test was published in France in 1905 and was then brought to the United States. This test assesses the mental capabilities of the child and compares set norms or expectations for each age. To determine a score, the mental age is divided by the actual age in years, and the total is then multiplied by 100. Children with attention deficit hyperactivity disorder (ADHD) may underperform due to the challenge of time restrictions and testing environment distractions (Sturner, 2009).

David Wechsler developed the Wechsler Intelligence Scale (WISC-V) for school-age children and adolescents aged 6–16, which offers more organized test items. The tests are not meant to be an overall test of general intelligence, but they can be used to predict school performance and to identify children who may need extra help or additional challenges. Psychological tests are available for multiple specific clinical issues and new intelligence tests are being developed based on modern knowledge of brain function. These tests should be administered by a licensed professional (Naglieri, 2020).

PSYCHOSOCIAL DEVELOPMENT

Task of Industry

Erikson believed the primary task for school-age children was to develop a sense of industry. A child can gain satisfaction from achieving even small goals. Praise is essential in this stage of development to build motivation to learn and achieve. A child who does not receive praise for achievements may feel inferior. Seven-year-olds may not have the attention span necessary to complete complex tasks. Nine-year-olds can usually work on a task to completion. By age 11, children are generally able to maintain work and motivation for a delayed reward.

Peer Relationships

School-age children begin to compare family values with the values of others. Friendships with peers are especially important for the school-age child. The reliance on and importance of the family can decrease, and sibling rivalry can cause some chaotic episodes. The child may become self-conscious about kisses and hugs from parents in public. Children who have difficulty separating from family and adjusting to school may be responding to the parents' difficulty in letting them go. Divorces, family violence, and other domestic problems can interfere with a child's achievement of age-appropriate developmental tasks with peers. The school-age child shifts away from egocentric thinking to understanding how friends and teachers see them and they appreciate the thoughts and feelings of others. The development of empathy is influenced by parental social behavior and digital media (Feigelman, 2016). Young school-age children may choose friends based on what they can offer and tend to protect their possessions from their friends; older school-age children make friends in order to be included and admired; while later friendship is more genuine and includes self-disclosure.

School-aged children should be given the responsibility of managing chores and money. However, allowances and family chores work best when kept separate from one another. Regular home chores help children gain a sense of responsibility and achieve a feeling that they are a member of a family group.

The home, the school, and the neighborhood each have an impact on the growth and development of the child. The culture of a school-age child involves memberships in groups of some kind. If parents do not provide access to a group, such as Scouts, a religious group, or a team, children will find their own group. The children may be influenced by that group to engage in socially unacceptable behavior to gain acceptance and to achieve a sense of belonging. Conformity to most groups is rewarding and enables social success with peers. When a child is labeled or is outcast by a peer, the identification may remain with the child and may be incorporated into his or her self-image.

Latchkey Children

Latchkey children are those who are left unsupervised after school because both parents work, and members of the extended family are not available to care for the children. Some children who are left alone at home enjoy the independence and develop maturity and problem-solving skills. Other children are at higher risk for feeling isolated and may be at an increased risk for accidents or getting into trouble. Without access to homework assistance, children often focus on electronic media and games that may limit progress in school performance. The emergence of Government grant-funded after-school programs has lowered the number of latchkey children, but government budget challenges continue to force some children to remain unattended. The latchkey child is not limited to low income families as some higher income families may feel their neighborhood is safe with neighbors close by and so they do not utilize available after-school programs (Box 9.2). In any case, a back-up adult should always be readily available close at hand in case of an emergency.

Sexuality

According to Freud, the child is in a period of sexual latency during the middle childhood years, and children often identify with same-sex parents. Modern children are often allowed to play with toys outside of their stereotypical gender roles. Research has shown that forcing children into traditional gender roles can have a detrimental effect of the

BOX 9.2   Guidance for Latchkey Families

TEACH CHILD ABOUT SAFETY

Do not enter the house if the door is ajar or if anything looks unusual.
Do not leave the house or yard without permission.
Never admit a stranger into the house.
Never agree to meet with someone you met online.
Never respond to messages on the computer that sound weird.
Do not display keys; keep doors locked.
Do not take shortcuts to school through alleys or across train tracks.
Walk to and from school with friends.
Never accept rides with strangers.
Know how to contact a trusted adult.
Teach first-aid techniques; know how to call 911.
Review fire-safety rules and the route of escape; walk through the procedure with the child.
Know and obey basic safety rules.

TEACH PARENTS TO

List emergency numbers and post them in the house.
Designate a neighbor who is usually home for help during emergency situations.
Teach the child his or her own name, telephone number, address, and parents' names.
Leave work number with the child.
Lock up firearms or remove them from the house.
Prepare a first-aid kit and keep it in a designated location.
Address with the child street safety when returning from school; include precautions with
    strangers.
Consider obtaining a pet for the child.
Be home on time or call the child.
Recommend specific home activities rather than electronic games or social media.
Help the child to feel successful and appreciated.
Assess the home and neighborhood for hazards specific to the locale.

Data from Leifer, G. (2019). *Introduction to maternity & pediatric nursing* (8th ed.). Elsevier Saunders; McClellan, M. (1984). On their own: latchkey children. *Pediatric Nursing, 10*(3), 198–202; American Academy of Child and Adolescent Psychiatry (2017). *Bulletin Facts for Families # 46 Home Alone Children.*

development of their skills and interests, thus minimizing later opportunities and perpetuating gender stereotypes (Kollmayer et al., 2018). Unisex toys and clothes are available, and families are choosing to raise children to have a subjective sense of gender identity regarding clothing, activities, and playmates that may be different from cultural norms for their biological sex at an increasing rate (Watkins, 2016). Gender neutral terms such as "theyby" have begun to appear to replace "boy" or "girl," as some parents attempt to reduce stigma and pave the way to a more tolerant society (Airton, 2019).

During middle childhood, an awareness of the body image develops along with a preference for modesty. Sensitivity of the hypothalamus and pituitary causes an increase in gonadotropin secretion that results in increasing interest in gender differences, and sexual interests begin to increase. Masturbation is common and children may engage in play activities that may involve viewing or touching the genitals. It is the parents who place sexual meaning on the activity, not the children. A negative body image may develop if parents shame their

TABLE 9.4   Sex Education of the School-Age Child

Intervention	Observation/Goal
Data collection; history taking Assess readiness to learn.	Readiness to learn is indicated by asking questions concerning sex, menstruation, "wet dreams," and pregnancy.
Analysis	Observe parent-child interactions and determine level of communication.
Assess interactions.	Observe peer interaction to determine the child's self-image, self-confidence, and ability to communicate about sensitive issues.
Assess parents.	Observe parents' knowledge and ability to discuss issues pertaining to sex education.
Assess child.	Determine child's understanding of sexual development and body changes.
Planning/Implementation	Discuss growth and development with the parents and child. Reinforce teaching techniques and opportunities with parents.
Evaluation	With each clinic or home visit, reevaluate parent-child interaction concerning sex education.

Modified from Leifer, G. (2019). *Introduction to maternity & pediatric nursing* (8th ed.). Elsevier Saunders.

children or imply that a part of the body is dirty or bad. Children often ask questions related to sexuality and should be given honest and accurate answers. They may be curious and are sensitive about developing secondary sex characteristics, and girls may eagerly await (or dread) signs of breast development. Interest in the opposite sex is often a sensitive topic and school-age children may be reluctant to admit this interest or to discuss it with parents. A new appreciation and insistence on privacy emerges as their awareness of "private" body parts increases.

Sex education is a lifelong process and may begin earlier than many parents believe. Parents convey their attitudes toward sexuality to the growing child, and sometimes parents need guidance in understanding their child's sexual curiosity. Sex education can be introduced in the context of normal anatomy and physiology. Values can be added and influenced by active parental and teacher participation and by encouraging questions and discussion. The Sex Information and Education Council of the United States (SIECUS), located in New York, advocates the idea that sex education programs should be taught from six basic aspects: biological, social, health, personal adjustment, interpersonal relationships, and developing values. Age-appropriate, culturally relevant, written information that treats sexuality as a healthy aspect of life should be included (SIECUS, 2020).

Table 9.4 reviews the interventions and goals for sex education for the school-age child.

ALCOHOL AND SUBSTANCE USE

Facts concerning alcohol and drug use are an important part of education in the school-age years. Children as young as 9 may begin to view alcohol in a positive way and children as young as 12 begin using marijuana. Approximately half of 12-year-olds obtain prescription pain relievers for nonmedical purposes (Substance Abuse and Mental Health Services

Administration, 2020). Early, open, and honest discussions between adults and children may prevent future high-risk behaviors if the child gains an understanding of the harm in trying alcohol and other substances. Many websites offer age-appropriate tips for parents to teach their children about drugs and alcohol.

TEACHING TECHNIQUES

Most school-age children have a natural curiosity and are therefore ready and eager to learn. Because the extended attention span of the school-age child is limited to a maximum of 45 minutes, teaching sessions should be planned for no more than this amount of time. All information should be presented in a truthful, factual, and age-appropriate manner. Step-by-step instructions are needed for children who are concrete thinkers. Encouraging verbal feedback from the child will ensure that the information provided was not misinterpreted. During any teaching process, periods of praise and occasional rewards reinforce learning accomplishments. Teaching techniques should encourage the child to accept responsibilities and should provide hands-on reinforcement whenever possible. Group instruction is effective in teaching positive health behaviors, because peer attitudes can influence learning and can enhance application.

Health Teaching

Health-teaching needs of healthy school-age children include prevention of injury; maintenance of adequate nutrition; the importance of regular dental care; screening for scoliosis, vision, and hearing deficits; and the need for immunizations. The recommended immunization schedule for school-aged children may be accessed at http://www.CDC.gov/vaccines/index.HTML. School nurses can be valuable resources for assisting preadolescents in making positive choices, developing interpersonal relationships, developing positive self-esteem, improving the ability to use problem-solving skills, and accessing community resources. School nurses should be aware that sometimes a school-age child will complain of minor health problems that have little evidence of pathology as a way of reaching out for help with psychosocial problems.

School-age children can understand the causes of illness and its consequences in terms of missing school and missing peer activities. Having to live with a long-term, chronic illness can slow cognitive learning. In most cases, illness causes more anxiety related to separation from peers, falling behind in school, and being left out of social activities than anxiety related to the illness itself. An important primary goal in the care of a school-age child is to foster normal growth and development even if some physical or intellectual disabilities are present. Teaching diabetic school-age children to test their own blood sugar and to administer their own insulin is an example of age-appropriate teaching.

DISCIPLINE

The word discipline is derived from the Latin word discipulus, which means "student." Discipline should be thought of as providing age-appropriate positive reinforcement of good behavior that plays an important role in the social and emotional development of children.

Punishment is only one aspect of discipline. Reward is another option. If punishment is used, it should be prompt, consistent, and fair. Parents often rely on culturally traditional disciplinary techniques. Some may shy away from asking for help because of the fear that their parenting skills may be criticized. It is through appropriate discipline that children learn self-control and a sense of parental caring. Whenever misbehavior occurs, the motivation should be investigated. Misbehavior often occurs if the child is bored or needs attention, or misbehavior may reflect a larger problem at home. Physical punishment can increase or reinforce misbehavior if it is the only way the child receives attention (Sege & Siegel, 2018).

Discipline should combine reward and redirection, be based on age-appropriate behavior expectations, offer the child information on alternative choices of behavior, and teach respect for others. Because the school-age child understands cause-and-effect relationships, discipline and rewards need to be immediate and consistent with the action so that the child understands that the behavior resulted in the reward or punishment. The school-age child can understand and respect rules. Therefore, behavior standards and social interactions can be guided and reinforced according to rules. Involving the child in designing an appropriate mode of punishment can help develop moral judgment and autonomy.

Including positive reinforcement in disciplinary efforts is crucial to the development of good behavior. Attention or praise from parents or teachers is an example of positive reinforcement. If only misbehavior results in getting extra attention from the parent or teacher, this may reinforce bad behavior. That means that in order to implement effective discipline, attention should be focused on behavior that is good. Rewards for good behavior can be in the form of extra attention, a smile, a hug, a word of praise, extra privileges, or a token reward such as a sticker or a star, and these token rewards can be collected and cashed in later for a material reward. As punishment for bad behavior, a child's stars can be removed.

Discipline should be used only for teaching and not for revenge, to vent anger, or to demand behavior that is beyond the child's ability. Time-outs (discussed in Chapter 8) are appropriate for the 18-month to 6-year-old age group. Time-outs for older children can be in the form of 15–20 minutes of calming down time. Removal of privileges such as an enjoyed activity, or television or Internet access, can be an effective deterrent. Verbal reprimands in the form of scolding can provide the needed correction for the child, but scolding, yelling, or shaming can escalate into shouting matches or can result in frustration or increased noncompliance and is not an effective method of discipline in the long run.

Corporal punishment is spanking, hitting, or inflicting pain to stop or alter behavior. There is a fine line between corporal punishment and child abuse. For this reason, many child experts discourage the use of corporal punishment. Spanking may be initially effective to stop a dangerous situation because of its shock value, but spanking may not be effective as a long-term disciplinary tool. Frequent spanking can teach violent behavior and can lead to decreased self-esteem, depression, and low educational achievement. Positive reinforcement (reward), removing privileges, or adding chores are other effective forms of discipline that clearly are nonabusive (Sege & Siegel, 2018).

Parent Teaching

Parents benefit from guidance in formulating effective disciplinary techniques. Every well-child visit should include a discussion of behavior management and discipline in the home. Teacher education programs also should include discipline techniques for classroom management. Discussion should include alternatives to corporal punishment, anger-control skills, and discipline that matches the developmental and educational needs of the school-age child. Community resources may include referral to parenting classes, support groups, or professional counselors. Online websites such as http://www.Healthychildren.org offer suggested positive discipline guidelines for children of different ages.

KEY POINTS

- Middle childhood includes school-age children between the ages of 6 and 12.
- In the school-age child, the body develops a lower center of gravity than it had in preschool years.
- The loss of primary teeth begins at about age 6, and approximately four permanent teeth erupt each year.
- Regular dental checkups are an important part of routine health care.
- Visual maturity is complete between preschool age and 6 years, and therefore large-print books are no longer necessary at this time.
- Excessive time spent with computer and video games can contribute to a sedentary lifestyle, which may result in obesity, poor health, and poor social development.
- By ages 9 and 10, an understanding of rules and teamwork enables the child to participate in competitive team games.
- School-age children, according to Piaget, are concrete thinkers, and hands-on learning is retained best.
- School-age children often tell jokes to entertain peers and to tease elders.
- School-age children are less egocentric than they were at earlier ages, and they can understand how their actions affect others.
- Moral behavior is based on logical understanding and feeling pride or guilt as a result of the behavior. Knowing a rule is right does not guarantee behavior according to that rule.
- In later childhood, the 10-year-old may enjoy creating new rules or changing the rules of a game.

- Kohlberg believed that moral reasoning develops as cognitive skills mature.
- A school-age child may have a maximum attention span of 45 minutes.
- School-age children use language as an effective communication tool in relationships with others.
- Some intelligence tests are designed for use in predicting scholastic ability and future performance.
- The primary developmental task of the school-age child is to attain a sense of industry by mastering skills and achieving goals.
- Belonging to a peer group is particularly important to a school-age child.
- The home, school, and neighborhood each affect the growth and development of school-age children.
- Creativity should be encouraged because it helps develop problem-solving skills.
- Information concerning sexuality should be age appropriate, culturally relevant, and treated as a healthy aspect of life.
- Discipline should be used for teaching and reinforcing good behavior, which plays an important role in social and emotional development.
- Strength, endurance, and coordination can be nurtured by daily physical activity. Physical activity can also decrease risk factors for illness in later life.
- The major health-teaching needs of the school-age child include prevention of injury; maintenance of adequate nutrition; providing regular dental care; screening for scoliosis, vision, and hearing problems; and developing an active lifestyle.

Clinical Judgment Case Study

A parent tells you that her child seems to spend a lot of time playing games on the iPad. She asks you what kind of play activity would be appropriate for her to introduce to the child that would be appropriate for his age and not involve screens. What suggestions would you offer her that would be appropriate for his developmental level?

REVIEW QUESTIONS

1. A parent and her 6-year-old child enter a supermarket to shop for items needed for dinner. After a few minutes, the child begins to repeatedly ask the parent to buy him various items and toys he sees on display and begins to scream and cry and hold the shopping cart back. Select the letters of the following responses of the parent that shows an appropriate response to manage this situation. (select all that apply)
   A. Ignore the behavior.
   B. Slap the child gently in the buttock area and tell him to stop screaming.
   C. Ask the child to help her pack the basket.
   D. Offer the child a bag of chips and tell him to be quiet.
   E. Tell the child to wait outside the store until she is done shopping.
   F. Tell the child he will be punished when he gets home unless he stops screaming.
   G. Tell the child you will destroy his iPad if he doesn't stop screaming.
   H. Warn the child his chores will be increased for today because of this behavior.
   I. Tell the child he can help pick out one item he would like for dinner tonight.
   J. Tell the child he should be ashamed of himself for acting this way and leave the store immediately to avoid embarrassment.
2. Which of the following are important benefits of participating in team sports for the school-age child? (select all that apply)
   A. Learning to manage conflict.
   B. Understanding teamwork.
   C. Trophies for all participants.
   D. Developing the ability to wait for a delayed reward.
   E. Mastering a skill.
   F. Improving physical fitness.
   G. Getting used to losing.
   H. Fostering social skills.
   I. Developing respect for authority.
   J. Collecting colorful uniforms.
   K. Learning to overcome symptoms of an asthma attack.
   L. Distracting children from academic responsibilities.
   M. Learning to imitate an injury to gain an extra point.
3. Interactive electronic media has largely replaced more passive forms of entertainment. Classify the following as positive or negative consequences of Internet use.

Consequence	Positive	Negative
Gamification of learning tasks		
Exposure to new ideas and different types of people		
Increased social contact and support		
Streamlined collaboration on projects		
Access to adult content		
Unsolicited social contact with strangers		
Sharing confidential information		
Increased sedentary behavior		
Eliminate need for use of verbal communication skills		
Easier access to health promotion information		

4. Identify which school-related tasks should be mastered by the child (A), and which by the child's parent (B).

    1. Compete with 30 or more peers for adult attention _____

    2. Communicate with teacher to maintain consistency in discipline ___

    3. Find satisfaction in school achievements ___

    4. Avoid comparisons to other children ___

    5. Learn behavioral self-control ___

    6. Cope with negative treatment from others in a constructive way ___

    7. Supervise peer activities ___

    8. Praise child's accomplishments ___

    9. Learn to accept criticism from peers and teachers without losing self-esteem ___

5. Select the appropriate term to complete each sentence.

    When children understand how their behavior might affect others, this is called (moral reasoning, social cognition, mnemonic technique).

    (Social cognition, moral reasoning, gamification) occurs when children can determine if an action is right or wrong.

    A pattern of reasoning is sometimes referred to as a (cognitive style, mnemonic technique, moral behavior).

Adolescence

http://evolve.elsevier.com/Leifer/growth

OUTLINE

OBJECTIVES

1. Define adolescence.
2. Describe the three phases of adolescence.
3. Discuss the physiological changes that occur during adolescence.
4. Define puberty.
5. Discuss how to determine the fertile period of a female.
6. Describe the physical activity guidelines for adolescents.
7. Identify the major developmental tasks of adolescence.
8. Discuss the adolescent's stage of development according to Erikson and Piaget.
9. Identify how culture affects adolescent behaviors.
10. Discuss the role of dating in the development of cognitive and social behavior.
11. Review sexual orientation and gender identity.
12. Discuss the role of parents in fostering the positive growth and development of the adolescent.
13. State two specific health risks in the adolescent age group.

KEY TERMS

abstinence
adolescence
asynchronous
clique
cultural competence
ejaculation
empathy

gender dysphoria
gender identity
gender nonconformity
menarche
menstrual cycle
nocturnal emissions

ovulation
puberty
secondary sex characteristics
sexual orientation
spermatogenesis
vigorous exercise

DEFINITION

The origin of the word adolescence is from the Latin word *adolescere*, which means "to grow and mature." Adolescence is considered to be the bridge between childhood and adulthood. It is a unique stage of development characterized by many physiological, cognitive, psychosocial, and sexual changes. The health habits and coping skills formed during this period last a lifetime, and mastery of developmental tasks during this period helps prepare the adolescent for adulthood.

DEVELOPMENTAL TASKS

Developmental tasks encountered during adolescence include establishing a stabilized sense of identity, separation from family, career planning, and establishing close peer relationships and intimacy.

Adolescence is separated into three phases: *early adolescence* (10–13 years), *middle adolescence* (14–16 years), and *late adolescence* (17–20 years). The 13-year-old adolescent differs greatly from the 18-year-old adolescent. Each of these three distinct phases of adolescence has its own set of challenges (Table 10.1).

PHYSIOLOGICAL CHANGES

Early adolescence (also called preadolescence) is characterized by physical changes in the structure and function of various parts of the body. Weight gain is normal and caused by an increase in musculoskeletal mass. However, growth is asynchronous, which means that different parts of the body mature at different times, possibly resulting in the temporary appearance of awkwardness. A growth spurt occurs during adolescence, and adult height is reached by approximately age 18. Because the sweat glands are more active, various skin problems such as acne can occur, which may have social consequences and may challenge teens' coping abilities. A facial pimple on the day of an important social event can cause chaos in the family.

The stomach and intestines increase in size and volume during adolescence, resulting in increased appetite and food consumption. The second and third molars, and often the wisdom teeth, erupt in early adolescence, and the jaw reaches adult size in mid to late adolescence.

The weight and volume of the lungs increase resulting in improvement of respiratory function. Improvements in eye-hand coordination and motor function enhance manual dexterity. Motor function also improves, and these factors contribute to the development of an interest and skill in sports activities and interactive computer games.

Puberty

Puberty refers to sexual maturity or having the functional ability to reproduce. Puberty involves physical and psychological changes.

Boys

For boys, puberty begins with hormonal changes between the ages of 10 and 13. Secondary sex characteristics are not involved in the reproductive process but appear at this time.

TABLE 10.1   Three Phases in the Growth and Development of the Adolescent

	Early (10–13 years)	Middle (14–16 years)	Late (17–20 years)
Physical growth	Appearance of secondary sex characteristics	Growth spurt in height	Growth slows
Body image	Self-conscious; adjusts to pubertal changes	Experiments with different images and looks	Accepts body image; personality emerges
Self-concept	Low self-esteem; denial of reality	Impulsive, impatient; identity confusion	Has positive self-image; empathetic; independent thinker
Behavior	Behaves for rewards	Behaves to conform	Shows responsible behavior
Sexual development	Sexual interest	Sexual experimentation	Sexual identity emerges; develops caring relationships
Peers	Unisex cliques of friends; has best friend; engages in hero worship; has adult crushes	Begins dating; has need to please significant peer; develops heterosexual peer group	Values individual relationships; begins partner selection
Family	Is ambivalent to family; strives for independence	Struggles for autonomy and acceptance; rebels/withdraws; demands privacy	Achieves independence; reestablishes family relationships
Cognitive development	Concrete thinking; here and now is important	Early abstract thinking, daydreams, fantasies; starts inductive and deductive reasoning	Abstract thinking; idealistic; thinks about their future.
Goals	Socializing is priority; goals may be unrealistic	Identifies skills/interests; becomes a super-achiever or dropout	Identifies career goals; enters work or college
Health concerns	Concerned about normalcy	Concerned about experimenting with drugs or sex	Idealistic; decision-making for lifestyle choice
Interventions	Convey limits; encourage verbalization	Help adolescents solve problems resulting from choices; use peer group sessions; provide privacy	Discuss goals; allow participation in decisions; provide confidentiality

Modified from Leifer, G. (2019). *Introduction to maternity & pediatric nursing* (8th ed.). Elsevier.

Increases in androgens (testosterone and androsterone) are responsible for producing the male secondary sex characteristics. These include growth of pubic, facial, and body hair; enlargement and darkening in color of the scrotum; and an increase in penis size. The vocal cords also lengthen and thicken, resulting first in voice instability (voice cracking) and then in a deepening of the voice.

An area in the brain called the hypothalamus secretes gonadotropin-releasing hormone (GnRH), which stimulates the anterior pituitary gland to secrete gonadotropins, follicle-stimulating hormone (FSH), and luteinizing hormone (LH). These gonadotropins stimulate the testes, located in the scrotum, to produce testosterone, and under normal conditions, a stable level of testosterone is maintained in the blood throughout most of the life span. FSH and testosterone stimulate spermatogenesis, the production of sperm. Sperm production starts during mid-puberty and continues throughout the male life span. Sperm production requires a temperature of about 5.4 °F (3 °C) below normal body temperature. This cooler temperature is possible because the testes are located outside the abdominal cavity in the scrotum, which hangs between the legs. Males of all ages should be counseled against wearing tight undergarments or sitting on enclosed plastic or leather seats for prolonged times, because fertility can be reduced if the temperature around the testes is too high.

Ejaculation is the release of sperm during an orgasm. This ability indicates the testes are mature. Most boys experience nocturnal emissions, also known as "wet dreams" when they ejaculate semen during sleep. This experience is part of normal sexual development and is not necessarily related to sexual activity.

Because of the enlargement of the scrotum and the penis during puberty, an athletic cup and/or athletic scrotal support (jock strap) should be worn by boys participating in sporting events to prevent injury to these vulnerable organs. Good personal hygiene is necessary to prevent friction rashes and fungal infections (jock itch). Sharing of athletic supporters creates a risk for spreading these infections and is strongly discouraged.

Girls

For girls during puberty, hormone secretions begin to establish a pattern within a monthly cycle. This pattern can typically be 28–32 days apart. Menstrual cycles begin at puberty and last about 40 years, at which time the hormone cycles stop, and menopause begins.

The hypothalamus gland produces a GnRH, which stimulates the pituitary gland to release LH and FSH. These hormones then stimulate the release of the female sex hormones (estrogen and progesterone) from the ovaries. Many thousands of eggs are present in the ovaries at birth. During ovulation, which typically happens once each menstrual cycle, one of the eggs reaches final maturity and is released from the ovary (ovulation) into the fallopian tube, which leads to the uterus. As the egg travels in the fallopian tube toward the uterus, it can be fertilized if sperm is present. If a sperm does not fertilize the egg, the egg enters the uterus and is expelled from the body with the blood and mucus that had thickened the walls of the uterus to prepare it for pregnancy. This blood, mucus, and unfertilized egg expelled from the body are called a menstrual flow (menstruation, or "period").

The very first menstrual period is called the menarche, which usually occurs between ages 10 and 15 years. The menstrual cycle consists of (1) maturing the egg in the ovary, (2) formation of blood and mucus in the lining of the uterus, (3) ovulation, and (4) expelling the unfertilized egg with the blood and mucous lining from the uterus. The menstrual flow typically lasts from 2 to 5 days, with a blood loss of about 1 ounce along with 1–2 ounces of serous fluid. This cycle repeats after approximately 28 days and continues until menopause.

Ovulation occurs about 14 days *before menstruation starts*, and the egg lives for 1 day. Therefore, this time is considered the most fertile period of a woman's cycle when pregnancy can occur if sperm is present. The best way to prevent an unwanted pregnancy is to avoid sexual intercourse, referred to as abstinence. Unwanted pregnancy may also be prevented using one of several methods outlined in Table 10.2.

Patient Teaching

In girls, secondary sex characteristics often become apparent before menarche. Hair develops in the pubic area and the axilla or underarms. Breasts begin to develop, fat begins to deposit more in the hips and thighs rather than being evenly distributed, and body contours change. At this time, adolescent girls are ready for their first bra to support their developing breasts. The bra straps should not fall from the shoulders but should not be too tight and the bra cup should support the fullness of the breasts near the underarms. Sports bras may be more desirable for girls who participate in athletics. A balance of diet, exercise, and maintenance of optimal weight is important for menstrual regularity and overall health.

Patient Teaching

Adolescence is the best time to teach preventative health measures to adolescents. Sex education classes should include information about safe sex, family planning, and prevention of sexually transmitted infections (STIs). The school nurse can be a valuable resource person to help locate family planning services, such as Planned Parenthood, that may be available in the local community.

The World Health Organization offers suggestions for world-wide self-care resources for sexual and reproductive health (WHO, 2020).

In early adolescence, teens often have emotional reactions and concerns about their changing bodies. Boys may have socially embarrassing erections, and comparison of penis size can be a normal part of social interaction and exploration. Girls are often concerned with their breast size and menstrual discomforts. Distorted self-image can be an issue at this time. Teen magazines often exploit the ideal female figure and the muscular male body with standards that are exceedingly difficult for the average teen to meet. Research suggests that males who sexually develop early may enjoy more social success and positive self-esteem, whereas girls who develop early may be at risk for lower self-esteem and a drop in school performance (Kleigman et al., 2016).

In many cultures a ritual rite of passage occurs at the onset of puberty. In the United States, sexual content in movies, television, and other media may influence the behavior of adolescents who are beginning to explore dating. Too often, teens obtain misinformation from peers or other unreliable sources and become vulnerable to unsafe practices or abuse. For example, some young girls falsely believe they cannot become pregnant the

TABLE 10.2   Birth Control Options*

Method	How Used	Protects Against STIs
MOST EFFECTIVE		
Abstinence	Avoid sexual intercourse.	Yes
HORMONAL		
Oral contraceptive ("the Pill")	Usually taken once daily. Extended dose regimens can delay menstruation up to a year.	No
Contraceptive injections (Depo-Provera)	Can take injection at specific intervals (e.g., every 3 months).	No
Implanon	Matchstick-sized capsules placed underneath skin of the arm provide contraception for up to 3 years. Can be removed by a health-care provider at any time.	No
Vaginal ring	Inserted monthly; stays in for a 3-week period and removed for 1 week (to allow for menstruation).	No
Intrauterine devices (IUDs)	Inserted into the uterus (to allow for menstruation) can be effective for 5 years, or a copper IUD effective for 10 years.	No
Skin patch	A new patch is applied to skin once weekly for 3 weeks, not worn for 1 week (to allow for menstruation).	No
NONHORMONAL		
Male condom	New condom must be applied before each act of coitus or sexual encounter.	Yes
Female condom	New condom must be inserted before each sexual encounter.	Yes
Spermicidal foams	Must be applied or inserted before each sexual encounter.	No
Cervical cap	Used with spermicide at every sexual encounter.	No
Fertility awareness planning	Must maintain records.	No
PERMANENT		
Vasectomy	One surgical procedure provides permanent prevention of pregnancy (can be reversed in some cases).	No
Tubal ligation	One surgical procedure provides permanent prevention of pregnancy (can be reversed in some cases).	No

*It is important to understand that a woman's fertile period (when pregnancy can occur if sperm is present) is 14 days *before the beginning* of the next menstrual period. This is not necessarily the same as 14 days after the last menstrual period if the cycle is fewer than or more than 28 days.

first time they have sexual intercourse, or believe pregnancy can be achieved through kissing.

Patient Teaching

Teens who become pregnant must cope with their own developmental tasks, as well as the tasks of parenthood. Counseling concerning their options and close health supervision are essential for a positive outcome in a teen pregnancy. Teens are at high risk for date rape and other sexual abuses, and therefore education concerning safe practices and preventative strategies is essential. Sex education is important before adolescence and must continue throughout adolescence. Accurate information from an authoritative source about the prevention of pregnancy and STIs can help teens make responsible and informed choices.

Patient Teaching

Adolescents who are homeless, abused, or disadvantaged may not be able to cope with the other developmental tasks of adolescence, such as dating, social development, or personal identity development, and they may act out in socially unacceptable ways.

Health-care professionals, educators, parents, school nurses, and counselors are challenged to provide guidance, support, and education that will help the teen develop coping strategies and promote healthy behaviors.

Physical Activity

The physical activity guidelines for adolescents are the same as those for children (60 minutes or more of physical activity every day). At least 3 days per week, the activity should include vigorous exercise, which is defined as movement using large muscle groups that causes elevations in heart rate, sweating, and breathing rate (Centers for Disease Control and Prevention, 2020). Structured exercise activities should include warm-up and cool-down components, but intermittent physical activity can also be beneficial. Physical activity should involve a combination of cardiovascular exercise, and exercises that improve muscle and bone strength. Muscle strengthening can include body weight exercises such as push-ups and pull-ups, or formal weight (resistance) training. Resistance training is beneficial, safe, and effective for adolescents, but it requires proper supervision. In addition to strengthening muscles, this type of training can reduce the risk of injury and play an important role in weight management throughout adulthood. Bone strengthening exercises are essential because bone mass peaks at the end of adolescence. Increasing bone mass typically involves some sort of impact, such as jumping. Because of decreased amounts of physical education opportunities in school, extracurricular physical activities become increasingly important during adolescence. Exercise activities can be performed individually or in groups and should be selected for personal enjoyment with consideration of individual capabilities and limitations.

COGNITIVE DEVELOPMENT

According to Piaget, young adolescents are in the *concrete phase* of thinking, which means they interpret words and concepts literally. By middle adolescence they begin to think more abstractly. This second stage of cognitive development is called the *formal operation stage*. Adolescents in this stage can process information quickly and efficiently, and their thinking becomes more complex. Adolescents can be self-absorbed and self-conscious. They may feel that everyone is looking at them and worry that others may notice even slight blemishes on their skin. They can spend hours examining and experimenting with hairstyles and dress, feeling they are on a stage with all the world as their audience (Figure 10.1).

Young adolescents fantasize about unrealistic career ideas, but by middle adolescence they may realize their true strengths and limitations and thus may set more realistic goals.

Kohlberg described the adolescent as moving toward the postconventional stage of moral judgment (Chapter 5). The early adolescent is motivated by the need to conform and to please others. As later adolescence approaches, moral principles are based on one's own individual priorities and beliefs.

Piaget's *post formal operational thinking*, the ability to consider multiple options and long-term consequences of actions, became more refined by the third stage of adolescence. Maturation of the neural system and myelination continues to the third decade of life (Holland-Hall & Burstein, 2016). The frontal lobes of the brain are the last to mature and that is the part of the brain responsible for complex thinking including impulse control and evaluation of risk and reward related to choices. In the middle stage of adolescence, the desire for immediate gratification may be explained by the delayed maturation of the frontal lobe of the brain (Holland-Hall & Burstein, 2016). For this reason, the adolescent needs assistance in making decisions while in a calm emotional state rather than making a quick decision under emotional stress. In late adolescence, decisions are usually more carefully thought out, with consideration of multiple options and possible consequences. This understanding helps explain why religious, political, or other types of organizations that imply easy answers to complex moral or social problems are often attractive to the teen in early or middle adolescence, and why guidance at that time is critical.

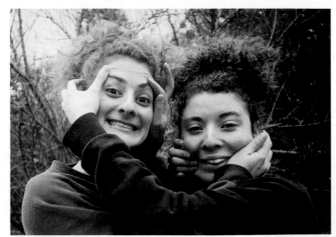

Figure 10.1 Best friends experiment with hairstyles, expressions, and make-up. Best-friend interaction supports growth and development.

Psychosocial Development

According to Erikson, one of the major tasks of adolescence is achieving a stable self-identity (Chapter 5). Psychosocial development is more closely related to physical maturation than to chronological age and is affected by culture and environment. Adolescents in the early stage of adolescence may try out various temporary styles and social roles in the process of finding their own individual identities. This process of identity exploration can lead to role confusion that can result in overcommitting to many causes. To achieve a sense of their own identity, adolescents must believe their identities are separate from their role as children in their families. The family can help secure a positive outcome in achieving this task by offering support and guidance and by giving adolescents freedom to discover their own interests. Close relationships with peers are helpful for adolescents exploring different roles and ideas. Close friendships develop mainly with same-sex friends in the early adolescent phase. They validate each other's thoughts and actions and may imitate each other's traits and habits. Group conformity is important. A feeling of abandonment may occur in early adolescence if one of two best friends leaves the other for a dating relationship.

Experimentation with sex and other social behaviors often occurs at this age, and a sense of omnipotence combined with curiosity may lead to risk-taking behaviors.

Debate is a healthy mental exercise that can sharpen cognitive and social skills and defuse intense emotions for most adolescents. School debate teams help teens express varying views in socially acceptable ways. Teenagers often daydream, which may be the imaginary acting out of what would be said or done in various situations. Daydreams help the adolescent think through how he or she might respond in situations and can be a safety valve for strong emotions. Daydreams in the adolescent are harmless unless they interfere with functioning in school or relationships.

As teens approach late adolescence, individual identity is discovered, and peer groups have less influence. In later adolescence, relationships may become less experimental, more affectionate, and longer lasting (Figure 10.2). School performance, interaction with

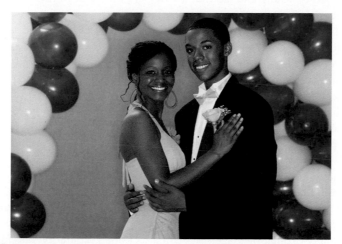

Figure 10.2 Dating is popular. Relationships may become less experimental, more affectionate, and longer lasting. (Courtesy Photos.com.)

teachers and counselors, and participation in extracurricular activities can positively influence the successful achievement of adolescents' career goals. Social skills and cognitive reasoning are aided by good coping skills to meet the challenges of achieving the many developmental tasks of adolescence.

Substance Abuse and Social Media

The major causes of death in the adolescent population are accidents, substance abuse, and violence. Substance abuse is bio-psycho-socially determined (Burstein, 2016). Alcohol, smoking, and drug use are frequently involved and engaging in these behaviors at an early age increases the overall risk of the activity. The challenge is to identify those at risk and provide early intervention because even after detoxification, substance abuse may leave long-lasting deficits in brain circuitry resulting in behavioral changes such as social impairment, inability to perform at school or work, and organ damage. A modern approach is to focus on harm reduction rather than complete abstinence (Stager, 2016). Electronic cigarettes (vaping) was initially introduced in 2006 as a tool to decrease cigarette smoking. It became popular with adolescents because it offered an increased nicotine "high" along with flavors, and a design that allowed more discreet use compared with the conventional cigarette. The electronic cigarette is battery operated and heats the nicotine dissolved in a solvent that is then pleasantly flavored. Toxic substances have been identified in the vapor (diethylene glycol) as well as carcinogens (nitrosamines) that may cause permanent lung damage. Secondhand exposure may also cause harm (Aoyama & McGrath-Morrow, 2020; Cherian et al., 2020).

Smokeless tobacco was also introduced in 2009 and involves flavored flat strips of finely ground tobacco placed in the mouth along the gumline or under the lower lip of the lower jaw, where it is slowly absorbed by the mucous membranes. There is no need to spit so it can be discreetly used throughout the day. It is most popular with 10th–12th grade adolescents who run the risk of developing serious complications such as oral cancer from use. Support for teen substance abuse is available on all cellphones, which most teens have access to via teen.smokefree.gov or by texting iQUIT (47848). There are many other substances abused by young and old that are beyond the scope of this text but well documented in other publications.

Social media exposure has its greatest influence in the pre-teen and teen population when access to sites is controlled by the individual rather than the parent (Chapter 9). Adolescents can benefit from online resources *personally*, with many online educational offerings, *socially* through use of social media platforms, texting, or twitter, and *physically* through telehealth care and fitness zoom classes. Many adolescents do not realize they leave a traceable "digital footprint" behind after using electronic media, which can prove harmful in their future. Potential employers often research a job candidate by reviewing their "online presence." It is essential that private, confidential, or otherwise damaging information is not shared and passwords remain secure.

Access to adult content, violence, and advertising for substances that can be abused are available, and many reach adolescents already addicted to screens. *Child porn* predators get access to the teen via social media, chat rooms, and online games and can lead to online grooming for sexual trafficking and sexual abuse. *Sexting* is the electronic transmission of sexually explicit messages that can affect one's reputation and lead to deviant sexual behavior. *Cyberbullying* is intentionally aggressive behavior via an online site against a victim. Teens cannot defend themselves and the messages can be spread rapidly through the Internet to others at school or in the community. Cyberbullying can result in difficulties in social, academic, and health consequences such as depression and suicide, substance use, or abuse. Social media experiences should be assessed at every health-care contact (ACOG, 2016).

Development of Responsibility

Adolescents look forward to challenges and often feel humiliated when placed in the dependent role. Independence in transportation can be achieved by riding a bicycle or driving a car. Babysitting or routine jobs to learn money management are important to the teenager. Using their own savings account, checking account, or debit or credit card to purchase some of their own clothes and supplies are important personal management skills that prepare adolescents for independence. It is important for the adolescent to be responsible for making decisions, especially those relative to career, politics, and religion. The role of parents should be to listen to and guide the adolescent rather than to mandate behavior. According to the behaviorist B.F. Skinner, teens will repeat behavior that is positively reinforced (Chapter 5). Bandura, a social cognitive theorist, suggests that setting a positive example for the teen will motivate positive behavior (Chapter 5).

Cultural Considerations

CULTURE AND THE ADOLESCENT

Culture plays a role in how adolescents think and interact. In some cultures, body piercing and tattoos are an accepted or expected practice, whereas other cultures view them as inappropriate or deviant. As global travel becomes more common, ethnic and economic diversity increases. There are generational differences between foreign-born parents and their American-reared adolescent children. This may result in decreased parent-child communication. Adolescents often form a cultural group of their own with people who share common values and experiences (Kaljee, 2016).

Health-care workers who interact with teens must be culturally competent. Cultural competence involves recognizing how your own values differ from those of other cultures and respecting the values and practices of others. Focusing on the cultural values and individual strengths of the adolescent, rather than the differences or variations, can help establish relationships to achieve positive health-teaching outcomes. Culture affects health-care practices and modes of communication. Health-care workers need to recognize accepted language and avoid responding to language commonly thought to be offensive in order to preserve patient-health care worker relationships. In most cases, the adolescent requires strict confidentiality. Maintaining this confidentiality can be a challenge when parents pay for the health insurance and control transportation access. It is important for nurses, health-care workers, and educators to be truthful, keep promises, and provide privacy for the adolescent. Cultural and religious traditions (Chapter 3) can help stabilize identity and involve rituals that celebrate the transition from childhood to the adult phase of life (Figure 10.3).

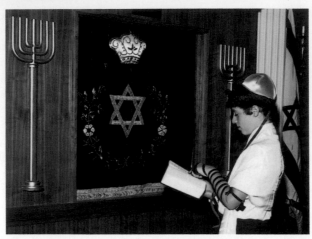

Figure 10.3 Cultural practice. Many childhood and religious traditions involve rituals that celebrate movement from childhood to the adult phase of life. Here a boy participates in the bar mitzvah ceremony marking his 13th birthday, when he is considered as entering adulthood.

PEER RELATIONSHIPS

Peer group affiliation has a major impact on adolescent growth and development. A clique is a social peer group with a fixed exclusive membership, whose members share similar interests, values, and tastes. Belonging to a group is of utmost importance to adolescents. From this social group, the adolescent chooses a best friend who enables the teen to experience mutual sharing of private thoughts and feelings. This may be helpful in normalizing and validating experiences and in forming successful relationships later in life.

During this period in adolescence, it is normal for openness and time spent with peers to increase and contacts with family to decrease. The teen may feel compelled to conform to peer pressures, which can cause problems and conflicts with the family if the values of the peer group conflict with family values or traditions. If the adolescent and the family relocate to a new neighborhood or a new state during this phase of the life cycle, the adolescent may experience more difficulty in joining an exclusive clique or group of friends in the new school. Failure to connect in a clique or a peer group can cause feelings of loneliness, loss, and interpersonal failure. This may contribute to lower self-esteem or to feelings of inadequacy. School performance may decrease as a result of social difficulty independent of academic ability, and the adolescent may become vulnerable to risky behaviors such as self-soothing with illegal substances or cutting classes. The dynamics of peer interaction are essential for the adolescent. Parents who accept and welcome peers into their homes can help encourage the formation of healthy peer relationships and may have fewer conflicts in their relationships with their adolescents. Peer counselors can be helpful in redirecting a troubled teen.

Erikson's sixth stage of psychosocial development, *intimacy versus isolation*, starts in late adolescence. After the middle adolescent establishes a fairly stable self-identity, the next developmental challenge is to share with another and develop a sense of intimacy. Empathy, understanding how others feel, is a quality essential to establishing a meaningful relationship with another person. This intimate relationship can be sexual, intellectual, or social. In late adolescence, a childlike dependence on the family is sometimes seen in times of illness or stress but relating to the adolescent as a young adult is the best means of supporting adolescent development.

SEXUALITY, SEX, SEXUAL ORIENTATION, AND GENDER IDENTITY

According to the World Health Organization the term *sexuality* encompasses sex, gender identification and roles, sexual orientation, eroticism, pleasure, intimacy, and reproduction. It is expressed in thoughts, fantasies, desires, beliefs, attitudes and values, behavior practices, roles, and relationships. Sexuality is influenced by the interaction of biological, psychological, social, economic, political, cultural, legal, historical, religious, and spiritual factors (WHO, 2020).

Biological sex refers to a male or female who is biologically identified at birth, primarily based on the presence of anatomical structures of the reproductive system. According to the American Psychological Association, one in every 1500 births are intersex, where genitalia are not easily classified. *Sexual orientation* refers to sexual attractions and preference for a sexual partner. This can include heterosexuality (an attraction to the opposite sex), homosexuality (an attraction to the same sex), bisexuality (an attraction to the same and opposite sex), and pansexuality (an attraction to any gender identity, including nonbinary and transgender). *Gender identity* refers to a feeling of how a person identifies themselves as feminine, masculine, or some combination of the two (nonbinary) (Lindsey, 2020). In 2017, "gender identity disorder" was removed from the *Diagnostic and Statistical Manual of Mental Disorders* (DSM) and replaced with "gender dysphoria." *Gender nonconformity*, in which a person identifies as their assigned gender but behaves in a nonstereotypical gender manner, is not a disorder. *Gender dysphoria* involves conflict between assigned sex and gender identity, and the presence of clinically significant distress associated with the feeling of mismatch, and how it is perceived by society, is important to address (American Psychiatric Association, 2016).

These feelings are often associated with increased levels of anxiety and depression related to the social stigma of gender nonconformity. These negative associations are mitigated in a more accepting social environment. One way a health-care worker can help to ease gender dysphoria is by asking for and using the adolescent's preferred pronouns (he, she, they).

Another role of the health-care worker is to help the adolescent understand how to cope with confused or prejudiced reactions of others towards the adolescent rather than to make attempts at changing behaviors. Nonstereotypical sexual orientation and behavior has been documented across cultures and historical periods and its acceptance varies greatly, but the process of "coming out" and revealing their sexual identity and attractions to family and peers is a significant step that is not easy. The adolescent faces the risk of family disapproval, peer bullying, harassment, and possible violent responses at a time in their life when acceptance is important. Therefore health-care workers must provide nonjudgmental support and open communication with the adolescent and the family and provide access to community resources and local support groups.

Developing a gender identity and a sense of sexuality is an important part of the *early adolescent's* sense of self (Adelson & Schuster, 2016). Masturbation is one way for an individual to explore and learn about his or her body. Mutual masturbation is a form of physical, erotic, and genital stimulation that teens may engage in with each other, and often does not include sexual intercourse (coitus). Manual stimulation can lead to orgasm and is a common sexual outlet for young teens. This type of experimental behavior helps the adolescent learn about sexual responses that are pleasurable and about behavior patterns that may contribute to later relationships. Sexual fantasy and experimentation are normal parts of sexual development and are not necessarily indicative of sexual orientation (Bockting, 2016).

Sexually active and exclusive relationships often develop during *later adolescence*. Health-care workers must be aware that many teenagers may not consider oral sex a sexual act, but the risk of STI transmission is high. Information concerning the risks of oral sex should be included in sex education programs, which should begin early because learning about sex 2 years too soon is better than 1 day too late.

The Sexuality Information and Educational Council of the United States (SIECUS) provides facts and guidelines about safe-sex practices and many other health topics for children from kindergarten through high-school age (http://www.siecusorg).

TEACHING TECHNIQUES

Teaching adolescents can be a challenge. There is enormous variability in the rates of physical, cognitive, and psychosocial maturity between early, middle, and late adolescence. Some adolescents pass slowly through the changes of puberty and cognitive development, yet may be advanced in physical development. The adolescent who appears physically mature but is not yet an abstract thinker does not learn or interact in the same way as an adolescent who is cognitively or emotionally mature. They therefore may be at high risk for destructive peer influences and may not make responsible decisions regarding these influences.

Patient Teaching

The health-care worker who understands the characteristics of each adolescent phase of development can be a highly effective teacher and source of information for teens and their parents. Identifying health risks of the adolescent is essential in planning teaching that is relevant to preventative health care. Rapid body changes can result in poor coordination that can result in sports injuries. Adolescents are capable of logical thought and abstract reasoning. They can understand cause and effect, health and illness, and disease prevention. However, healthy teens may have difficulty picturing themselves as vulnerable to illness or injury with an "it will never happen to me" attitude and may engage in high-risk behavior.

The first step in effectively teaching adolescents involves establishing a trusting relationship. Communication must be supportive and not threatening to adolescents' sense of independence or autonomy. If they are informed in a respectful way and understand the value of healthy behavior, they are more likely to use the information wisely. This approach is better than just telling them what they need to do. Providing privacy and one-to-one consultation can open up communication and reduce defenses. However, peer group teaching sessions may be more helpful and practical for discussing common problems such as smoking, sexual activity, substance abuse, and other health-related challenges. Discussion of options and decision-making must be shared, and options that support the adolescent in thinking and acting as an adult and staying open to learning should be offered. Confrontation should be avoided. Often the health-care worker, counselor, or nurse can help guide the family concerning parenting strategies relating to their teens. Setting realistic limits without damaging the sense of independence is a delicate balance and a learned skill for most parents.

Health Promotion

The Society for Adolescent Medicine identified seven characteristics critical to providing effective health education and care for adolescents: *availability, visibility, quality, confidentiality, affordability, flexibility, and coordination.* One of the goals of *Healthy People 2030* is to provide community resources with these characteristics to increase access to health care and education for all adolescents.

KEY POINTS

- Adolescence is the bridge between childhood and adulthood.
- Adolescence is divided into three phases: *early adolescence* (10–13 years of age), *middle adolescence* (14–16 years of age), and *late adolescence* (17–20 years of age).
- The major tasks of adolescence include establishing a sense of identity, separation from family, establishing intimacy and peer relationships, and career planning.
- The physical, psychological, cognitive, and emotional aspects of development may mature at different rates.
- Puberty refers to sexual maturity.
- The reproductive system is controlled by hormones regulated by the hypothalamus and secreted by the anterior pituitary glands and the ovaries or testes.
- Ovulation occurs 14 days before the menstrual period begins.
- The changing body plays a role in the adolescent's development of self-image, self-esteem, and social interactions.
- Adolescents should engage in at least 60 minutes of physical activity every day and activity of vigorous intensity at least 3 days per week.
- Adolescents engaging in competitive sports can benefit from strength training.

- Young adolescents are in the concrete phase of thinking, but teens in late adolescence use abstract thinking to assess realistic outcomes of decisions.
- Daydreaming can be developmentally appropriate and a useful safety valve for strong emotions.
- By middle adolescence, career goals may become more practical and realistic.
- In late adolescence, moral principles are based on the adolescent's own beliefs.
- Culture plays a role in how adolescents think and interact, and traditions can help stabilize identity.
- It is important to allow adolescents to begin to behave independently and to make their own decisions.
- Peer groups have a major impact on the social and emotional growth and development of adolescents.
- In late adolescence, intimacy with a peer can be sexual, intellectual, or social.
- Gender identity and sexual orientation are important components of developing sexuality during adolescence.
- Effective health education and care include *availability, visibility, high quality, confidentiality, affordability*, and *flexibility*.

Clinical Judgment Case Study

You are preparing to teach a group of young adolescents about sexuality and menstrual health. Sexual topics are an important part of adolescent teaching. Outline a plan that will discuss menstrual health, help the adolescent girl understand her "fertile period," and create an awareness of birth control options and sexuality.

REVIEW QUESTIONS

1. Put the events of the menstrual cycle in the proper order:

   A. ovulation.

   B. maturing the egg in the ovary.

   C. expulsion of the egg from the uterus.

   D. thickening of the uterine lining.

2. Classify the following hormones and secondary sex characteristics as typical for males, females, or both, by placing an X in the appropriate column.

	Boys	Girls	Both Boys & Girls
Spermatogenesis	☐	☐	☐
GnRH	☐	☐	☐
Pubic hair	☐	☐	☐
Voice deepening	☐	☐	☐
Menarche	☐	☐	☐
LH	☐	☐	☐
Nocturnal emissions	☐	☐	☐
Estrogen & progesterone	☐	☐	☐
Androgens	☐	☐	☐
Menstruation	☐	☐	☐

3. Select the proper terms to complete the sentences.

   According to Piaget's cognitive theory, young adolescents are in the -----1----- stage of thinking. This means they are likely to -----2-----. The middle adolescent is on the -----3----- stage and will often -----4-----. An older adolescent is in the -----5----- stage and will -----6-----.

   1. Formal operational, postformal operational, concrete.

   2. Use literal interpretations, use more complex thinking, consider long-term consequences.

   3. Formal operational, postformal operational, concrete.

   4. Use literal interpretations, use more complex thinking, consider long-term consequences.

   5. Formal operational, postformal operational, concrete.

   6. Use literal interpretations, use more complex thinking, consider long-term consequences.

4. Choose the most appropriate plan of action for the following case study.

   A father brings in his 15-year-old son, complaining that the boy is homosexual and would like to enter him into some type of medical or psychological therapy. The boy avoids eye-contact and looks only at the floor, and bruises are apparent on his left arm and cheek. When separated from his father, the boy becomes animated and engaging, with a bright smile. He states that he is bisexual and out among his friends. He recently told his family.

Which of the following would be the most appropriate course of action?

A. Refer the boy to a psychiatrist for suspected gender identity disorder.

B. Refer the boy to a family physician for blood tests to check for STIs.

C. Refer the boy to a psychologist for suspected gender nonconformity.

D. Refer the father and son to local resources and community support groups.

5. Identify whether the birth control options are hormonal, nonhormonal, or permanent. Also identify whether they are protective against STIs by indicating 'yes' or 'no.'

	Hormonal	Nonhormonal	Permanent	Protects against STI
Oral contraceptive				
Male condom				
Vasectomy				
Intrauterine devices				
Injections				
Tubal ligation				
Spermicidal foam				

Young Adulthood

http://evolve.elsevier.com/Leifer/growth

OBJECTIVES

1. Define young adulthood.
2. Discuss the developmental tasks of young adulthood.
3. Describe the physiological changes that occur in young adulthood.
4. Discuss at least four priority health issues related to the young-adult stage of the life cycle.
5. Use knowledge of men's and women's health needs in applying gender appropriate care and guidance.
6. Review health-screening preventative programs that are important during young adulthood.
7. Discuss the role of schools in helping individuals adjust and cope with tasks and challenges of young adulthood.

8. Describe the psychosocial tasks of young adulthood as described by Erikson.
9. Explain Piaget's theory of cognitive thinking in young adulthood.
10. Describe Kohlberg's theory of moral development in the young adult.
11. Discuss Piaget's formal operational thinking as it applies to the young adult.
12. Trace the growth and development of a parent and helpful guidance interventions.
13. Design teaching techniques that will contribute to successful learning in the young adult.

KEY TERMS

ectopic pregnancy
exercise
hysterectomy
intimacy
intimate partner violence (IPV)
pelvic inflammatory disease (PID)

physical activity
postformal operational thought
sexually transmitted infections
   (STIs)
structure
transitional phase

trial of labor after cesarean
   (TOLAC)
vaginal birth after cesarean
   (VBAC)
young adulthood

DEFINITION

Young adulthood is most often defined as the age between 20 and 40 years. The stage may also be referred to as *early adulthood*. The legal age of adulthood in the United States is 18 years, when the individual can vote, be drafted into the military, and enter into marital relationships without parental consent. Until an individual reaches age 21, however, there may still be legal limitations on some activities, such as the use of alcohol.

DEVELOPMENTAL TASKS

According to Erikson, the major developmental task or crisis of young adulthood is *intimacy versus isolation*. The young adult makes the transition from the safety of the parents' home and the structure of the high school to achieve the tasks of self-support, independence, developing intimate relationships, and establishing a stable family and lifestyle. By age 21, some adults live separately from parents, establish a commitment to a work identity, and develop an adult social role of their own design. Others do not take on these adult roles and responsibilities until after they pursue a college education to achieve a career goal. In some cases, social and political events such as war or an economic crisis can interrupt the progress toward career goals or financial or social independence. The developmental process from adolescence to adulthood is most often a gradual one, but in many cultures, there are traditional expectations during this transition.

PHYSIOLOGICAL CHANGES

Physical growth in height and weight and organ and sexual maturation are generally complete by young adulthood. Physical health, motor coordination, and physiological performance typically peak between the ages of 20 and 30 (Figure 11.1). The epiphyses of the

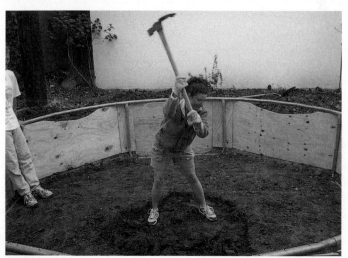

Figure 11.1 Physical health, motor coordination, and physiological performance are at their peak in young adulthood. Hard physical work and exercises are often enjoyed and are productive.

long bones fuse by the early twenties, and muscular strength is at its peak. The heart and lungs are also at their peak capacity during young adulthood. Lifestyle choices made during the young-adult years will dramatically affect heart and lung health in middle age and beyond.

Health Promotion

By age 30, muscle mass and body water may naturally decrease, and fatty tissue increases, resulting in increased vulnerability to injuries. Efforts toward maintaining good physical fitness can prolong peak functioning or reestablish good health and fitness at an older age (Piercy, 2018). Poor health habits can compromise health at any age.

PHYSICAL ACTIVITY

The benefits of physical activity throughout adulthood are numerous and undisputed. Among the benefits of regular exercise are decreased risk of heart disease, stroke, and diabetes; decreased cholesterol levels and blood pressure; increased insulin sensitivity; and increased muscle and bone mass. Active adults also display higher energy levels, improved cognitive function, and less anxiety and depression. Physical activity is also a key component of weight control. These benefits can be achieved through moderate levels of exercise, and there is a dose-response relationship so that more exercise leads to even stronger benefits.

According to the *Physical Activity Guidelines for Americans,* second edition (USDHHS, 2018), adults should perform at least 2.5 hours (30 minutes/day for 5 days/week or broken into shorter sessions of as little as 10 minutes at a time) to 5 hours (60 minutes/day for 5 days/week) of moderately intense aerobic exercise every week. Vigorous-intensity exercise of 1.25–2.5 hours per week or a combination of moderate and vigorous intensity will also provide substantial health benefits. Additional benefit is gained if exercise exceeds these suggested time periods.

Muscle-strengthening activities such as weight training, body-weight calisthenics, and manual labor provide additional health benefits. These types of exercises should be moderate to high intensity, involve all major muscle groups, and be performed 2 or more days per week.

Exercises involving balance and coordination such as backward walking, standing on one foot, and stretches for flexibility in all major muscle groups should be performed 2 or more days per week. In all cases, types of physical activity should be appropriate for current fitness level and health, and intensity should be gradually increased over time. A sedentary adult should begin to increase activity levels slowly, with light to moderate intensity for a short duration (e.g., 10 minutes of walking). This can be gradually increased in *duration, intensity,* and *frequency* until minimum guidelines can be met. Appropriate safety gear should be used, and a health-care provider should be monitoring health status particularly if any chronic conditions are present.

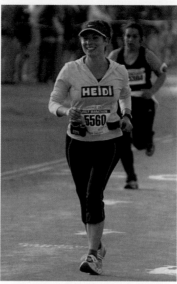

Figure 11.2 Young adults benefit from regular physical exercise such as running.

Health Promotion

Wise food choices provide optimum nutrition, and regular exercise can help maintain health and prevent obesity or cardiovascular disease (Figure 11.2). **Physical activity** is the daily actions that use energy such as dog walking or gardening, whereas exercise consists of specifically planned and structured repetitive activities designed for a level of calorie burning that aids *endurance* (dancing, jogging, or swimming) (Table 11.1), *balance* (Tai Chi, heel-toe walk), *strength* (weight lifting), or *flexibility* (yoga or Pilates). *Moderate physical activities* include walking at 3 mph, golf, water aerobics, or dancing. *Vigorous activities* include aerobics, walking at 4 mph, competitive basketball, or bicycling at 10 mph (USDHHS, 2018).

MyPyramid was developed in 2005 by the U.S. Department of Agriculture (USDA) as a guide for healthy daily food choices and was replaced in 2011 with MyPlate (Figure 11.3A). MyPlate reflects healthy food choices and does not include foods that supply empty calories such as cookies, cakes, sugary drinks, and most fast foods. Dietary guidelines for Americans, 8th edition can be accessed at https://www.dietaryguidelines.gov/sites/default/files/2019-05/2015-2020_Dietary_Guidelines.pdf (Figure 11.3B).

Health Promotion

Smoking, vaping, or substance abuse can contribute to a more rapid decline in health, beginning when the habit originates and extending throughout the lifespan. The eruption of the wisdom teeth and the development of gum disease are potential dental problems that commonly arise in this age group, and they must be addressed during the young-adult years. Conscientious brushing, flossing, and regular preventive dental care can help ensure good dental health. As the individual approaches

(Continued)

Health Promotion (*Cont.*)

age 30, gastric secretions may decrease, resulting in increased gastric discomforts. Junk foods, highly spiced foods, foods high in fat, and irregular eating habits established in adolescence may be more difficult to tolerate as a young adult progresses toward middle age. Visual acuity may begin to decline as the individual approaches middle age, and corrective lenses may be needed for reading or driving. Visual habits, such as taking breaks from reading to focus eyes on a distant point, can minimize visual decline associated with reading and frequent computer work.

Healthy People 2030 (Chapter 1) has identified priority areas for health promotion during the young adulthood years. The priority areas include maintaining physical activity, fitness, and nutrition; decreasing the use of tobacco and alcohol; encouraging positive mental health practices; and providing adequate information concerning family planning options. It is easier to develop positive health habits at a young age than to change or compensate for bad habits later in life. Most lifestyle choices and health habits are made during the young-adult years.

TABLE 11.1   Approximate Energy Expenditure for Levels of Activity Expressed as Multiples of Resting Energy Expenditure (REE)

Activity Category	Energy as Multiple of REE	kcal/min
Resting (sleeping, reclining)	REE × 1.0	1–1.2
Very light (seated and standing activities, painting trades, driving, laboratory work, typing, sewing, ironing, cooking, playing cards, playing a musical instrument)	REE × 1.5	Up to 2.5
Light (walking on a level surface at 2.5–3 mph, garage work, electrical trades, carpentry, restaurant trades, house cleaning, childcare, golf, sailing, table tennis)	REE × 2.5	2.5–4.9
Moderate (walking 3.5–4 mph, weeding and hoeing, carrying a load, cycling, skiing, tennis, dancing)	REE × 5.0	5.0–7.4
Heavy (walking with load uphill, tree felling, heavy manual digging, basketball, climbing, football, soccer)	REE × 7.0	7.5–12.0

Data from Rowe, D., Welsh, G., & Hell, D. (2011). Stride rate recommendations for moderate intensity walking. *Medicine and Science in Sports and Exercise, 43*(2), 312–318; Troino, R. P., et al. (2008). Physical activity in the US measured by accelerometer. *Medicine & Science in Sports & Sports Exercise, 40*(1), 181–188; Dong, L., Block, G., & Mandel, S. (2004). Activities contributing to total energy expenditure in US: Results of NHAPS Study. *International Journal of Behavioral Nutrition and Physical Activity, 1*(4), 1–4; Ainsworth, B., et al. (2000) Compendium of physical activities: an update of activity codes and MET intensities. *Medicine and Science in Sports and Exercise, 32*(9 Suppl), S498–504.

The major causes of death in young adulthood are most often related to accidents, drugs, or violence, which often are preventable. Typically, entrance into college provides the final opportunity for parents to initiate a health checkup and to provide education concerning lifestyle choices. After the pre-college physical examination, the young adult often does not

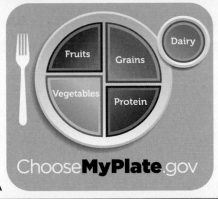

A

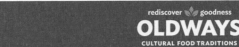

Latin American Diet Pyramid
La Pirámide de La Dieta Latinoamericana

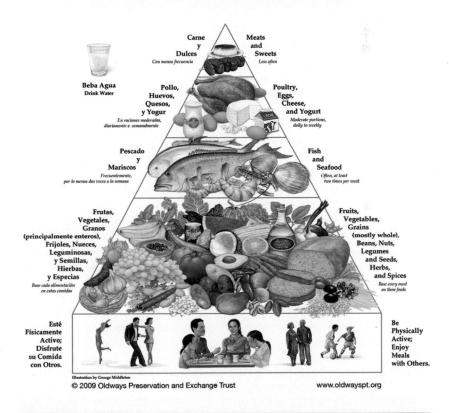

Carne y Dulces
Con menos frecuencia

Meats and Sweets
Less often

Beba Agua
Drink Water

Pollo, Huevos, Quesos, y Yogur
En raciones moderadas, diariamente a semanalmente

Poultry, Eggs, Cheese, and Yogurt
Moderate portions, daily to weekly

Pescado y Mariscos
Frecuentemente, por lo menos dos veces a la semana

Fish and Seafood
Often, at least two times per week

Frutas, Vegetales, Granos (principalmente enteros), Frijoles, Nueces, Leguminosas, y Semillas, Hierbas, y Especias
Base cada alimentación en estas comidas

Fruits, Vegetables, Grains (mostly whole), Beans, Nuts, Legumes and Seeds, Herbs, and Spices
Base every meal on these foods

Esté Físicamente Activo; Disfrute su Comida con Otros.

Be Physically Active; Enjoy Meals with Others.

Illustration by George Middleton

© 2009 Oldways Preservation and Exchange Trust

www.oldwayspt.org

B

Figure 11.3 MyPlate. (A) MyPlate.gov offers guidelines for good nutrition. *(From U.S. Department of Health and Human Services/U.S. Department of Agriculture, 2015–2020.)* (B) The traditional healthy Latin-American food pyramid has daily physical activity as its base and includes foods common to the Latin-American diet. The Latin-American Diet Pyramid can be accessed at https://oldwayspt.org/traditional-diets/latin-american-diet/latin-american-diet-pyramid. *(Courtesy Oldways Preservation and Exchange Trust).*

BOX 11.1   Recommended Preventative Health Screenings for Adults Aged 20–40 Years

- Blood pressure every 2 years
- Cholesterol level repeated every 5 years if remains within normal range
- Screening for diabetes if overweight (body mass index over 25)
- Cervical exam and Pap smear (screening for cervical cancer) for females beginning age 21 every 3 years; at age 30, if all previous exams have been normal, the Pap smear should be done every 5 years
- Mental health and substance abuse screening at each health-care provider visit
- Dental exam and cleaning every 6 months
- Eye exam every 2 years or yearly if the adult has been diagnosed with diabetes
- Influenza vaccine yearly
- TdAP booster (tetanus, pertussis, acellular pertussis) every 10 years
- Varicella vaccine (chickenpox) and HPV (human papilloma virus) vaccine if the adult was not immunized in childhood

Modified from U.S. Preventive Services Task Force (2020). *A and B recommendations*. https://www.uspreventiveservicestaskforce.org/uspstf/recommendation-topics/uspstf-and-b-recommendations.

---

seek health assessment unless a problem arises. Box 11.1 lists the recommended preventative health-screening points for young adults aged 20–40 years in order to maintain good health.

WOMEN'S HEALTH

Women have a great influence on childrearing and early learning. Maintaining women's health, therefore, may enable women to influence a generation of children to practice good health habits and to choose healthy lifestyles. Education concerning women's health issues and access to care have increased dramatically in the past few years. Women's health clinics and women's health specialists are available at most health-care facilities.

Cultural Considerations

Wide variations exist in cultural practices (Figure 11.4). Health-care workers must be alert to individual differences within a cultural group and must avoid stereotyping patients from specific cultural backgrounds. A strong belief in fate may prevent some women from seeking health care early. Diet, religious objects, and the use of folk medicine also play roles in preventing illness in some cultural groups. Modesty can influence the desire to avoid genital examinations; maintaining privacy is particularly critical during examinations. Communication between the health-care worker and the patient is important because eye contact, touch, and use of personal space influence the rapport between patient and caregiver. Some women prefer to receive health care from female providers. Cultural response to a change in gender function may influence a women's acceptance of contraception or sterilization practices. In some cultures, women who are menstruating are considered unclean. They may be isolated and forbidden to have contact with males. In some cultures, women consider menopause as a nonevent and do not suffer from anxieties related to aging (Chapter 3).

Cultural beliefs concerning women's health care influence preferred labor management, position for birth, location of delivery, and the role of family members during labor and delivery. Ethical issues also influence women's health care. Ethical issues include abortion, surrogate parenting, infertility treatment techniques, adoption, stem cell research, gene therapy, cord blood banking, and organ transplantation. Social issues such as homelessness, access to health care, and poverty also need to be considered as issues related to women's health care.

Pregnancy

Because a unique risk to health occurs during pregnancy, providing family planning services and birth control options for the young adult is essential (Chapter 10, Table 10.2). Maternal mortality rates have continued to decline during the past decade thanks to the availability of health care. The major risk factors contributing to mortality include lack of prenatal care, inadequate knowledge of health needs, and poor nutrition. The death rate for young mothers obtaining legal abortions in the United States is low, but those performed outside an accredited facility have higher rates of negative outcomes. The healthcare worker can play an important role in referring the young adult to available community resources. Recommended exercise during pregnancy is discussed in Chapter 6.

 ### Health Promotion

Healthy People 2030 goals include reducing the rate of cesarean births by the year 2030. According to research, the **trial of labor after cesarean (TOLAC)** in order to achieve **vaginal birth after cesarean (VBAC)** shows 60%–80% of women have a successful vaginal delivery, but VBAC is not right for everyone (Barbieri, 2017).

Ectopic pregnancy (pregnancy in the fallopian tube instead of the uterus) can be the result of malformation of the fallopian tube or from damage caused by pelvic inflammatory disease (PID). Sexually transmitted infections (STIs) are the major causes of PID. Therefore, promoting healthy behaviors related to safe-sex practices during adolescence and young adulthood can reduce maternal morbidity and mortality.

Hysterectomy (removal of the uterus) is the most common surgery performed on women during the reproductive years. The increasing use of laser techniques to treat uterine fibroids and other causes of excessive menstruation may decrease the need for this surgery.

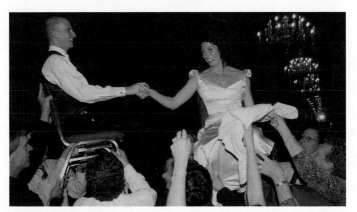

Figure 11.4 A typical cultural practice in a Jewish religious wedding ceremony. Cultural beliefs and practices are learned in childhood and can be carried throughout generations.

Papanicolaou (Pap) smears are encouraged for sexually active young women, because human papillomavirus (HPV) is also known to be a cause of cervical cancer, and both Pap and HPV tests are done at the same time (see Box 11.1). However, the HPV vaccine, introduced in 2006, has decreased the incidence of HPV infections by as much as 86% (Centers for Disease Control and Prevention, 2020). Encouraging routine breast self-examinations and mammograms at appropriate intervals can lead to early detection and early intervention for breast cancer (Box 11.2).

BOX 11.2   Breast Self-Examination

Perform breast self-examination monthly. If you are menstruating, do the examination 1 week after the beginning of your period, because your breasts are softer and less tender at this time. If you are not menstruating, choose any day that you can easily remember, such as the first day of each month. Examine your breasts in three ways: in front of a mirror, lying down, and in the shower.

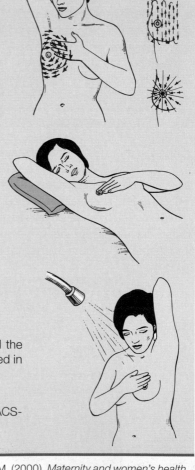

IN FRONT OF A MIRROR
Inspect your breasts in four steps:
1. With arms at your sides.
2. With arms over your head.
3. With your hands on your hips, pressing them firmly to flex your chest muscles.
4. While bending forward. Note any change in shape or appearance of your breasts and note skin or nipple changes such as dimpling of the skin. Squeeze each nipple gently to identify any discharge.

LYING DOWN
Place a small pillow under your right shoulder and put your right hand under your head while you examine your right breast with your left hand. Use the sensitive pads of your fingers to press gently into the breast tissue. Use a systematic pattern to check the entire breast. One pattern is to feel the tissue in a circular pattern, spiraling inward toward the nipple. Another method is to use an up-and-down pattern. Use the same systematic pattern to examine the underarm area, because breast tissue is also present here. Repeat for the other breast.

IN THE SHOWER
Raise your right arm. Use your soapy fingers to feel the breast tissue in the same systematic pattern described in the "Lying Down" section.

FOR ADDITIONAL INFORMATION
Contact the American Cancer Society at 1-800-ACS-2345 or visit www.cancer.org.

Illustrations from Lowdermilk, D. L., Perry, S. E., & Bobak, I. M. (2000). *Maternity and women's health care* (7th ed.). Mosby.

Stress, Coping, and Domestic Violence

The multiple roles of women in the young-adult phase of life can contribute to stress and the potential development of depression or anxiety. A single working mother may have the combined responsibilities of running a household, earning enough money to cover basic expenses, finding adequate and affordable day care for young children, and caring for an elderly parent. These responsibilities may cause the young woman to delay seeking health care for herself, which can lead to devastating results.

Violent behavior against women is an epidemic that contributes to the morbidity and mortality statistics of young adult women (Figure 11.5). Domestic violence can include psychological, physical, sexual, financial, and social abuses between intimate partners. The result is often social isolation and physical trauma. The Centers for Disease Control and Prevention (CDC) now refers to domestic violence as intimate partner violence (IPV). IPV involves all ethnic, racial, socioeconomic, and educational levels of the population (Box 11.3).

Health Promotion

Many communities have programs to address domestic violence and other crimes targeting women. *Healthy People 2030* lists specific objectives related to prevention and treatment programs (Chapter 1).

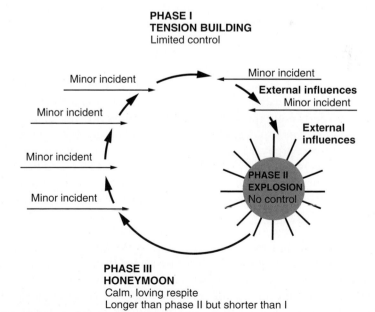

Figure 11.5 Cycle of violence. (From Rawlins, P., Williams, S., & Beck, C. (1993). *Mental health psychiatric nursing.* Mosby.)

> **BOX 11.3   Signs of Intimate Partner Violence**
>
> - Erratic prenatal care
> - Erratic child health-care appointments
> - Bruises and lacerations in various stages of healing
> - Self-blame for marital or relationship problems
> - History of alcohol or drug abuse in partner
> - History of abuse as a child (cycle of violence)
> - History of minor battering incidents

MEN'S HEALTH

Men currently do not have gender-specific health-care providers as women do. Men's health as a specialty may be a future trend but is not yet established in most health-care facilities. Young male adults appear to seek health care or guidance less frequently than women within this age group. Although they may accompany their pregnant partners to the obstetrician, unless they have fertility issues, men rarely seek medical assistance until a specific problem presents itself, but it is important to seek regular preventative care visits (see Box 11.1).

The high testosterone levels in males may contribute to a lower cholesterol level compared with women, but as the high levels of male hormones begin a natural decline with age, combined with poor diet, sleep, and exercise habits, cholesterol levels can begin to increase (Tambo et al., 2016). Statistically, men may be at a higher risk for injury because of their work environment. Men may also smoke and drink alcohol more often than women, contributing to the development of many health problems. The most common solid malignancy among men 20–40 years of age is testicular cancer (Seigel et al., 2019) and one of the few with reliable serum markers for diagnosis, but most often symptoms are not detectable until the advanced stage; therefore, the American Cancer Society and the U.S. Preventative Task Force in 2020 no longer have a policy concerning regular testicular self-examination (TSE) for all men (Gilligan et al., 2019).

Free clinics are available within many communities for STI testing and treatment, and human immunodeficiency virus/acquired immunodeficiency syndrome (HIV/AIDS) counseling. Physical examinations have become routine requirements at colleges before a student can enter sports programs and can be the initial access route to health care. Education concerning the harmful effects of smoking, alcohol, substance abuse, and obesity and ways to reduce these problems have increased awareness of health in men. Health and fitness clubs have become popular and lucrative businesses and have led to improvements in the health status for men and women. However, health-care workers must caution men concerning the adverse effects of overtraining and misuse of body-building supplementation, which are manifested by body and muscle fatigue, joint or muscle injury, dehydration, intestinal upset, and liver damage (Martin et al., 2018).

Increasing access, within the community and workplace, to health education and screening can be very advantageous. Studies have shown that community education and federal intervention concerning issues such as the need for seat-belt use, the dangers of smoking and drinking, and the use of condoms may have contributed significantly to healthier behavior choices. Many colleges and community groups host health fairs where blood pressure checks and education concerning various lifestyle choices are offered.

PSYCHOSOCIAL DEVELOPMENT

Schools play significant roles in helping the adolescent prepare for the developmental tasks and challenges of young adulthood. Parenting and family-life classes and money-management workshops are examples of courses that can help prepare for the transition into adult life. Students who plan to attend college often do not participate in these preparatory courses, because their focus is on college prerequisite courses. Some colleges have designed survival programs that help freshman students adjust to their new environments and adult responsibilities. Most colleges also offer career counseling and support services for young adults to help them achieve their educational goals. Work-study courses introduce young adults to the work environment and help them adapt to the expectations.

There are many developmental tasks and challenges that occur during the young-adult years. These tasks include developing a mature sense of right and wrong, successful separation from family control, initiating a preferred lifestyle, establishing friends and intimate relationships, deciding on marriage, pursuing career goals, and developing parenting skills. The sense of identity should be formed and stable by young adulthood and will start the individual on a path toward specific goals. These specific goals can change in later stages of the lifespan, when unexpected events, further self learning, or periods of transition allow time for reflection and reevaluation of accomplishments, and new goals can be formulated.

Intimacy

Erikson described establishing intimacy as one of the major tasks of young adulthood (Chapter 5). Intimacy involves more than sexual behavior. It includes the ability to develop a warm, trusting, honest relationship with another person with whom it is safe to be open and to express and share private thoughts. If a clear sense of identity has not been achieved during adolescence, then the young adult may feel guarded and only form casual relationships. Eventually this may contribute to isolation or difficulty in forming deep, long-term commitments.

Cognitive Ability

Intellectual and creative skills and abilities peak during young adulthood and improve with expanded education and experience. Piaget was a theorist (Chapter 5) who believed that the development of the formal operation as a method of thinking begins in adolescence and extends into young adulthood. The level of abstract thinking and logical reasoning is enhanced by the technology that is available in everyday life. The formal-operation type of thinking is necessary in the techniques of effective problem solving.

The young adult's cognitive process involves realizing that knowledge is the integration of multiple points of view. This process of integrating various points of view to develop knowledge and understanding is sometimes referred to as Piaget's fifth stage of development, known as postformal operational thought (Berger, 2020). Postformal operational thought uses tension from two conflicting approaches to a problem in pursuit of new and innovative outcomes. Individuals who have a well-developed postformal thought process are best able to problem solve in general, including choosing between multiple-choice answers on a test. Therefore, school performance may be best in the young-adult age group.

Levinson was a psychologist who described four seasons of life (Chapter 5). He believed that each season had a structure that is separated by transitional periods. During the structure period of young adulthood, significant choices such as a marriage partner and commitment to a career are made. During the following transitional phase, those choices are reviewed and reevaluated, and changes may be made. During one of the later transitional phases, individuals may reflect on past activities and may become unhappy because of missed opportunities or what they perceive as wrong choices. This may contribute to a midlife crisis experience.

Moral Reasoning

Kohlberg was a theorist who believed that the individual must be capable of the formal operational level of thought before achieving mature moral reasoning. Life experiences in an adult role or a college environment can enhance the development of moral reasoning. Taking responsibility for the care of others, handling the differing points of view of others, and understanding how their own actions affect others all contribute to the development of mature moral reasoning.

Sexuality

Young adults who are significant in a child's life can model positive displays of affection. Having young children see loving and joyous contact, such as hugging and kissing between parental role models and close family members, can help a child understand caring behaviors. Although allowing nudity in the home is a personal choice for parents, the concept of demonstrating comfort with their own bodies helps children to develop a positive body image. Treating one part of the body as dirty or naughty may result in having to readjust these beliefs when the child reaches maturity in order to achieve a sense of comfort in intimacy, and therefore the mature child's mastery of this task of attaining intimacy may be delayed.

Sexual intimacy in young adulthood differs from that in adolescence. By young adulthood, identity and cognitive function have reached the level that allows intimate sharing, controlled but honest emotional expression, caring about the partner, and the ability to make compromises and commitments. Sexual behavior and expectations are influenced by culture, customs, and environment. However, the ability to develop a sense of intimacy and the attachment required for a long-term commitment is closely related to the individual's experience when he or she was an infant seeking attachment with a parent (Augustyn et al., 2009). Healthy parent-child bonding produces a sense of security and trust. If relationships with parents in the early years did not produce a healthy, secure attachment, then achievement of a secure and stable intimacy with others in the young-adulthood phase of life may be more difficult or delayed.

Marriage

Many young adults who pursue higher education in college either postpone marriage or choose careful family planning or childcare arrangements that allow them to continue to pursue their goals. See Table 10.2 in Chapter 10 for contraceptive options available for effective family planning. Marriage most often occurs during the young-adult phase of the life cycle. However, many individuals delay marriage and/or childbearing until they are established in their careers. Today childbearing can be achieved at a later age due in large part to the advances in research and technology. The mean age at the birth of a woman's first child in the United States is on the rise from 24.9 years of age in 2000 to 26.4 years of age in 2015 (CDC, 2016; CIA, 2019).

People often select partners who are similar to themselves in interests, values, religious beliefs, and education. Family pressures or cultural traditions may also play a role in choosing a marriage partner (Smock & Schwartz, 2020). Partner choice is thought to be based on a three-stage process (Murstein, 1982). The first stage is the *stimulus stage*, which involves initial impressions and awareness of characteristics that attract each partner in the couple to each other. The *value-comparison stage* follows and involves getting to know one another better. The *role stage* involves evaluating long-term compatibility and deciding on a long-term commitment.

Gender roles and career issues play an important part in early adjustment to marriage. Balancing work, marriage, family, and parental roles is a challenge for young adults. This period is known as the beginning task of *generativity*, as described by Erikson (Chapter 5). It should be noted that generativity can be achieved by means other than parenting, such as involvement in a career, close interactions with family, or participation in community activities.

Parenting

Not all adults achieve or desire marriage and family. Some pursue careers that are fulfilling, thereby leaving little time for the responsibilities that marriage and parenthood require. Others choose to be in long-term, committed relationships without children, and some choose to delay marriage and childrearing until later life stages. However, this chapter will include the development of parenting skills as one of the tasks of young adulthood (Table 11.2).

The most proactive development of parental skills begins at the time conception is confirmed. When parents learn they are to have a baby, both positive and negative feelings are normally evoked. Parents may want the baby and want to be perfect parents. However, they may worry about being inadequately prepared for the parental role, the time commitment, and the impact on their careers and lifestyle. In the second trimester of pregnancy, when parents begin to feel the fetus move, their focus turns to the baby and what it might be. By the beginning of the third trimester of pregnancy, parents ascribe personality traits to the fetus and are receptive to teachings about parenting and childcare.

If the newborn arrives as a welcomed guest in the home, and the parents are supportive of one another, healthy parenting styles can be easily learned. At least 6 months of maternity leave, from work or from other routine activities, may be ideal in fostering attachment between parent and child, but often financial or career pressures require a shorter adjustment time. Close parent-child interactions during the early months of life can help in the formation of healthy attachments and positive parenting styles. Stepparents or parents who adopt older children may need extra time and effort to develop parent-child attachment and relationships.

The infant soon learns to associate the presence of the mother with feeding and relief of hunger and discomfort, and the baby soon calms whenever the mother is present. This behavior in turn strengthens the mother's sense of adequacy and effectiveness as a

TABLE 11.2   Growth and Development of Parents

Child's Task (Erikson's Stages)	Parents' Task	Intervention
FIRST PRENATAL TRIMESTER		
Growth	Develop attitude toward newborn. "Happy" about child? Parent of one disabled child? Unwed mother? These factors and others will affect the developing attitude of the mother.	Develop positive attitude in both parents concerning expected birth of child. Use referrals and agencies as needed.
SECOND PRENATAL TRIMESTER		
Growth	Mother focuses on infant because of fetal movements felt. Parents picture what infant will look like, what future he/she will have, and other ideas.	Parents' focus is on childcare and needs and providing physical environment for expected infant. Information concerning care of the newborn should be provided at this time.
THIRD PRENATAL TRIMESTER		
Growth	Mother feels large. Attention focuses on how fetus is going to get out.	Detailed information should be presented at this time concerning the birth process, preparation for birth, breastfeeding, and care of sibling at home.
BIRTH		
Adjustment to external environment	Elicit positive responses from child and respond by meeting child's need for food and closeness; if parents receive only negative responses (e.g., sleepy infant, crying infant, difficult feeder, congenital anomaly), positive development of the parent may be inhibited.	Encourage early touch, feeding, and other practices. Explain behavior and appearance of newborn to allay fears. Help parents to identify positive responses. (Use infant's reflexes, such as grasp reflex, to identify a response by placing mother's finger into infant's hand.)
INFANT		
Trust	Learn "cues" presented by infant to determine individual needs of infant.	Help parents assess and interpret needs of infant (avoid feelings of helplessness or incompetence). Do not let in-laws take over parental tasks. Help parents cope with problems such as colic.

TABLE 11.2   Growth and Development of Parents (*Cont.*)

Child's Task (Erikson's Stages)	Parents' Task	Intervention
TODDLER		
Autonomy	Try to accept the pattern of growth and development. Accept some loss of control but maintain some limits for safety.	Help parents cope with transient independence of child (e.g., allow child to go on tricycle, but do not yell "Don't fall," or anxiety may be radiated).
PRESCHOOL		
Initiative	Learn to separate from child.	Help parents show standards but let go so child can develop some independence. A preschool experience may be helpful.
SCHOOL AGE		
Industry	Accept importance of child's peers. Parents must learn to accept some rejection from child at times. Patience is needed to allow children to do things for themselves, even if it takes longer. Do not do the school project for the child. Provide chores for child appropriate to his/her age level.	Help parents to understand that child is developing his/her own limits and self-discipline. Be there to guide child but do not constantly intrude. Help child achieve results from his/her own efforts to perform.
ADOLESCENT		
Establishment of identity Acceptance of pubertal changes Development of abstract reasoning Examination of career choices Investigation of lifestyles Controlling of feelings	Parents must learn to let child live his/her own life and not to expect total control over the child. Expect at times to be discredited by teenager. Expect differences in opinion and respect them. Guide but do not push.	Help parents adjust to changing role and relationship with adolescent (e.g., as child develops his/her own identity, child may become a Democrat if parents are Republican). Expose child to varied career fields and life experiences. Help child to understand emerging emotions and feelings brought about by puberty.

Modified from Leifer, G. (2019). *Introduction to maternity & pediatric nursing* (8th ed.). Elsevier.

parent. Parent-infant attachment is best observed during feeding, when both mother and infant should be focused on each other. If either is preoccupied or inattentive, parent-infant bonding may not be successful. If the parent is an adolescent, some developmental tasks of adolescence may interfere with the developmental tasks of parenthood. Special interventions by the health-care worker can be helpful in prioritizing behaviors and in meeting the major needs of the infant and adolescent parent. Refer to Chapter 10 for more information on the adolescent stage of development.

TEACHING TECHNIQUES

Successful learning for adults always involves relating the information they are learning to the appropriate developmental tasks they are experiencing. For example, a new parent will likely be very receptive to information concerning parenting skills. An adult in a managerial position at work may be most receptive to learning about managing styles and techniques. The knowledge and skills learned should be applicable to the learner, should be realistic, and should help solve the problems currently encountered by the learner. Concepts presented to young adults should build on their previous knowledge and skills, rather than beginning below their level of understanding, or they will be "turned off." Teaching goals should be clear and should outline how the new knowledge can be applied and how it will benefit the learners' current life roles. Learning is a lifelong process. Teaching techniques for young adults should be interactive, problem oriented, and related to daily psychosocial tasks at work, home, or school.

KEY POINTS

- Young adulthood is most often defined as being from 20 to 40 years of age.
- Physiological performance has a natural peak between 20 and 30 years of age.
- Proper nutrition and exercise can prevent obesity and can contribute to health during the young-adult years and beyond.
- Most lifestyle patterns are established during the young-adult years.
- It is easier to develop positive health habits as a young adult to achieve a positive health status than it is to change habits later in life.
- The major causes of death in the young-adult age group are related to accidents, drugs, and violence, all of which are preventable.
- Promoting healthy behaviors relating to safe-sex practices during adolescence and young adulthood can reduce the incidence of sexually transmitted infections.
- Health and fitness spas have become lucrative businesses that help improve the health status of men and women.

- Developmental tasks of young adulthood include developing a stable sense of identity and a mature sense of right and wrong; successful separation from family control; establishing adult friendships and intimate relationships; choosing marriage partners and career goals; developing parenting skills; and initiating a preferred lifestyle.
- Piaget's formal operational thinking begins in adolescence and extends into young adulthood.
- Formal operational thinking is necessary for the establishment of effective problem-solving skills.
- Postformal operational thought involves integrating various points of view.
- In most cultures there are established expectations of adulthood.
- The task of generativity can be achieved by a means other than parenting.
- Development of a parent accelerates when conception is confirmed.
- When teaching young adults, the goals and how the new knowledge can be applied in the lives of the learners should be made clear.

Clinical Judgment Case Study

A 20-year-old female presents to the emergency department with severe left-sided abdominal pain, nausea, and dizziness. Although she usually has a regular menstrual cycle of 28 days, her last menstrual period was 6 weeks ago, but she has had light intermittent vaginal bleeding for 1 week. She is sexually active but does not use birth control and has a prior history of an STI 2 years ago. Given she has missed a menstrual period, what do you think a pregnancy test result might be? Given she has a prior history of an STI, what is she at risk for? What are some priorities for her nursing care?

REVIEW QUESTIONS

1. Match each activity with its proper frequency and example.

Activity	Frequency	Example
Moderate/vigorous-intensity physical activity		
Muscle/bone-strengthening activity		
Balance activity		
Flexibility activity		

Frequency options: 1. 2–3 days/week, 2. 3–5 days/week

Examples: 1. backward walking, 2. weight training, 3. jogging, 4. hamstring stretch

2. Match each theorist with their focus during young adolescence, and an example of each.

Theorist	Focus	Example
Erikson		
Piaget		
Levinson		
Kohlberg		

Focus choices:

1. Many decisions are made during the season of young adulthood that may be regretted during later transitional phases.
2. Postformal operation thought improves problem solving.
3. Developing intimacy is the major task of young adulthood.
4. Experiences in adulthood help form moral reasoning.

Examples:

A. Deciding to get a job instead of attending college and later wishing you had made a different choice.
B. Seeing your mother treated badly and deciding to be extra nice to her.
C. Helping your 2-year-old twins figure out how to share a toy.
D. Deciding to take your significant other away for a weekend trip.

3. You are caring for a 22-year-old male with a body mass index in the obese range. Blood work indicates abnormal liver function and increased blood sugar. He also

admits to daily use of vaping tobacco. Based on the information provided, what are some appropriate items to add to his plan of care? (Select all that apply)

A. Develop a physical activity plan.

B. Provide information on regular testicular self-examination.

C. Provide tobacco cessation program information.

D. Initiate a consult with a nutritionist.

4. You are caring for a 30-year-old female in the emergency department who presented with bruises to her face and swelling to her left eyelid. Green-tinged bruises are noted on her right upper arm. She states her husband has "anger issues when he drinks, but it's usually because I've done something I shouldn't do." Which of the following signs of intimate partner violence are represented in this scenario? (Select all that apply)

A. Erratic prenatal care.

B. Erratic child health-care appointments.

C. Bruises and lacerations in various stages of healing.

D. Self-blame for marital or relationship problems.

E. History of alcohol or drug abuse in partner.

5. Major causes of death in young adults are: (select all that apply)

A. drug use.

B. violence.

C. chronic illness.

D. accidents.

E. infections.

Middle Adulthood

http://evolve.elsevier.com/Leifer/growth

OUTLINE

OBJECTIVES

1. Define middle adulthood.
2. List the physiological changes that occur during middle adulthood.
3. Define the major developmental tasks and challenges of middle adulthood.
4. Define midlife transition compared with midlife crisis.
5. Define the "sandwich generation."
6. Discuss sexuality in the middle-adulthood phase of the life cycle.
7. State the complexities of the menopausal experience in women.
8. Discuss the male climacteric.
9. List preventative health-care measures appropriate for middle adulthood.
10. Describe the benefits of regular exercise during middle adulthood.
11. List teaching strategies that may be effective for the patient in the middle-adult phase of the life cycle.

KEY TERMS

climacteric
"empty nest" syndrome
generativity
hot flashes
identity accommodation

menopause
middle adulthood
midlife crisis
midlife transition
reproductive health

sandwich generation
sexuality
stagnation

DEFINITION

Middle adulthood is defined as the period of development after the early adult years but before retirement (Levinson et al., 1978). Middle adulthood is often referred to as the period between 40 and 65 years of age. An individual's behavior during this period is influenced by genetics and the environment, and an interaction of biological, psychological, and social changes occurs. By middle age, the adult has established roots in a community with ties to culture, religious groups, schools, neighborhood centers, and friends. Some culture-specific influences affect development, but the greatest current environmental influence is the worldwide political dynamic that reaches across oceans to influence life and lifestyles in the United States. Some theorists suggest that developmental changes are gradual and progressive, but others express the concept of passing through distinct stages (Chapter 5).

 Lifespan Considerations

Metabolic needs decrease during middle adulthood, and if diet and exercise are not part of a healthy lifestyle, excess weight begins to accumulate. A decrease in energy and perceived physical attractiveness may occur. A loss of muscle tone and skin elasticity may result in a less firm appearance of body contours. Body fat may redistribute to the stomach and hip area. Impacted wisdom teeth may now begin to cause issues requiring extraction, and periodontal disease is a risk if oral care is not meticulous. Hair may begin to gray and thin. Eye changes common to middle age can be easily corrected with glasses, contact lenses, or laser surgery. Diet, smoking, and lack of exercise influence cardiovascular changes that occur during midlife, but hormonal changes also influence risk factors for cardiovascular disease.

DEVELOPMENTAL TASKS

The main task or crisis of middle adulthood is generativity versus stagnation (Erikson, 1994). *Generativity* has been defined as contributing in a positive way to family, community, or the world. This contribution that includes creating relationships with friends and family or mentoring others that results in positive changes that are of benefit to society improves self-image and promotes subjective well-being. Failure to achieve generativity results in *stagnation*, which is total self-absorption, being unproductive, or failing to get involved with others including family, community, or world and placing personal concerns above all else (Newton et al., 2016). Generativity can be achieved in many ways and is not necessarily limited to having children and a family of one's own. There are many opportunities to achieve generativity through career and personal activities and achievements. Other developmental tasks of middle adulthood include managing a career and finances, managing a household, and nurturing marriage and family relationships.

Maintaining a positive self-image is important to the middle-aged adult. When individuals deny they are aging and cannot view themselves as middle aged, they often experience difficulty in adjusting to necessary changes, and depression may develop. Maintaining a positive self-image is a challenge when society and the media place high importance on looking and acting young. Another important task of middle age is identity accommodation, which is changing the concept of one's own identity to fit reality, rather than what was dreamed.

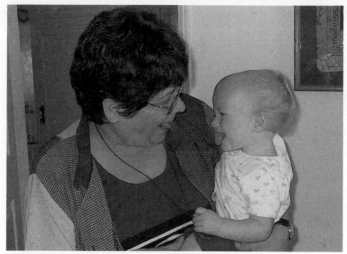

Figure 12.1 A grandparent enjoys remaining involved with the family and values interaction with grandchildren.

The effect of the spouse or significant other on continued development and life stability is important. The feedback of a spouse or significant other influences self-image in the midlife stage. New social experiences challenge the middle-aged adult. Involvement with childcare, athletic events, parents of school friends, and parent-child relationships can also influence psychological well-being (Figure 12.1).

CHALLENGES

Midlife is a time of life filled with transitions. New relationship dynamics are being set with spouses in a home no longer with young children, with aging parents and their changing requirements, with children becoming young adults, and with new grandchildren for some. Financial vulnerabilities are considered with an eye toward retirement amid an environment with market volatility, increasing health-care fees, and rising college education tuition or the often enormous cost of weddings. Internal transitions are occurring as well, as the body responds to changing hormone levels.

Maintaining optimum cognitive functioning is necessary to prevent a decrease in problem-solving skills. Adjusting to changes in relationships with coworkers, friends, and family is also important to maintaining psychological well-being. Many middle-aged adults find time to continue their education, which may have been interrupted by marriage and childrearing. The stresses of middle adulthood often include marital separation, divorce, major illness or injury, loss of a spouse or loss of income, unplanned pregnancy, and the challenge of caring for aged parents while helping teen children into adulthood. The "empty nest" syndrome that can occur when grown children start to leave home for the first time can additionally lead to feelings of social isolation and stress.

Midlife Transition Versus Midlife Crisis

Middle adulthood is a time of self-reflection, reevaluation, and prioritization. Looking back, the adult may grieve lost youth and missed opportunities. Looking ahead, adults

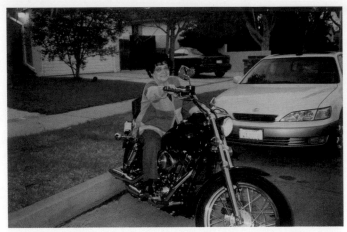

Figure 12.2 It is never too late to learn and to enjoy the skills of a new activity.

may become aware of the inevitability of their own mortality, which may lead to despair. The process of aging is felt. Some adults experience this as a midlife transition as they are able to realign themselves with this next stage of life in a healthy way (Figure 12.2). Other adults experience this as a midlife crisis as they try to make up for lost opportunities of the past or challenge the inevitability of the future (Malone et al., 2016). They may start to engage in reckless or unhealthy behaviors that are atypical for their character. Sometimes reflection and reinterpretation of past experiences bring new insights and may serve as turning points in self-perception.

The Sandwich Generation

Middle adults are said to be in the sandwich generation, which means they must handle increased financial and emotional responsibilities related to their children and their older and possibly dependent parents. Many men feel overextended, but mothers in this age group feel more stress than any other age group as they balance caregiving demands, with approximately 40% reporting extreme levels of stress affecting their personal relationships and capacity for self-care (APA, 2020). Fulfilling relationships will help validate positive self-esteem, whereas divorce, separation, conflicts with adult children, or aging parents may impact the psychological functioning of middle-aged adults in a negative way. Healthy ways to reduce stress such as regular exercise, eating a healthy diet, engaging in social contact with friends, and getting adequate sleep should be emphasized as important to self-care but also as a positive model for the rest of the family.

SEXUALITY

Sexuality is multifaceted and according to the World Health Organization (WHO, 2006, as cited in WHO, 2020) it encompasses sex, gender identity and orientation, intimacy and eroticism, desires and pleasure, attitudes and values, behaviors, roles, and relationships. It is a central aspect of being human and is a part of every phase of the life cycle. Sexuality involves beliefs and behaviors that surround physiological and psychological responses, religious, spiritual, and sociocultural values. Communication, a sense of closeness, and mutual comfort are key aspects of sexuality. Middle adulthood is a time when the adult may be struggling with self-perception due to changes in weight or other aspects of appearance. Middle adults may also be focused on career goals and financial stability, and little time or energy may be set aside to fulfill sexual needs. The middle-aged woman may be at the peak of sexual desire as they feel more empowered to communicate their sexual needs to their partners and have a better understanding of their bodies (Thomas et al., 2018). For some, decreases in testosterone and other sex hormones for both men and women during this phase can lead to decreased sexual desire. Men may find difficulty achieving or maintaining an erection, often related to diabetes, high blood pressure, or medication side effects.

A significant percentage of the population in the United States is living as single adults. The reasons can include postponing marriage for a career, divorces, or never entering into a long-term relationship. Options for sexual lifestyles for the single person can include celibacy, a sexually exclusive companion, or a long-term relationship with one or more partners. Less common situations that people engage in to satisfy sexual needs include open marriages, group marriages, and swinging (i.e., mate swapping) (Masters et al., 1986). Studies show that in midlife, more emphasis is placed on other aspects of sexuality such as emotional closeness and quality communication rather than physical sensations (Thomas et al., 2015).

The climacteric refers to the time in life in which hormonal changes result in cessation of the reproductive ability in the female and a corresponding decrease in sexual activity in the male. Gradual hormonal changes in the woman occur before menopause and may start as early as age 35, although the age for actual menopause is on average closer to 50. Each woman responds to subtle menopausal changes in a unique way, and sexuality can be affected by these changes. Estrogen-sensitive skin can lead to vaginal dryness. Breasts flatten and hair thins as estrogen-to-androgen ratios change.

The absence of children in the home, who may have left for college or marriage, may provide time to renew relationships between partners. A self-assured attitude, developed as a result of experience and age, may limit inhibitions and can create many enjoyable close moments with partners at this stage of life.

Women's Health

Menopause is the cessation of the menstrual period caused by hormonal changes in the body. Menopause usually begins between 45 and 55 years of age and is genetically controlled. The menstrual cycle becomes shorter and more irregular. Hot flashes may result when capillaries dilate and blood rushes to the skin surface. The body feels warm, the woman may sweat, followed by vasoconstriction and the woman feels cold. This can occur several times a day and is uncomfortable and distracting. Hormone replacement therapy (HRT) may be prescribed but is not appropriate for all women because of the risks of its use (NCI, 2018). Complementary and alternative medicine (CAM) therapy is popular with many women during menopause. Health-care workers must assess any interactions between CAM therapy used by the woman and prescribed medicines or treatments.

The onset and experience of menopause is unique for each woman, and health-care approaches must be tailored to each (Box 12.1; see also Chapter 13). A detailed and accurate personal-health interview can uncover problems that require interventions.

BOX 12.1   Signs of Menopausal Changes in Women

- Hot flashes
- Heart palpitations
- Headache
- Decreased vaginal lubrication
- Fatigue
- Insomnia
- Emotional lability (happy one minute, crying the next)

Recent medical advances have prolonged the physical reproductive capabilities of some women. The psychosocial issues involved in childbearing at a later age, and the advantages and disadvantages of the middle-aged or older adult becoming a new parent, present new challenges to the parents, the child, and the health-care worker.

Men's Health

Indicators of health, as outlined in *Healthy People 2030*, include rates of longevity, morbidity, and mortality. Although longevity rates have increased for both men and women, women still generally live longer than men. In each leading cause of death in adults, men have a higher rate of mortality and are more burdened by illness during life. A contributory factor may be that men perceive themselves as healthy and therefore delay seeking medical care and preventative care. Research has shown that there are explanations for gender differences in health and illness. Genetically, males have a shorter Y chromosome paired with the longer X chromosome which can increase his risk for sex-linked genetic disorders. Men are more likely to have heart disease, stroke, and diabetes (Crimmins et al., 2019). Men still suffer more from alcohol and substance abuse, but both sexes smoke in equal numbers (Harvard Men's Health Watch, 2019).

The male climacteric involves a gradual decline in the blood concentration of testosterone and other hormones. This results in a decrease in muscle mass and strength, a decrease in sex drive and erectile function, and a decrease in a sense of well-being. Testosterone-replacement therapy has recently been studied and has been found to have positive influences on improving strength, decreasing fat accumulation, and increasing libido and sense of well-being. Testosterone-replacement therapy does not increase erectile function, because it does not specifically affect blood circulation. Androgen therapy is used with caution in older men with enlarged prostates and urinary symptoms. Medications are available for use for specific symptoms related to the male climacteric. Many drugs decrease testosterone levels, such as chemotherapy, ingestion of lead and exposure to certain insecticides, alcohol, and many illicit drugs. Diseases such as cystic fibrosis, sickle cell anemia, obesity, diabetes, sleep apnea, liver disease, and kidney failure also decrease testosterone levels (Adlin, 2020).

Generally, men remain in the workforce longer than women and may partake in activities that pose a higher potential for injuries. Men engage in sports and leisure activities that also have a high risk for injury, and some may use illegal substances to prove their masculinity. Young boys are often socialized to ignore symptoms of illness and therefore may postpone seeking medical advice as adults until the problem is more advanced.

Middle-aged men who fear the aging process may begin to experience alteration in sexual performance, but the ability to procreate, or father children, remains intact.

Health Promotion

Gender-appropriate health education is important to provide vital information without damaging sex-role-stereotyped self-images. Men typically contact the health-care system via a pediatrician when young, a school nurse when school age, and a military doctor or company physician when a young adult. Men often do not choose a personal doctor until middle age. Middle-aged adults should be counseled concerning healthy lifestyles, preventative medicine screening exams, sexually transmitted illness prevention, anticipated role changes, and job retraining when necessary. Expanded health promotion and early detection activities help achieve the goals of *Healthy People 2030* (Box 12.2). The current immunization schedule for adults can be accessed at http://www.CDC.gov/vaccines//index.HTML.

PHYSICAL ACTIVITY

In middle adulthood, the purpose of regular physical activity shifts from increasing fitness (as in young adulthood) to maintaining fitness and avoiding disease. Cardiovascular endurance, muscle strength, and bone mass all decrease naturally beginning around age 35, but regular physical activity can slow these changes. As in younger adulthood, middle adults should continue to strive for a minimum of 2.5 hours of moderate physical activity per week and can benefit from additional vigorous exercise. Care must be taken to avoid

---

BOX 12.2	Essential Health Screening for Middle-Aged Women and Men

Healthy, middle-aged women and men should have the following screening tests performed at regular intervals (interval may vary depending on risk factors):

- Vision testing at least every 2 years
- Dental checkups once or twice yearly
- Blood pressure monitoring at least yearly
- Lipid (cholesterol, triglycerides) and blood glucose check
- Colorectal cancer screening beginning age 45
- Flu shot yearly, Shingles immunization after age 50

WOMEN

- Breast examination and mammogram every 2 years aged 50–74
- Osteoporosis screening between ages of 50 and 70
- Papanicolaou (Pap) testing every 3 years for ages 21–29 and every 5 years for ages 30–65

MEN

- Prostate cancer screening at age 45–50 if African American

Data from U.S. Preventive Services Task Force (2020). *Screening recommendations* https://www.uspreventiveservicestaskforce.org/uspstf/topic_search_results?category%5B%5D=All&searchterm=screening.

injury if a previously sedentary middle adult begins an exercise routine in response to the signs of aging.

Exercise can also be a social outlet for an otherwise isolated person. During middle age, people often are busy with work and family and may find it difficult to find time for exercise or socializing. Exercise groups, gyms, and personal trainers can all provide access to physical activities among peers.

It is important for middle-aged adults to find enjoyable activities to ensure regular participation. Hiking, outdoor bootcamps, group exercise classes, and recreational sports such as soccer or basketball are all examples of physical activities with a social component. Activity trackers can provide immediate feedback on progress and create competition and collaboration among similar-minded individuals within their social group (Brickwood et al., 2019).

TEACHING TECHNIQUES

Teaching plans should be related to the problems and concerns of the individual and the age group. Successful teaching of middle-aged adults relies on understanding their typical concerns and potential sources of stress. Stress can inhibit learning or be the motivational force for learning. Misconceptions concerning changes that come with aging are common, and many adults desire information related to the prevention of chronic illnesses. Middle-aged adults are often interested in learning about menopause and the teaching of coping styles that will help maintain a positive health status. Middle-aged adults may be concerned about the lives of their grown children, require assistance adjusting to the role of grandparent, or need help with designing strategies to care for their own older, frail parents.

Teaching strategies should incorporate the independence and competencies of the adult learner. An understanding of adult learning theories may be helpful in selecting the best instructional strategies, learning objectives, assessment and evaluation approaches, and learning environment (Mukhalalati & Taylor, 2019). Table 12.1 summarizes adult learning theories used in health-professional education. As with all age groups, a simple compliment (validation) concerning their learning competencies can also provide the reward needed to support motivation for further learning.

TABLE 12.1   Adult Learning Theories Used in Health-Professional Education Programs

Learning Theory	Sub-Category	Originator(s) (Year)	Summary of Concepts
Instrumental learning theories: focus on the learner's individual experience	Behavioral theories	Thorndike (1911), Pavlov (1927), Skinner (1954)	Focus on stimulus leading to change of behavior. Positive consequences enhance learning while negative consequences weaken learning.

Learning Theory	Sub-Category	Originator(s) (Year)	Summary of Concepts
	Cognitivism	Piaget and Cook (1952), Bruner (1966)	Focus on internal environment of the learner. Associated with cognition elements such as insight, perception, reflection, and memory.
	Experiential learning	Kolb (1984)	Learning is facilitated through interaction with the environment: concrete experience, reflective observation, abstract conceptualization, and active experimentation.
Humanistic theories or facilitative learning theories. These theories promote individual development and are more learner-centered	Self-directed learning	Rogers (1963), Maslow (1968), Knowles (1988)	Focus is on human freedom and dignity. Learning is self-directed and adults can plan, manage, and assess their own learning. Student-centered and personalized learning. Educators are facilitators.
Transformative learning theories	Critical reflection	Mezirow (1978, 1990, 1997)	Learners identify and challenge the validity of embedded assumptions. Confusing problem promotes reflection and critical evaluation. Action is taken based on this reflection.
Social theories of learning: focus on context and community	Some of proximal development	Vygotsky (1978)	Focus on social interaction, person, context, community, and desired behavior for learning. Observation and modeling are fundamental.

(Continued)

TABLE 12.1   Adult Learning Theories Used in Health-Professional Education Programs (*Cont.*)

Learning Theory	Sub-Category	Originator(s) (Year)	Summary of Concepts
	Situated cognition	Lave and Wenger (1991)	
	Communities of practice	Wenger (1998)	
Motivational models	Self-determination theory	Ryan and Deci (2000)	Motivation and reflection are fundamental to learning. Focus on intrinsic motivations.
	Expectancy valance theory	Weiner (1992)	Incorporates expectancy of success.
	Chain of response model	Cross (1981)	Focuses on self-evaluation, attitude toward education, and importance of goals and expectations.
Reflective models	Reflection on action	Schön (1987)	Learning through reflection after an activity occurred.
	Reflection in action	Schön (1987)	Learning through reflection during the activity.
Constructivism	Cognitive constructivists	Ausubel and Robinson (1969), Piaget and Cook (1952)	Learners construct new knowledge through interaction between previous knowledge and skills, and knowledge gained from social interaction with peers, teachers, and social activities.
	Sociocultural constructivism	Vygotsky (1978)	

Modified from Mukhalalati, B., & Taylor, A. (2019). Adult learning theories in context: A quick guide for healthcare professional educators. *Journal of Medical Education and Curricular Development, 6.* doi: 10.1177/2382120519840332.

The health-care worker can also assist middle-aged adults with finding activities to support their need for generativity. This can provide the patient with great personal satisfaction as they contribute to the community or begin to take up new activities in preparation for their alternative lifestyles during retirement (Figure 12.3).

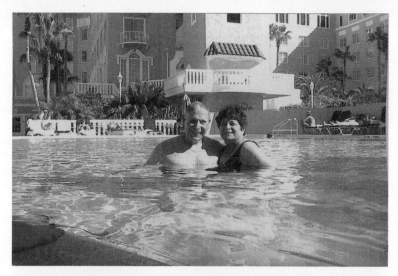

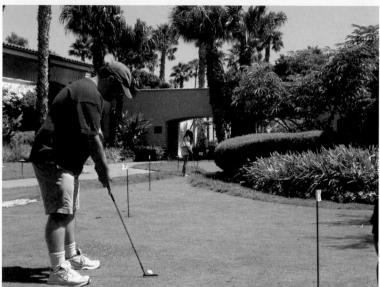

Figure 12.3 Finding active and enjoyable leisure activities is an important step in preparation for successful retirement.

KEY POINTS

- Middle adulthood is the period after the early adult reproductive years and before retirement. It includes the period between 40 and 65 years of age.
- Erikson's developmental task of middle adulthood is generativity versus stagnation.
- Other developmental tasks of middle adulthood include managing finances and a career; nurturing marriage and family relationships; managing a household; and maintaining a positive self-image.

- Middle adulthood is a time of self-reflection, reevaluation, and prioritization.
- Gradual hormonal changes occur before menopause; these changes may begin as early as age 35.
- The climacteric is when hormonal changes result in cessation of menstruation in women and decreased muscle mass and sex drive in men.
- Concerns of middle-aged men are typically related to role changes, work-related stress, decreased physical fitness, and performance anxiety.
- Preventive health care for men includes dental examinations, blood pressure and blood-lipid levels, and prostate and colorectal cancer screenings.
- Middle age is referred to as the *sandwich generation*, where responsibilities include the care of children and older parents.
- Physical activity is important for maintaining fitness and preventing illness. Exercise with a social component can provide a social outlet for the busy middle-aged adult.

Clinical Judgment Case Study

Mrs. B. is a 53-year-old female who is seeking counseling for stress. When reviewing her current situational stress factors, she states her youngest child is going to college soon and her parent's health is declining. She is noticing changes in her body that she is struggling to feel comfortable with. Her spouse is supportive, but both are feeling overwhelmed and that leads to disagreements. What is unique about the stress encountered in this period of life? What stresses might Mrs. B. and her spouse be feeling differently? Discuss what role the health-care worker can play in helping them to manage their stress and increase their health status.

REVIEW QUESTIONS

1. Identify the examples below as either generativity (A), stagnation (B), or identity accommodation (C): (circle one)
   A. Feeling depressed when your son can beat you in a 100-meter race. A B C
   B. Acceptance and appreciation of the home you own, even though it is not fancy. A B C
   C. Feeling a sense of pride for donating a large sum to your alma-mater. A B C
2. Which of the following are typical goals of physical activity in middle adulthood?
   A. Improve marathon time.
   B. Reduce blood pressure.
   C. Engage socially with peers.
   D. Slow down the loss of bone mass.
   E. Prepare body for pregnancy.
   F. Weight control.
   G. Slow down decreases in cardiovascular endurance.
   H. Avoiding cardiovascular disease.

3. Place the following behaviors into the appropriate column:

Midlife Transition Behavior	Midlife Crisis Behavior

A. Joining a gym to manage midlife weight gain.

B. Asking for a new hair style and color from their stylist.

C. Starting to smoke marijuana regularly with a new group of friends.

D. Engaging in an extramarital affair with a much younger partner.

E. Taking out a loan to purchase an expensive sports car that the person cannot afford.

F. Beginning to engage in extreme sports without training.

G. Going back to college to complete a new degree.

H. Making time to write a novel that they have been dreaming of for years.

I. Having a tummy tuck or breast lift surgery.

J. Having extensive expensive plastic surgery that significantly alters the appearance.

4. Fill in the blanks from the word bank: (not all words will be used)

Sandwich Generation	Empty Nest Syndrome	Stagnation	Climacteric	Midlife Crisis	Identity Accommodation

Joe, a single parent, is having difficulty dealing with stress since his last child moved away to college. This syndrome of feelings is known as _____ and can lead to social isolation. He is trying to find a new concept of himself which previously had been parent, cook, housekeeper, taxi driver, disciplinarian, and friend. This task of middle age is known as _____. Joe is concerned about financing his child's college education, concerned about the safety and continued maturation of his child when they leave his immediate care, and also concerned about the safety and well-being of his aged parents whom he has been helping to care for in their home in a neighboring community. Joe is in the _____ generation handling responsibilities of both his children and his parents and the health-care worker should evaluate all sources of stress for Joe in order to provide comprehensive care.

5. Mrs. A. is a 50-year-old female who has been experiencing symptoms that could indicate she is going through menopause. Choose the symptoms below that are *commonly* associated with this hormonal change: (select all that apply)

A. heavy vaginal bleeding.

B. headache.

C. significant weight loss.

D. hot flashes.

E. insomnia.

F. vomiting.

G. fatigue.

H. emotional lability.

Late Adulthood

http://evolve.elsevier.com/Leifer/growth

OUTLINE

OBJECTIVES

1. Discuss the major goals of *Healthy People 2030* as related to late adulthood.
2. Identify common health concerns of late adulthood.
3. Describe challenges and developmental tasks of late adulthood.
4. Discuss lifestyle changes that may be necessary for late adulthood.
5. Discuss the relationship of physical activity to the aging process and cognition.
6. Define elder abuse and describe one means by which it can be prevented.
7. Discuss the ways menopause may affect women in the late-adulthood phase of the life cycle.
8. List the learning needs of later adulthood.
9. Select appropriate teaching techniques to promote effective learning and coping for late adulthood.

KEY TERMS

assistive devices
autonomy
CAM therapy
competence

disengagement
elder abuse
HRT therapy
late adulthood

polypharmacy
relatedness
teaching moment

DEFINITION

For statistical and public administrative purposes, the U.S. government has traditionally defined old age as over age 65 or 67, when full Social Security benefits become available, retirement usually occurs, and a leisurely lifestyle is adopted (Britannica, 2020). It is interesting that definitions of old age are not consistent across all societies and countries who regard old age as occurring anywhere from the mid-40s to the 70s (Britannica, 2020) and Merriam-Webster (n.d.) does not place a specific chronological age in its definition of senior citizen, but rather defines it as "an elderly person especially one who has retired."

The Western default definition of late adulthood is considered as encompassing the ages between 65 and 74 years. This focuses on chronological age only and does not take into consideration the biological, employment and retirement, and sociological dimensions of older age (Britannica, 2020). Increased technology and improved health-care practices have enabled people to live longer and to remain active and productive. Today many people in the late-adulthood phase of the life cycle postpone retirement and remain active in the workforce as senior employees or part-time consultants.

Some health concerns of someone in late adulthood include:

- Development of osteoporosis
- Risks for falls and fractures
- Insufficient awareness of healthy behavior options
- Increased risk of influenza and pneumonia
- Development of cataracts
- Reduced hearing acuity

Health Promotion

Some of the major goals of *Healthy People 2030* for older adults are to increase the lifespan and the quality of life by focusing on wellness and healthy behaviors, prevention of illness, and treatment of disease. Reducing the number of illnesses and deaths related to vaccine-preventable illness, reducing the occurrence of hip fractures from unintentional injuries, and early diagnosis and management of dementia are priority goals for late adulthood.

Maximizing health as much as possible promotes mobility and independence. The older adult can develop meaning and enjoyment in life despite increasing physical limitations. *Healthy People 2030* goals related to independence include increasing the availability of certified specialists to care for the elderly, promoting housing and transportation services, and understanding and studying elder abuse.

STATISTICS

Americans are having fewer children and living longer. According to the Department of Health and Human Services (USDHHS, 2018), the number of Americans aged 65 or older grew by 49.2 million between 2006 and 2016, an increase of 33%. It is estimated that this population will continue to increase to 77 million by 2034 when older adults will outnumber children under the age of 18. Additionally, by 2060 we expect to have over 98 million people in this age group. In less than 15 years, the graying of America will be inescapable (Vespa, 2019). Table 13.1 shows population and poverty level statistics for the elderly population in the United States according to the 2016 Population Survey and American Community Survey.

Income

The income sources for older persons in the United States include Social Security, pensions, income from assets, and earnings. Approximately 18.8% or 9 million Americans older than 65 years of age are still actively employed. More older Americans in this age group are working than at any time since the turn of the century (Pew Research Center, 2020). Approximately 4.6 million persons above age 65 were below poverty level with this increase being attributed to out-of-pocket medical expenses, and the 3% of this group requiring caregiver assistance in 2017. In the year 2017, 93% of persons above 65 years of

TABLE 13.1   2016 Age 65 and Over Population by State, Percent Increase 2006–2016, and Percent Below Poverty Level

State	Number of Persons 65 and Over	Percent of All Ages	Percent Increase from 2006 to 2016	Percent Below Poverty 2016
US total (50 States + DC)	49,244,195	15.20	32.50	9.30
Alabama	784,551	16.10	28.00	10.00
Alaska	77,206	10.40	65.60	4.20
Arizona	1,170,924	16.90	50.00	9.00
Arkansas	486,734	16.30	24.00	10.50
California	5,346,635	13.60	38.10	10.30
Colorado	743,524	13.40	55.00	7.60
Connecticut	577,403	16.10	21.20	6.50
Delaware	166,950	17.50	44.20	6.90
District of Columbia	78,691	11.60	19.40	13.40
Florida	4,094,917	9.90	36.30	10.40
Georgia	134,566	13.10	49.40	10.10
Hawaii	243,962	17.10	37.30	8.90
Idaho	254,989	15.10	48.70	10.00
Illinois	1,871,264	14.60	22.80	9.20
Indiana	991,563	14.90	25.90	7.70
Iowa	514,215	16.40	17.10	6.90
Kansas	436,993	15.00	21.70	8.00
Kentucky	690,717	15.60	28.30	11.10
Louisiana	674,443	14.40	30.90	13.00
Maine	257,683	19.20	32.40	9.10

TABLE 13.1   2016 Age 65 and Over Population by State, Percent Increase 2006–2016, and Percent Below Poverty Level (*Cont.*)

State	Number of Persons 65 and Over	Percent of All Ages	Percent Increase from 2006 to 2016	Percent Below Poverty 2016
Maryland	876,210	14.60	35.60	8.20
Massachusetts	1,074,964	15.80	26.30	8.50
Michigan	1,611,755	16.20	27.00	8.10
Minnesota	834,228	15.10	31.80	7.20
Mississippi	450,941	15.10	26.00	12.30
Missouri	978,021	16.10	24.80	8.20
Montana	185,040	17.70	39.50	8.90
Nebraska	286,744	15.00	21.60	7.80
Nevada	441,142	15.00	57.30	8.70
New Hampshire	226,804	17.00	39.90	4.60
New Jersey	1,372,612	15.30	22.10	8.30
New Mexico	342,426	16.50	40.40	11.50
New York	3,032,509	15.40	21.80	11.40
North Carolina	1,569,465	15.50	43.10	9.40
North Dakota	109,999	14.50	16.00	7.90
Ohio	1,886,629	16.20	22.40	8.10
Oklahoma	590,138	15.00	24.20	8.60
Oregon	688,878	16.80	42.80	7.50
Pennsylvania	2,223,721	17.40	17.50	7.80
Rhode Island	173,964	16.50	17.40	9.10
South Carolina	830,232	17.60	49.50	8.60
South Dakota	138,805	16.00	25.10	10.90
Tennessee	1,047,052	17.50	35.30	8.90
Texas	3,353,240	12.00	44.00	10.50
Utah	321,164	10.50	44.80	6.70
Vermont	112,932	18.10	35.20	8.70
Virginia	1,228,744	14.60	39.70	7.80
Washington	1,081,063	14.80	47.20	7.60
West Virginia	343,517	18.80	21.00	9.50
Wisconsin	928,418	16.10	26.70	7.60
Wyoming	87,812	15.00	38.00	8.50
Puerto Rico	645,887	18.90	26.30	38.10

Data from United States Department of Health and Human Services (USDHHS) Administration for Community Living (2018). *2017 Profile of older Americans*. Retrieved July 3, 2020 from https://acl.gov/sites/default/files/Aging%20and%20Disability%20in%20America/2017OlderAmericansProfile.pdf.

age were covered by Medicare with 53% having private health insurance. A total of 1% of persons over 65 had no health coverage (Pew Research Center, 2020). These statistics will undoubtedly change due to alterations to U.S. health-care laws that are continuously under debate for future implementation.

Education Level

As of 2015, approximately 84% of people over 65 years of age were high-school graduates and 34% of those were college graduates. In comparison, in 1965, only 5% of people 65 and older had completed a bachelor's degree or higher (Mather et al., 2019). This percentage varies somewhat by race and ethnic origin: 89% of Whites (not Hispanic), 89% of Asians (not Hispanic), 87% of African American (not Hispanic), and 67% of Hispanics had a high-school diploma (Ryan & Bauman, 2016).

LIVING ARRANGEMENTS

In 2017, 70% of men and 46% of women over 65 years of age were married, but widows accounted for 33% of all older women and there were three times as many widows as widowers. Half of noninstitutionalized persons over 65 live with their spouse, and 28% live alone. The percentage of persons who live alone increases with advancing age, with almost half of women over 75 living alone. One million grandparents over the age of 60 were primary caregivers of their grandchildren (Administration for Community Living, 2018). With the growing population of elderly adults, there is a need for living arrangements that promote safety and comfort, such as hallways and doorjambs wide enough to accommodate wheelchairs, handrails or grab bars and bath seats in bathrooms, elevated toilets, and single-story homes without staircases (Vespa, 2020). This increase in population of this age group will also lead to a greater than 50% increase in the number of Americans over 65 requiring assisted living or nursing home care (Mather et al., 2019).

Understanding these statistics enables the health-care worker to plan for the needs and limitations of the elderly population they serve in the twenty-first century. The living arrangements, support systems, income, and educational levels all influence the plan of care for the older person. The health-care worker can refer to the U.S. Department of Health and Human Services Administration on Aging for elder-care resources and other information concerning the geriatric population. The World Health Organization (WHO) has urged governments around the world to consider the health needs of the older adult in the general health programs of their countries.

CHALLENGES AND PROBLEMS

Several factors influence the health and well-being of older adults:
- *Access to health care:* Access to health care to maintain optimum physical and mental health may be blocked by lack of transportation or knowledge of community resources. When access to health care is blocked, preventive care is neglected, and health care is only obtained after an illness or disease develops.
- *Reduced income*: Reduced income is a problem for many older adults. Social security and pension incomes may not cover daily living and health-care expenses. Working past retirement age is a potential solution for some older adults. In 1986, age-based

mandatory retirement was abolished, but age discrimination remains a problem for those seeking new jobs.

- *Changes in living arrangements:* Adjusting to changes in living arrangements can also influence the physical and mental well-being of the older adult. Evidence suggests that living with extended family, or near family members, is optimal. As another option, assisted-living communities help the older adult maintain independence, social interaction, and a positive self-concept. Rent in these communities is much higher than the average rent in the surrounding area and may exceed the capacity of someone on a fixed income. Some older adults may live in inadequate housing, whereas others may be institutionalized in nursing homes and may lose independence and control over their lives.

- *Caregiver assistance:* According to the Centers for Disease Control and Prevention (CDC), the most common activities of daily living that require assistance by home health-care aides include body hygiene, bed-to-chair transfer, toileting, shopping, meal preparation, and light housework. Ambulatory-care clinics and home-care organizations can be helpful to the older adult.

- *Altered nutritional needs:* Dental problems, inability to cook, dislike of eating alone, pain or malaise because of a medical condition, or lack of accommodation for special needs related to cultural or religious food traditions may be causes for altered eating habits. Attention to diet and nutrition improves and maintains good health in the older adult. Caloric needs may decrease with age, but a balanced nutritional intake remains essential. Assessment of the nutritional needs of the older adult is vital, and community resources such as "Meals on Wheels" can be used.

- *Assistive devices:* Assistive devices may be needed to help the older adult maintain independent living. Assistive devices include such items as walkers, canes, respiratory equipment, hearing aids, and electronic emergency-response devices.

- *Preventing falls:* Preventing falls becomes more important as the older adult develops vision or hearing problems and slower response times. It is estimated that more than 25% of people aged 65 and older fall each year and medical costs of fall-related injuries total more than $50 billion annually (Burns & Ramakrishna, 2018). The use of certain medications can cause dizziness or imbalance that can also increase the vulnerability of the older adult to falling. The health-care worker can assess the older adult's environment and can help with securing loose rugs, improving tracking on slippery floors, clearing general clutter, and improving lighting, especially near stairways. Installing handgrips in showers and tubs can also be instrumental in preventing accidents. Reaching for items on high shelves, changing light bulbs, going up and down stairs, and opening simple medicine bottles are some activities that may require assistance or improved safety strategies.

- *Polypharmacy:* The problem of polypharmacy arises with the use of medications by older adults. Polypharmacy is the ingestion of multiple medications in 1 day. Medications may be prescribed for various medical conditions or may be purchased over the counter. Drug-drug interactions, drug-food interactions, and drug-environment interactions (such as increased sensitivity to sun exposure) can occur. In older adults, the decreased ability of the liver and kidneys to excrete drugs from the body can result in an accumulation of the drugs to toxic levels. The older adult may forget to take a dose of medication or may accidentally take an extra dose and therefore may be undermedicated or overmedicated and prone to undesirable side effects. Patient monitoring and education are essential. The use of memory aids such as notebooks, electronic reminders, or labeled pill boxes may be helpful. Many older adults receive referrals to specialists resulting in multiple physicians managing their care rather than one who manages all their prescriptions. The use of the electronic health record is one measure to ensure all physicians caring for a person are aware of what medications have been prescribed.

- *Elder or dependent abuse:* Elder abuse affects more than 2 million older adults each year. Elder abuse is defined as the infliction of harm or neglect through actions or acts of omission. Abuse can be physical, emotional, or financial and can include neglect or obstruction of personal rights. The family or health-care worker can observe interactions between older adults and the caregivers and alert other family members to potentially abusive situations. Referral of the caregiver to community agencies for respite care may decrease the stress that can often lead to abuse.

PSYCHOSOCIAL DEVELOPMENT

There are many developmental tasks and related challenges for the older adult (Box 13.1). Older adults with healthy attitudes and coping skills typically do not mourn their lost youth but are able to find fulfillment and meaning in their lives despite health limitations. However, weight gain, dental problems, diminished eyesight and hearing, decreased mobility, and changes in body image are some issues that create difficulty. Older adults may show a readiness for learning if they recognize old age is near and they realize that physical health and life circumstances may change. Developing a healthy lifestyle and healthy behaviors with access to preventative care is a primary goal in the education and care of the older adult.

PSYCHOSOCIAL ISSUES

The social network of friends usually narrows for the older adult because of the death of peers. This may result in fewer social experiences unless older adults live in retirement communities or are connected with organized social activities specific for their age group. Remaining an integral part of an extended family provides valuable social activities and relationships, but family relationships are different than peer relationships.

Basic needs for autonomy (self-direction), competence (effective interactions), and relatedness (a sense of belonging) motivate social activities that enhance general well-being. An environment that helps meet these basic needs enables the older adult to maintain positive social interactions (Figure 13.1).

Complete dependency often does not support *autonomy, social competence,* or *relatedness* in satisfying ways unless the situation is specifically designed to aid in achieving these

---

BOX 13.1   Tasks and Challenges of the Older Adult

Older adults must adjust to the following:
- Menopause
- Retirement and redirection of goals and energy
- Decreased income
- Grandparenting
- Reentry into the job market

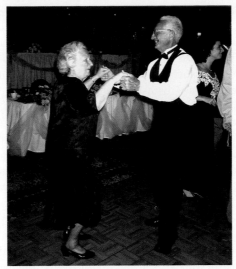

Figure 13.1 Social activities and positive social interactions enhance a feeling of well-being in the older adult.

goals. Many assisted-living facilities for older adults are designed to offer assistance while allowing the fulfillment of these three basic needs.

Grandparenting

The grandparenting role can be satisfying for the older adult, because it enhances self-image, increases activity level, creates feelings of self-worth and usefulness, and contributes to the meaning and quality of life. Many older adults may enjoy their grandchildren more because they know the children's parents will take over when they tire. Some older adults serve as volunteer adoptive grandparents to children in need or seek useful volunteer activities in the community. The role of the grandparent in the home can be a positive experience for grandchildren when healthy relationships between all generations are maintained.

It is when grandparents become ill or disabled that the roles can reverse, and the older adult needs more assistance. This role reversal can result in family stress and financial strain. Many families are not aware of community programs available for assistance with older adults and for caregiver support. Family education concerning the older adult's limitations and abilities can increase compassion and motivation to assist and improve verbal communication and the quality of the relationship. Health-care workers can educate and guide families concerning resources available to them before emotional stress, financial strain, caregiver burnout, and older adult alienation occur.

Postmenopause

Adjusting to the postmenopausal phase of life is an important developmental task of the older woman. Menopause is defined as the absence of menstruation for a period of at least 1 year (due to decline or cessation of hormonal production and function).

Menopause is not a disease or illness; it is a natural occurrence in the life cycle. Most women eventually adjust to the changes in estrogen levels that occur during menopause, but for those whose symptoms persist, discomforts and risks associated with the post-menopausal phase can be averted with healthy lifestyles and access to preventative medical care. Some discomforts associated with postmenopause include genital atrophy, vasomotor instability, heart disease, breast cancer, or osteoporosis. Hormone replacement therapy (HRT) was designed to relieve some of these discomforts, but controversy exists concerning the safety and advisability of routine HRT. Complementary and alternative medical (CAM) therapies are also available when HRT is not recommended. *Complementary therapy* refers to nontraditional therapies, such as relaxation or biofeedback, which are used with traditional therapy. *Alternative therapy* refers to nontraditional therapy, such as herbs and oils, which are used instead of traditional therapy. A healthy lifestyle is essential. See Chapter 3 for cultural aspects of aging. The *Physician's Desk Reference for Herbal Medicines* can be used as a guide in helping the older patient evaluate complementary therapies that they may choose to use.

Simple lifestyle changes for women experiencing menopausal and postmenopausal symptoms include the use of water-based gels or lubricants. The use of CAM therapy such as herbal supplements to prevent the development of depression requires close evaluation for possible interaction with prescribed medicines or other treatments.

Decreases in estrogen often cause vaginal wall thinning and urine leakage when sneezing or laughing. Panty liners, pads, and adult protective undergarments can be of help in handling these embarrassing problems that can otherwise cause the woman to self-isolate.

Driving Safety

Many adults over age 65 may have early undetected impairments that can affect their safety on the roads. Occupational and physical therapy can help maintain driving safety and delay loss of their driver's licenses, but when driving is no longer safe, the license must be relinquished. Counseling concerning other methods of transportation available within their community is essential. Isolation, loneliness, stagnation, inadequate nutrition, or depression may occur if alternative transportation options are not offered.

Health Screenings

Health screenings can identify developing health issues in early stages and can lead to early interventions and prevention of greater difficulties. Screenings should include dental and eye checkups and a general physical evaluation. It is useful to assess for substance abuse, overmedication or polypharmacy, sexual dysfunction, urinary incontinence, and other indications that lifestyle changes are necessary. Referral for dental care or community services such as "Meals on Wheels" may be an option to assist in the maintenance of nutrition if transportation is an obstacle. Screenings currently recommended by the United States Preventative Services Task Force (USPSTF) (2020) for this age group with a grade of A or B (A: The USPSTF recommends the service with high certainty that the net benefit is substantial. B: The USPSTF recommends the service with high certainty that the net benefit is moderate or there is moderate certainty that the net benefit is moderate to substantial) are:

- Screening for depression, elder abuse, and/or intimate partner violence
- Screening for high blood pressure

- Screening for fall risk and need for exercise interventions to prevent falls
- Asking questions about unhealthy drug or alcohol use or smoking in adults age 18 or older
- Screening for hepatitis C in adults aged 18–79
- Screen for the need for interventions for weight loss if body mass index is 30 or higher
- Abnormal blood glucose up to age 70 for those who are overweight or obese
- Screen for the need for cholesterol reducing medications if age 40–75 and have a risk factor for cardiovascular disease
- Screening for osteoporosis with bone measurement testing in women 65 and older
- Screening for colorectal cancer until age 75
- Biennial screening mammography for women until age 74
- One-time screening for abdominal aortic aneurysm with ultrasound in men aged 65–75 years who have ever smoked
- Screening for lung cancer in adults aged 55–80 with a 30 pack-year smoking history and have smoked within the past 15 years
- Screening for prostate cancer in men up to age 69 years is based on individual preference

Health Promotion

Assessing for alcohol abuse is an important aspect of health screening. A quick and simple assessment tool for alcohol abuse is the CAGE questionnaire, which includes four simple, nonjudgmental questions regarding the patient's feelings about his or her drinking or drug-specific habits. Two affirmative answers to the specific questions related to alcohol intake may indicate a need for further evaluation or follow-up (Ewing, 1984). The National Council on Alcohol and Drug Dependence states that up to 11% of elderly hospital admissions are related to drug and alcohol-related issues and 10%–15% of people do not start to drink heavily until they are at an older age (National Council for Aging Care, 2020). Persons in this age group are already at increased risk for falls or traffic accidents and the use of alcohol compounds that risk since it slows reaction times, decreases coordination, interferes with eye movement, and slows the processing of information (NIH, 2017). Additionally, persons in this age group often take more than one type of medication, and alcohol can be dangerous or even deadly when added to this mix (NIH, 2014). Because seniors often have less muscle mass, slower intestinal transit time, and less body water content, they are more susceptible to the effects of alcohol that can damage the liver, increase overall blood pressure, weaken bones, worsen diabetes, and memory or mood disorders (National Council for Aging Care, 2020).

Sexuality

As people age, specific changes in sexual responses occur. However, the notion that the older adult is sexually inactive is untrue. Some older adults may feel guilty or abnormal because they continue to have sexual feelings. The most common cause of sexual dissatisfaction is the lack of a partner. In this age group, divorces, widowhood, or ill or disabled spouses are common problems. Men may develop erectile dysfunction, which is now treatable with a high rate of success. Painful intercourse (dyspareunia) for women may be the result of atrophy of the vaginal wall and a decrease in natural lubrication. Both problems can be easily overcome.

Health Promotion

HRT or CAM therapy can alleviate menopausal symptoms that interfere with sexual pleasure. A health-care provider must evaluate the suitability of HRT for individual patients before determining the appropriate approach to care. Sex therapy is available and can be helpful. The main obstacle in maintaining a healthy sexual lifestyle is the tendency to avoid talking about it because of embarrassment. Therefore, it is the health-care worker's responsibility to assess sexual functioning in older men and women as part of routine screening and preventative care.

Memory Loss

The older adult experiences memory changes, particularly in remembering names and faces of people. Normal memory loss can be associated with aging, and temporary memory loss can be caused by depression or anxiety. Preclinical manifestations of Alzheimer disease are a common worry when normal memory loss becomes increasingly noticeable (Boxes 13.2 and 13.3).

Health Promotion

Active lifestyles that routinely exercise memory skills are thought to help maintain memory function. Perhaps this is another "use it or lose it" phenomenon. However, studies have shown that older adults need more time to process thoughts and perform tasks than younger adults (APA, 2020). Knowledge or information that is deeply processed rather than superficially memorized will be remembered longer. There is a growing trend of adults over 65 adopting technology, particularly those who are younger, more affluent, and more highly educated. About 40% of seniors own smartphones and 32% own tablet computers (Anderson & Perrin, 2017). Along with the adoption of technology comes the use of the Internet and social media to find news and information, connect with friends and family, learn new skills, read books, and play memory games (Anderson & Perrin, 2017). Declines in memory are not necessarily inevitable; see Table 13.2 for a summary of memory decline resulting from normal aging compared with depression or dementia.

BOX 13.2   Warning Signs of Problematic Memory Decline

- Memory loss affecting job functioning
- Difficulty remembering steps in familiar tasks
- Disorientation
- Lack of awareness of time, place, or date
- Decrease in abstract thinking (increased need for concreteness)
- Associated problems with mood, language, or personality changes

BOX 13.3 Preventable Causes of Memory Problems

- Drug toxicity
- Depression
- Metabolic problems (kidney or liver dysfunction, hypoglycemia)
- Sensory problems (difficulty hearing, seeing, or sensing information)
- Nutritional deficiencies (dehydration, vitamin B12 deficiency, iron deficiency)
- Illness (pneumonia and other infections)

TABLE 13.2 Memory Decline Resulting From Normal Aging, Depression, or Dementia

Normal Age-Related Memory Decline	Depression-Related Memory Problems	Dementia-Related Memory Problems
Onset age specifically identifiable	Onset with depression	Difficult to establish onset
Slow progression of symptoms	Rapid or sudden progression of symptoms	Slow or stepwise progression
History of depression less common	History of depression less common	History of depression less common
Complains about memory loss	Complains about memory loss	Usually unaware of memory loss
May emphasize disability	May emphasize disability	Conceals disability
May decrease or increase efforts to perform	Decreases effort to perform	Struggles to perform
Uses notes and other memory aids	May not try to keep up	Needs instruction to use memory aids
No lasting mood change associated	Consistent depressive mood	Emotional lability and shallowness
Behavior may or may not change	Behavior change is greater than impairment	Behavior change may be appropriate for the impairment
Nocturnal drop in performance unusual	Nocturnal drop in performance unusual	Nocturnal drop in performance common
"Don't know" answers common	"Don't know" answers common	Guesses or "near miss" answers common
Recent and remote memory losses are equal	Recent and remote memory losses are equal; memory gaps for specific events common	Recent memory impaired, remote is intact; memory gaps for specific events unusual

Emotional Health

Emotions and emotional control develop during the growth and development process, as a person copes with the challenges in each phase of the life cycle. Earlier theorists believed disengagement was a task of the older adult. This implies that removing emotional attachments to people, places, and objects is part of the natural aging process. This may be true of the depressed older adult but is likely not a natural or healthy process. The aging healthy adult does not naturally disengage. Instead he or she continues emotional learning and emotional competencies. Past experiences from the long lives of older adults may influence their expression of emotional responses.

Cultural Considerations

Culture and expectations play a role in the emotional status of the older adult. In cultures with close families, more respect and inclusion in the lives of their families, or maintenance of communication and relationships with their families, will encourage and maintain emotional competencies and enhance quality of life for older adults.

Depression

Depression should not be automatically expected to appear in the older adult. In some older adults, depression occurs as a continuation of a negative attitude from young adulthood. A young person who looks at life's events in a pessimistic way may be vulnerable to developing depression as an older adult. However, late-onset depression (or a change in personality) may be attributed to changes in the brain itself. The traditional symptoms of depression as listed in the *Diagnostic and Statistical Manual of Mental Disorders, Fifth Edition (DSM-V)* criteria for diagnosis of major depression are more accurate for older adults than they were in previous editions of the DSM, but care must still be taken to note differences in this population (Khoury et al., 2020). Older adults may be taking medications for various medical conditions that have side effects that mimic depression. Several factors increase the vulnerability of the older adult to depression. Chronic poor health can lead to stress, decreased activity, and fewer social interactions, which can trigger depression. Prescribed treatment of the medical conditions can induce changes that result in a deepened depression. Depression itself in turn can also trigger physical illness.

Patient Teaching

Helping the older adult manage stressful life events, strengthening coping strategies, and providing social support can help avoid the development of depression for many older adults. Any person who first develops depression as an older adult usually has experiences and coping styles that can be used by a professional therapist in individual or group sessions to help treat the depressive symptoms. Providing access to mental health care and early screening for the presence of risk and depressive symptoms can empower older adults to be in control of their own emotions.

The American Psychiatric Association (APA) Division of Clinical Psychology and the American Association of Geriatric Psychiatry have developed evidence-based practice guidelines that recommend specific treatments for a variety of psychological problems. Evidence-based practices for treatment and services to improve outcomes for older adults experiencing depression are available for download at https://store.samhsa.gov/product/Treatment-Depression-Older-Adults-Evidence-Based-Practices-EBP-Kit/SMA11-4631.

Obstacles in accessing or using available mental health-care resources have led to the emergence of self-help techniques that are available to all at low cost. Self-help resources include books and support groups led by clergy, peer counselors, and others who advertise their successes. Many psychologists recommend CAM therapy treatments to supplement their therapies such as breathing exercises, use of music, Qi gong, Tai Chi, meditation, acupressure, and mindful yoga. The combination of various types of interventions has been embraced by the interdisciplinary Society for the Exploration of Psychotherapy Integration (SEPI). This and other professional networks, such as the Association for Behavioral and Cognitive Therapies (ABCT) and Anxiety and Depression Association of America (ADAA) organizations, offer conferences and newsletters on effective mental health care. The American Association of Retired Persons (AARP) is also an advocate for the older adult regarding education for healthy living.

CLINICAL DISEASE

Good health in older people is often defined as the absence of disease or disability. However, normal body changes resulting from aging, such as ovarian failure or menopause, place a risk on the cardiovascular, skeletal, and metabolic systems. This occurs at a time when emotional stress may increase because of other life changes. Most older persons have at least one chronic condition and many have multiple conditions. In 2015, the top five reported chronic conditions were hypertension (58%), hyperlipidemia (48%), arthritis (31%), heart disease (29%), and diabetes (27%) (USDIHIS, 2018).

 Lifespan Considerations

The combination of subclinical cardiovascular changes associated with aging and the response to stressful life events can affect the risk factors for the development of a clinical disease. Individuals who characteristically suppressed their emotions in young adulthood and held a pessimistic view toward life events may be at a higher risk for clinical disease as they age. This may indicate that prevention of disease in the older adult lies partially in the development of positive attitudes and coping skills.

PHYSICAL ACTIVITY

Numerous changes occur with age including metabolic function, cardiac function, muscular strength, and bone structure. Many of these changes occur regardless of physical-activity levels, but exercise can significantly slow the aging process, increase life expectancy, and reduce mortality (Mandsager et al., 2018).

Resting metabolic rate decreases with age, so fewer calories are burned during a resting state. Without adjustments in food intake and energy output (exercise), this metabolic shift is likely to result in weight gain. Regular aerobic exercise increases caloric expenditure, which helps maintain a caloric balance. Examples of light-to-moderate intensity aerobic activities for seniors include walking, swimming, dancing, bicycling, tennis, and various aerobic exercise classes.

Muscle-strengthening exercises can increase the amount of metabolically active muscle tissue, or at least slow the decreases in muscle mass that often come with age and a sedentary lifestyle (Butler-Browne et al., 2018). Decreases in muscle mass during aging impact daily functioning and eventually impede independence and reduce quality of life. Regardless of age or initial strength level, improvements can be achieved through regular muscle-strengthening activities. Muscle-strengthening exercises for seniors can include carrying groceries, yoga, Tai Chi, heavy gardening, and exercises with weights or exercise bands. Regular balance exercises such as practicing walking backward and sideways in a safe environment can result in fewer falls, which is a significant danger for the elderly population. Stronger muscles and joints reduce the risk of falling and decrease the likelihood and severity of injury if there is a fall, which is a significant danger for the elderly population.

There is evidence that physical activity has a protective effect on cognitive function in the older population (Reas et al., 2019). Habits of physical activity may be used in the future to aid in the battle of causes of cognitive decline such as Alzheimer disease and other types of dementia.

An active person entering late adulthood can and should continue his or her level of physical activity. Older adults should continue, when possible, to achieve the same guidelines as those in middle adulthood. A total of 2 ½ hours of moderate-to-vigorous physical aerobic activity spread throughout the course of a week is a baseline goal for adults of all ages. When that baseline is achieved, the guidelines shift to encourage 5 hours per week, with vigorous exercise counting as double (1 minute of vigorous exercise equals 2 minutes of moderate exercise). More benefits can be achieved with more vigorous activity levels.

Many people entering late adulthood have spent years or even decades at varying levels of a sedentary lifestyle, and as a result have a very low level of fitness. As the aging process begins to threaten their independence, physical activity becomes an essential component for an elderly person to maintain cardiac and muscle function, balance, and range of motion. A combination of aerobic training and resistance training can slow the aging process and maintain good quality of life.

Seniors with extremely low levels of fitness can achieve a significant training response even from low-intensity training. Improvements can be seen even when the heart rates reach only 100 beats per minute during periodic 10-minute exercise sessions. Higher exercise heart rates will elicit stronger training responses.

TEACHING TECHNIQUES

Human growth and development occur in a sequential pattern, and developmental tasks are often related to the phases or stages within these patterns. Therefore, within any stage or phase of development there can be a wide variation of abilities that are mastered. A person's ability and readiness to learn depends on his or her stage of development; physical, psychological, and social health; support systems and environmental stress; and personal motivation. It must be noted, however, that chronological age is not a specific indicator of stage of development.

A *teaching moment* has been defined as the point at which the learner is most receptive to change or growth within a situation (Havighurst, 1974). The learner must be motivated to learn, and the teaching must be relevant to the learner and appropriate to the developmental stage and abilities of the learner. For the older adult, learning is enhanced if mutual respect exists between teacher and learner. The teacher should recognize and appreciate the lifelong accomplishments of the older adult, should be nonjudgmental, and should foster an environment conducive to learning. Visual aids should include large print in a bright color. Visual decline in the older adult often causes color distortions, so medications or pills should not be referred to by color.

Hearing loss in the older adult usually affects perception of high-pitched sounds or rapid speech. Shouting or raising the volume is not helpful. With use of face coverings in the community and within health facilities, people of all ages find speech reception to be an increased challenge. Masks degrade speech quality. This, in combination with ambient noise and the absence of visual cues that are a large part of speech recognition, can make speech close to unintelligible for seniors with existing reductions in hearing (Goldin et al., 2020). Speaking clearly and slowly, making eye contact while speaking, wearing lipstick (to assist visual perception) when a mask is not being worn, intentional use of body language, and using an interactive style to obtain feedback from the older adult will assist with communication and confirm that the information conveyed was received and understood.

Scheduling short teaching sessions enables the older adult to concentrate and absorb all the information throughout the session without losing concentration due to fatigue or other interference, such as having to use the restroom. During educational sessions, the teacher can counteract avoidance or denial of the need to change lifestyle practices by validating the older adult's experiences and needs and by limiting topics to those related to here and now. Relating learning topics to autonomy, social acceptability, and strong coping skills can boost learning effectiveness. Repetition of information helps encode information into long-term memory, especially if memory skills are in decline. Presenting information in different ways, visually, verbally, and experientially (hands-on), can also be an important aid to learning. However, repetition of material already known by the older adult can discourage him or her from feeling motivated to learn.

Health Promotion

Important goals in managing the aging process include preventing illness and disability, maintaining cognitive functioning, and maintaining an active and healthy lifestyle. Assessment for cardiovascular risks; nutritional needs; bone density; visual, hearing, and memory loss; depression; and specific concerns of the individual are helpful in developing a meaningful teaching plan for the individual. Decreasing stress and maintaining a positive attitude are essential to successful living (Figure 13.2).

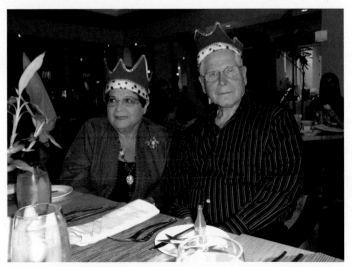

Figure 13.2 Older adults find pleasure in celebrating holidays and life events with others.

KEY POINTS

- A *Healthy People 2030* goal for the older adult is to increase the lifespan and quality of life by focusing on wellness and preventive care.
- Some health challenges for the older adult include managing on a reduced income, adjusting to changes in living arrangements, accessing preventive health care, maintaining nutrition, and preventing accidents.
- Elder abuse is the infliction of harm or neglect through actions or acts of omission and can be physical, emotional, financial, or include omission of personal rights.
- Menopause is not a disease; it is a natural occurrence in the life cycle.
- Health screenings for the older adult may include dental and vision checkups; screening for breast or prostate cancer; checking blood glucose and lipid levels; weight and blood pressure monitoring; and alcohol and depression screening.
- The most common cause of sexual inactivity in the older adult is loss of a partner.
- Keeping an active mind and lifestyle can enhance memory performance in the older adult.
- Exercise prescriptions for older adults should include aerobic exercise, muscle-strengthening exercise, flexibility exercise, and exercise to improve balance to prevent falls.
- Seniors with low levels of fitness can achieve a significant response from low-intensity exercise. The frail elderly can achieve benefits of exercises performed in a chair.
- An older adult can benefit from the use of memory aids such as lists or calendar notes.
- Basic needs for autonomy, social competence, and relatedness in the older adult motivate continued social interactions and prevent isolation and disengagement.
- Several factors cause older adults to be vulnerable to developing depression.
- Providing access to mental health care, early screening, and a combination of social and psychological interventions can help avoid the development of depression in the older adult.
- Specific teaching techniques can enhance the learning process for the older adult.

Clinical Judgment Case Study

Mr. Smith is a 72-year-old widower. He is generally in good health, but his eyesight is declining from complications related to adult-onset diabetes. His primary care doctor has recommended that he have a screening colonoscopy that requires sedation. Because of the sedation requirement, Mr. Smith will need someone to drive him home from the appointment and stay with him until he is fully recovered. Mr. Smith does not have any friends or neighbors willing to do this and his children live out of state. What are some challenges people face in this stage of life that make preventive health-care practices more difficult? Would you also be concerned about the effects of social isolation on Mr. Smith? Why or why not?

REVIEW QUESTIONS

1. Which of the following people would be considered to be in late adulthood? (select all that apply)

   A. A 50-year-old woman who has just become a grandmother.

   B. A 70-year-old man who is actively working at a large company.

   C. A 45-year-old man who had a stroke and relies on a wheelchair.

   D. A 72-year-old woman who is bedridden.

   E. A 55-year-old man who is retired.

2. Older adults face many challenges. Write the letter corresponding to the appropriate description for each challenge.

Challenge	Description
Access to health care	
Reduced income	
Changes in living arrangements	
Caregiver assistance	
Altered nutritional needs	
Assistive devices	
Preventing falls	
Polypharmacy	
Elder abuse	

   A. Using a hearing aid.

   B. Retired and struggling to live on Social Security.

   C. An emergency room (ER) doctor prescribes a medication that interacts with a medication she is already on.

   D. Cannot drive herself to a doctor's appointment.

   E. A caregiver is stealing jewelry from a drawer.

   F. Having a nurse come in daily to help with showering.

   G. Moving in with an adult son for help with self-care.

   H. Unable to chew fibrous food.

   I. Removing loose rugs and small objects from the floor.

3. Identify which case study (A, B, or C) belongs in each column.

Normal Age-Related Memory Decline	Depression-Related Memory Problems	Dementia-Related Memory Problems

   A. Mrs. G. is a 73-year-old female who lives at home with her spouse. Her children visited her for her birthday and took her to her favorite restaurant where they celebrated with food and cake. Later that evening, the family was discussing the event and Mrs. G. became upset. When asked why, she stated she was "mad that everyone went to her favorite restaurant without her."

   B. Mr. C. is a 68-year-old who was recently asked to retire from his long-term job. His job performance had been declining since his wife of 34 years passed away 6 months prior. He had been missing work days and not meeting deadlines, complaining that he "forgot" when they were due.

C. Mr. P. is a 74-year-old retired life insurance salesman. In his career, he was successful due to his ability to remember names, faces, and life circumstances of his customers, which made them feel comfortable doing business with him. He became aware of a slow decline in this ability beginning 5 years prior and compensated by keeping little notes in his pocket with details about a person he met so he could refer to them before meeting with them again.

4. Match the causes of falls and ways to prevent them.

Cause of Falls **Ways to Prevent Falls**
Dizziness or imbalance
Living environment
Slipping or tripping during toileting or bathing
Tripping on staircases

A. Install safety ramps in exterior entryways or mechanical lifts.

B. Assess flooring for loose rugs, clutter, or poor lighting.

C. Assess medication side effects and explore alternatives with reduced effect on balance.

D. Install handgrips, shower chairs, elevated toilets, and increased lighting.

5. For each blank, select all appropriate options from the list.

Mrs. A. lives alone in an apartment with few neighbors her age. She has been losing weight recently. A home health visit may reveal common causes of weight loss in the older population as related to (1)_____. _____. Her caloric needs are (2)_____. _____ with age, but intake based on (3)_____. _____ diet is essential for health and wellness. Suggestions to assist Mrs. A. maintain her nutritional status might be (4)_____. _____.

1. A. depression; B. dental problems; C. social isolation; D. medical conditions

2. A. increased; B. decreased; C. unchanged

3. A. a nutritionally balanced; B. an exclusively high protein; C. an exclusively low residue

4. A. to arrange a consult with a nutritionist; B. to contact Meals on Wheels; C. provide references to local senior groups in her area; D. suggest she see her primary care doctor to assess for medical conditions or dental problems

Advanced Old Age and Geriatrics

http://evolve.elsevier.com/Leifer/growth

OUTLINE

OBJECTIVES

1. Explain the concept of geriatrics.
2. Discuss the anticipated future increase in the advanced old-age population as related to the development of geriatrics as a specialty.
3. Discuss theories of the aging process.
4. State four normal physiological changes that occur in the geriatric adult.
5. Discuss the sexuality needs of the geriatric adult.
6. Name three psychological changes or challenges that occur in the geriatric adult.
7. Discuss three specific psychosocial problems associated with aging.
8. List the major developmental tasks of the geriatric adult.
9. List four specific health-promoting activities for the geriatric adult.
10. Discuss the role of diet, exercise, and stress management in achieving the goals of *Healthy People 2030* in relation to the older adult.
11. Discuss various modifications of the environment necessary for the geriatric adult.
12. State four factors to consider when helping to select a nursing home for placement.
13. Discuss alternatives to nursing-home care.
14. Define activities of daily living.
15. Discuss principles of elder care and the role of the health-care worker.
16. Discuss the teaching needs of the geriatric adult.

KEY TERMS

activities of daily living (ADLs)	atrophy	geriatrics
aging in place	biological clock	immune theory
ageism	disengagement	osteoporosis
Alzheimer disease	elder abuse	senescence
apoptosis	free radical	wear-and-tear theory

DEFINITION

Some define advanced old age according to chronological age or physiological decline. Others define advanced old age as a time when psychological changes occur. For the purposes of statistics, old age is defined as above the age of 65–67, although there is variation in this definition as noted in Chapter 13. The term "seniors" is often preferred to the term "elderly," which carries connotations of fragility and dependency.

Senescence is described as a period in an older adult's life in which the body begins to age and weaken. It is considered a signal of the final stage or end of the lifespan. Senescence is a gradual process, and people age in different ways and at different rates. The health needs of advanced old age may differ slightly from those of late adulthood. For example, the incidence of chronic disease increases markedly after age 80. Social gerontologists have defined senescence in years, and it had been categorized into three periods (Dodig et al., 2019):

- Early-old: 60–75
- Middle-old: 76–90
- Late-old: 90 and older

Since aging is not a disease, the definition of old age varies as people live longer and health care improves. The ages in categories of old age are changing rapidly, and the long-standing standard definitions no longer reflect reality. Modern gerontologists list old age as when the prospects of living less than 15 more years is evident (Sanderson et al., 2017). The term *advanced old age* as used in this chapter refers to people over the age of 75 years.

Geriatrics is the study of a rapidly expanding age group and has become a specialty in the health-care field. Geriatrics includes the biological, psychological, physiological, and sociological aspects of aging. The goal in the care of an advanced old-age adult is to maximize the ability to function and to live independently and to shorten the period of illness and disability. *Healthy People 2030* topic areas and goals for the aged adult are listed in Box 14.1.

The United States Census Bureau (2011) reported that in 2010 there were 1.9 million Americans above the age of 90, which is triple the number from 1980 with projections to quadruple over the next four decades. By 2019, there were already 6.61 million Americans of age 85 and over (2.38 million males, 4.23 females) (Duffin, 2020). The 90-and-older population is growing and the majority report one or more disabilities, residency in a nursing home or living alone, and possession of a high-school diploma. They are more likely to be women (2.5% of the population 85 years old and over are female compared with 1.3% male) (U.S. Census Bureau, 2017) and have higher widowhood, poverty, and disability rates than people just under 90.

BOX 14.1   *Healthy People 2030* Topics and Goals for the Aged

The following *Healthy People 2030* goals are designed to increase the number of healthy, aged people who continue to enjoy life and to contribute to society:
- Provide access to preventive health services
- Manage chronic illnesses such as diabetes and heart disease
- Diagnose and manage dementias
- Encourage health-promotion activities such as increasing engagement in physical activity
- Reduce the use of nonessential medications
- Reduce the rate of hospital visits for pneumonia, urinary tract infections, diabetes, falls, and pressure ulcers
- Increase hearing and vision screening and care
- Train caregivers for the elderly
- Improve housing, transportation, and coordination of care

Data from United States Department of Health and Human Services (2020) *Healthy People 2030*. Retrieved from https://health.gov/healthypeople

---

There are many who make significant contributions and achievements in their old age, including Nola Ochs who earned her master's degree in history at the age of 98. Yuichiro Miura summited Everest at the age of 80, and Leonid Hurwicz received the Nobel Prize in economics at the age of 90 (Coxwell, 2017).

THEORIES OF THE AGING PROCESS

The process of aging occurs as a result of multiple factors, including the genetic life-span of cells. The past lifestyle, level of activity, dietary practices, and social support all play roles in the process of aging as well. Selected theories concerning the aging process follow.

CELLULAR CHANGES

Free Radicals

Ions travel in pairs within cells and are stable. For example, sodium and chloride are paired in the cell as sodium chloride (salt). Oxygen atoms are similarly paired to make O_2. When one ion breaks off and is no longer paired, it becomes a free radical. Free radicals are unstable and seek other atoms or molecules to bond to. Oxygen, in particular, will bond to other molecules and create what is known as a reactive oxygen species or ROS. This begins a process called oxidative stress that damages the body's cells, DNA, and mitochondria, which cannot be repaired. The numbers of free radicals in people increase as they age (Gladyshev, 2014).

Biological Clock (Programmed Cell Death)

Also known as apoptosis, the membrane surrounding a cell starts breaking down. As this process continues, the debris is phagocytized (eaten) by surrounding cellular materials.

This biological clock process dictates the occurrence of menopause in women and contributes to the body changes that ultimately result in death. Interestingly, the ovary is the only organ that appears to have a "programmed senescence in adult life that leads to predictable complete loss of function during aging in all human populations" (Patton, 2018).

Wear-and-Tear Theory

The wear-and-tear theory can be equated with a machine. Just as the parts in a machine begin to wear out or break down, so too does the human body. With humans, not all parts are so easily replaced or repaired. An example would be the ease and frequency of hip or knee replacement surgery versus heart transplantation (Vanhaelen, 2019).

Immune Theory

As one ages, the body finds it more difficult to tell the difference between healthy and defective cells, and the body responds by destroying both types. Immune theory states that the end result is that the body's immune response is impaired, which causes the aging person to be more susceptible to a variety of illnesses or infections as well as being susceptible to the body's immune cells attacking normal body cells (autoimmune response) (Queen et al., 2020; Trzewikoswki de Lima & De Gaspari, 2019). Decreased immune function of the thymus gland, lymph nodes, spleen, and bone marrow are also thought to be contributing factors to immune-system impairment (Zugich, 2018).

There are additional theories of aging such as the disposable soma theory, the historical theory of aging, the telomere shortening theory, and antagonistic pleiotropy theory (Vanhaelen, 2019), which are all beyond the scope of this text. Regardless, aging occurs not because of one of these events, but a combination of many.

Cellular damage or decline during a number of years results in the activation of the stress responses in the body in an attempt to repair what it can. When the body is unable to repair itself as efficiently as it did in the past, changes occur in the various body systems.

PHYSIOLOGICAL CHANGES

Bones and Cartilage

The loss of body water and bone mass and the degeneration of spinal disks result in a decrease in height during the aging process. A decrease in muscle mass, loss of body water, and increase in fat deposits occur after age 65 as a result of the aging process as well as from decreased physical activity (Amarya et al., 2018). Collagen in the body becomes rigid, and elastin in the body becomes brittle. These substances facilitate regeneration, support, and transport of material between cells, and the changes that occur during the aging process result in decreased function of the cells.

The loss of estrogen decreases the ability of the body to use calcium to maintain bone density. Loss of bone mass can result in osteoporosis, which is a thinning of the bone. This predisposes the geriatric adult to bone fractures. Posture and balance may change, and falls become a common problem.

Blood Vessels

Arterial walls thicken with fatty deposits and connective tissue resulting in a narrowing of the arteries. As a consequence, coronary arteries provide less oxygenated blood to the heart muscle. The heart muscle and muscle lining in the arteries become less elastic, making them stiffer and less resilient (Alvis & Hughes, 2016). Oxygen exchange slows, and blood pressure may rise to compensate for the lowered oxygen supply. These processes predispose the geriatric adult to the development of high blood pressure and blood pressure cannot adjust as quickly with position changes, which can result in dizziness, fainting, and stroke. It takes longer for the heart to beat faster in response to activity or stress, and therefore the observable response to pain, stress, or anxiety may be delayed. This means that the health-care worker cannot rely on observing changes in the vital signs to determine the presence of pain, stress, or anxiety (Alvis & Hughes, 2016).

Lungs

The ribs and cartilage become more rigid, and thus the respiratory muscles have to work harder. Age-related osteoporosis and reduced height of the vertebrae result in a smaller chest cavity. Lung tissue loses elasticity, which adds to a decrease in lung volume. Surface area within the lung is also decreased, which impairs oxygen exchange. Geriatric adults may not breathe as deeply or cough as effectively and have decreased ability to swallow, making them more vulnerable to respiratory infections (Alvis & Hughes, 2016).

Kidneys and Bladder

Due to decreased blood flow and scarring that occurs over time, the kidneys filter the blood more slowly. This can result in a toxic accumulation of medication and other biological waste products in the blood. The kidneys are more susceptible to failure since their overall filtering capacity is reduced (Alvis & Hughes, 2016). Bladder capacity decreases, with urinary frequency as a common result. Urine leakage can happen when physical activity puts stress on the bladder causing incontinence. In men, an enlarged prostate may block the urethra, resulting in urinary frequency or complete obstruction of urinary flow. This obstruction of urinary flow is known as urinary retention and requires prompt medical intervention.

Metabolism

Many changes in metabolism that occur with aging can lead to retention of glucose (sugars) and lipids (fats). In addition, as muscle mass decreases, body fat tends to increase with aging, even if overall weight does not increase. This may causes changes in glucose and lipid metabolism (Chia et al., 2018). These changes place the geriatric adult at risk for developing cardiovascular disease and diabetes with elevated lipid and glucose levels (Leung et al., 2018), and over 50% of persons over 80 years of age develop impairments in glucose tolerance (Alvis & Hughes, 2016).

Digestion, Taste, and Smell

The decreased motility of the gastrointestinal system results in difficulty with swallowing, slower emptying of the stomach, and delays in movement of waste through the large intestine (Alvis & Hughes, 2016). Digestive enzymes also decrease, which can result in poor appetite and digestive disturbances. The replacement of taste buds with connective tissue leaves only about 40% of taste buds present by 75 years of age (Patton, 2018). Declining perception of salt, increased detection of bitter, and declining quantities of saliva make eating less interesting, which results in the loss of appetite (Amarya et al., 2018). More than 75% of people over the age of 80 have major impairment of their sense of smell. This decreased sense of smell can affect the quality of life and add to the loss of appetite (Amarya et al., 2018).

A reduced gag reflex increases the risk of choking, so the geriatric adult should cut their food into small bites, chew thoroughly, and eat slowly while sitting upright. Decreased *peristalsis* (a wavelike motion that causes intestinal contents to be moved through the gastrointestinal tract) can cause constipation and discomfort from gas. This discomfort often leads the older person to use laxatives and antacids, which may decrease nutrient absorption and contribute to other health problems.

Teeth

Tooth loss is common as the jawbone gradually shrinks and circulation to the gums decreases. The membranes inside the mouth become thin, smooth, dry, and less elastic. The remaining teeth often do not provide adequate chewing ability, as lifelong wear reduces cutting and grinding effectiveness (Lee et al., 2017). This influences nutritional intake and may also negatively affect self-image. As time passes, receding gums can lead to ill-fitting dentures and gum lesions (sores). Regular follow-up with a dentist is essential. Providing nutritious foods that are attractively prepared and easy to chew will help meet the nutritional needs of the geriatric adult.

Skin

As the body ages, the repair and replacement of skin cells takes longer. Because of the loss of subcutaneous fat and collagen, the skin becomes thinner, and *turgor* (elasticity) is poorer (Shanbhag et al., 2019). This makes the geriatric person more vulnerable to skin injury, and healing of skin wounds is slower. The thin, dry skin develops wrinkles and spotty pigmentation. The ability to perceive cold and hot sensations also decreases, and geriatric adults are at an increased risk for burns. Decreased sense of touch affects motor skills, hand grip strength, and balance (Amarya et al., 2018). A decrease in the number and function of sweat glands in the skin results in difficulty adjusting to changes in environmental temperature. Chilling (hypothermia) and heat exhaustion occur more easily.

Eyes

Loss of elasticity of the eyelids and reduction in fat around the eyeballs can result in lashes rubbing on the eye and watery irritated eyes. Reduction in tear production may also cause eye irritation. Cholesterol deposits may form a yellowish ring around the iris of the eye. A loss of cells in the optic nerve makes it more difficult to see details. Degradation to the eye's rod cells that perceive size, shape, and brightness reduces the ability to detect contrast making night driving difficult (Levine, 2019). The pupil of the eye opens and closes more slowly, so more time is needed to adapt visually to the surroundings when moving from light to dark areas. Cataracts develop in the lens of the eye, which further decrease vision in advanced old age (Fernandez et al., 2018). Cataract surgery is common for this age group and is successful in restoring vision in most cases.

Advancing age and diabetes are two of the risk factors for the development of glaucoma, which is atrophy of the optic nerve and increased intraocular pressure. Glaucoma is the leading cause of blindness, and the condition affects more than 60 million people in the world (Mancino et al., 2019). All adults should be periodically screened for the development of glaucoma. Diabetes can also contribute to the development of diabetic changes in the retina (the lining on the back of the eye) where the blood vessels become damaged from poor circulation (NIH, 2019). Age-related macular degeneration is a retinal degeneration that causes the loss of central vision in the geriatric adult. Some peripheral vision may be retained, and total blindness is rare.

Ears

Degenerative changes in the bones of the middle ear result in a decrease in hearing ability, and a significant loss of hair cells in the organ of corti in the inner ear results in difficulty in hearing certain frequencies of sound, especially the high tones (Patton, 2018). Untreated hearing impairment can have negative effects on mental, physical, and social well-being and therefore should be treated early; although loss is usually so gradual, many people do not realize the extent of their disability (Lohler et al., 2019).

Teaching Tip

When teaching patients with hearing loss, it is wise to ask them to repeat what was heard to ensure that clear communication and understanding is taking place.

Nervous System

Loss of brain function is one of the biggest concerns among seniors (Amarya et al., 2018). Neurons atrophy (decrease in size) and the brain's volume shrinks at a rate of approximately 5% per decade after the age of 40 (Alvis & Hughes, 2016). The transmission of impulses to the brain becomes sluggish. Because of the fatty deposits within the walls of the blood vessels, blood flow to the brain slows. Motor responses and reaction time to stimuli are delayed, and maintaining environmental safety is a challenge.

SEXUALITY

As people age, specific changes in sexual responses occur. However, it is a myth that the aged person ceases to desire or experience sexual intimacy or pleasure (APA, 2020). Part of the reason for this myth is that the concept of love and romance, as portrayed in the media, focuses more on the young adult and the relationship of sex to having children. People of advanced age may even feel guilty or abnormal because they recognize that they continue to have sexual feelings. Ageism is prejudicial attitude and discriminatory practices against older people, and assuming older people are asexual and have no interest in sexual pleasure is false (Dhingra, 2016). Aging without protest is becoming more popular today, with the older woman taking pride in maintaining her physical and mental competencies while allowing her face and body to show the natural consequences of age and experience.

Health Promotion

Medications are often prescribed for the geriatric patient without considering or educating the person about potential effects on sexual performance. Many medications prescribed for conditions common to the aged have inhibitory effects on sexual interest, arousal, and performance. To ensure compliance with the medication regimen, appropriate education about these effects must be an integral part of the overall provision of health care in the aging population. It is also important to instruct the aging adult about the prevention of sexually transmitted infections (STIs), which are on the rise in this age group. They are at risk because their immune systems are less able to combat infection, they are less likely to use condoms, may be dating more than one partner after divorce or death of a spouse, and often are reluctant to discuss the issue with their doctors (Harvard Health, 2018).

Personality and behavior are important dimensions in sexuality. According to the World Health Organization (2020), key conceptual elements of sexual health when viewed holistically are:

- Sexual health is about well-being; it involves respect, safety, and freedom from discrimination and violence.
- Sexual health depends on the fulfillment of certain human rights.
- Sexual health is relevant throughout the individual's lifespan including the young and the elderly.
- Sexual health is expressed through diverse sexualities and forms of sexual expression.
- Sexual health is critically influenced by gender norms, roles, expectations, and power dynamics.

Box 14.2 provides some details concerning the aging process and its effects on sexuality.

BOX 14.2   Factors That Influence Sexuality in the Geriatric Adult

ATTITUDE/INTEREST
- Previous life experiences
- Body-image perception
- Mental function
- Self-expectations and image promotion
- Social contact/isolation
- Environment/privacy

SEXUAL HEALTH
- Incontinence, urinary/fecal devices
- Reduction in mobility
- Impotence and menopause
- Chronic or terminal illness
- Medications and their side effects

Sexual Responses in the Aging Woman

Menopause, or climacteric, in women does not decrease sexual response. Because of varying hormone levels, women will notice dryness in the vaginal mucosa, hot flashes, and other assorted hormone-related body changes (Dhingra et al., 2016). Frequent sexual activity, use of creams and water-soluble lubricants in the vagina, exercise, proper nutrition, and soy supplements can be alternatives to hormone replacement therapy (HRT); HRT may be contraindicated in some women (NIH, 2017). Although the erotic responses of the nipple and clitoris do not decrease, the intensity of vaginal lubrication and tissue expansion during sexual arousal does decrease with age and can make sexual activity uncomfortable. This is primarily because of decreased levels of estrogen. The ability to achieve multiple orgasms continues, although the intensity is decreased. As part of a health-maintenance plan, women should continue to obtain regular health screenings.

Sexual Responses in the Aging Man

Testosterone production decreases between the ages of 40 and 60 but remains stable thereafter. This leads to a decrease in the size and firmness of the penis and reduced production, motility, and lifespan of sperm, although sexual interest remains (Dhingra et al., 2016). The ability to attain an erection may be delayed and requires increased physiological stimulation as men age. Anxiety may also contribute to increased delay or sexual dysfunction. After the erection is achieved it can be maintained for a longer period when compared with earlier years, but loss of erection after orgasm happens more quickly (NIH, 2017). The intensity of orgasm may be decreased, but the pleasurable response is usually retained.

A decrease in men's sexual function is similar to that in women and is referred to as the male climacteric. Some men experience similar symptoms of hot flashes, feelings of suffocation, and depression. These symptoms can usually be treated with hormonal replacement, such as testosterone, synthetic androgens, and in some cases estrogen (Patton, 2018).

The Impact of Illness on Sexuality

Cancer of the prostate is a risk, and preventive screening via periodic examinations, which may include prostate-specific antigen (PSA) blood levels and professional guidance, is recommended in this age group. Hormone treatments for cancer of the prostate can interfere with achieving and maintaining penile erection. Some men who have had surgery of the prostate gland experience retrograde ejaculation into the urinary bladder rather than out through the urethra.

After a heart attack, the aged patient is given extensive information about necessary dietary changes, but rarely are they or their partner educated about when to resume sexual activity (Illiades, 2019). Hospitals and nursing homes do not often address the sexual needs of the aged, and sexual opportunity, privacy, and programs are often absent from care plans (Metzger, 2017). Postoperative instructions concerning surgery that involve reproductive organs should include an understanding of the effects on sexuality and the options available to cope with these effects.

Patient Teaching

Health-care workers have the opportunity to discuss with patients the discomforts or problems with sexual functioning in the aging patient, in the postoperative patient, and in the perimenopausal and postmenopausal woman. Patients should be taught that maintaining physical activity can help them to enjoy erotic activity. Studies by Masters and Johnson (1976) explain that regular sexual activity with a partner, or through masturbation, also contribute to maintaining the capacity for sexual pleasure. Overeating, drinking alcohol, and a sedentary lifestyle all negatively affect sexual vigor (NIH, 2017). The normal alterations of aging may decrease, but they do not eliminate the ability to enjoy a satisfactory sex life.

The health-care worker should help the aged understand the normal changes and responses in their bodies to avoid misinterpretations. Intimacy is a lifelong need. For some, cuddling and caressing is all that is needed, whereas others prefer to form an increased intellectual and emotional closeness with friends and to develop interests that will meet their intimacy needs. Sexual concerns in the geriatric adult can be discussed with the health-care provider for assessment and intervention.

PSYCHOLOGICAL CHANGES

Throughout the life cycle, attractiveness and independence have a high value. The media and the marketplace encourage appearing eternally young at any cost. This, and other societal factors, can foster a negative self-image. Fortunately, the aging process is a gradual one that provides time for coping and adaptation to the physical changes that are evident as one grows older. Although aging is gradual, role changes may be abrupt. One partner may become the caregiver, decision-maker, and homemaker if the other becomes disabled. Major changes can be stressful and lead to feelings of insecurity or loss of self-worth. These various role adjustments require adaptation and acceptance. The health-care worker should assess for anxiety or depression in response to changing life situations. Geropsychology is a growing field within psychology that focuses on providing psychological interventions specific to this age group (APA, 2016).

Cultural Considerations

Culture also affects the aging process. In cultures where people of advanced old age are valued and respected, the feeling of self-worth contributes to general health. In cultures where people of advanced old age are avoided (ageism), a feeling of usefulness declines and depression can set in. Geriatric persons usually fear loss of independence and fear disability that will make them a burden to their families (APA, 2020).

The loss of friends, siblings, and spouse can result in loneliness. Disengagement is the process in which an older adult withdraws from social contacts and relinquishes independence and control to others (Crossman, 2020). A decline in income or self-care abilities may require relocation, and a new environment may intensify the feeling of loneliness. Some guidance may be needed to help the older person seek new relationships and

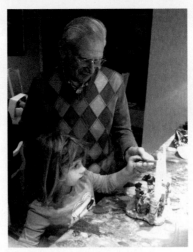

Figure 14.1 Grandparenting can be a source of satisfaction for the geriatric adult. The interactions benefit both the child and the grandparent.

activities that are enjoyable. Grandparenting can be a source of satisfaction if the children and grandchildren live nearby (Figure 14.1). People of advanced old age may take longer to learn new skills, because concentration and memory decline with advancing age (APA, 2020).

The development of dementias that involve cognitive impairments, including memory loss, loss of ability to communicate, and decreased functioning in social situations (such as Alzheimer disease) often leads to complete dependence on others. There are several organizations and resources that address the needs of older Americans and can aid with the diagnosis and management of persons with dementias, including the American Association of Homes and Services for aging and the Gerontological Society of America (GSA).

A White House Conference on this topic, held in 2005, focused on the theme of *The Dynamics of Aging: From Awareness to Action*, which suggested policies to Congress and the President concerning the needs of the aged population. A year later, the Older American Act of 2006 was passed, which provided services such as long-term care strategies, assistance with nutrition, interventions to combat social isolation, elder abuse prevention, and transportation assistance. This act was extended for an additional 5 years in 2020 (NCOA, 2020).

DEVELOPMENTAL TASKS

Mastering the crisis of ego integrity versus despair is the challenge of the older adult (see Chapter 5). Mastering the crisis of immortality versus extinction is the major task of advanced old age. Reflecting on their own accomplishments and legacies brings ego integrity and satisfaction to geriatric adults and implies successful mastery of the developmental tasks from previous stages of the life cycle.

Reminiscing about past experiences is therapeutic. If reflection about life's experiences brings feelings of unresolved conflicts and failures, then a feeling of despair will prevail, resulting in anxiety, bitterness, and perhaps even stress and illness. Ego integrity

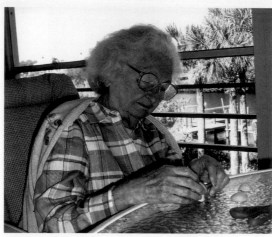

Figure 14.2 Older adults can engage in hobbies or activities that bring them pleasure and help maintain an active mind and body.

is achieved when reminiscing reveals satisfaction with past achievements and a sense of leaving a positive legacy or memories behind (Westerhof et al., 2017). If geriatric adults can focus on prioritizing activities that bring them pleasure, they can enjoy daily life.

A major developmental task of old age and sometimes advanced old age is adjusting to retirement. The work setting is no longer the center for maintaining a feeling of self-worth, so having a hobby or interest to pursue that offers a sense of fulfillment and satisfaction is essential in maintaining good mental health (Figure 14.2). Another developmental task for the advanced old age group is adjusting to and accepting the frailties of aging and the accompanying changes in physical appearance and lifestyles.

 Lifespan Considerations

Today better foods, safer surroundings, and high-tech medical care have extended lifespan expectations. However, lifestyle modifications that include exercise, a healthy diet, and stress management are essential to achieve this goal.

PHYSICAL EXERCISE

"Use it or lose it" is an old adage, and it is true. The losses in physiological functioning may be related to a lack of activity (Patton, 2018). Regular exercise promotes mental and physical health. In accordance with *Healthy People 2030* goals, regular exercise should be maintained as long as possible. With guidance, regular physical activity can be safe for healthy and frail older people and it reduces the risks of developing disease, muscular weakness, falls, and cognitive impairments (McPhee et al., 2016). Guidelines for physical activity for older adults are discussed in Chapter 13.

HEALTHY PEOPLE 2030 GOALS
OCCUPATIONAL ACTIVITIES

Adjusting to retirement from the life's work, and finding fulfillment and self-worth from part-time employment, volunteer activities, hobbies, or travel, can help maintain an active mind and body. This is often referred to as the *activity theory* and is related to a positive transition in the aging adult (HRF, 2020).

Nutrition

Maintaining adequate nutrition intake is important for health maintenance. There are challenges to overcome, such as dental loss, adaptation to dentures, slowed digestion, constipation, and a decline in the ability to buy or prepare nutritious meals. Many communities offer a Meals on Wheels service that delivers one meal a day to geriatric residents. Senior centers within the community often serve one meal a day as well, and this environment has the added advantage of providing socialization for older adults.

Prevention of Illness

Providing regular health checkups and follow-up for abnormal symptoms is essential for health maintenance. Immunizations recommended by the Centers for Disease Control and Prevention (CDC), such as the pneumococcal vaccine (pneumonia) and flu shots, are also advisable. For a list of recommended immunizations refer to the CDC's website at https://www.cdc.gov/vaccines/schedules/downloads/adult/adult-combined-schedule.pdf (CDC, 2020). Close monitoring of chronic illnesses such as heart disease, high blood pressure, arthritis, and visual disturbances is important. Providing access to regular medical care is often a challenge due to immobility, lack of transportation, and other factors. Most preventative health-care screenings are not routinely offered past the age of 75 since the likelihood of developing a new onset of a disease that might be detected by the screening exam often is less than the risk of the exam itself. However, with advancing medical technology and increasing opportunities to retain good health well into the eighth decade and beyond, health-care providers should weigh the benefits versus risks in offering screenings for breast, lung, skin, and colon cancer; osteoporosis; cardiovascular disease; and diabetes (USPSTF, 2020).

Mental Health

Late-life depression is the most common mental health problem in the geriatric age group. It is typically brought on by isolation from social contacts, change in environment, low self-esteem, loss of loved ones, and general loss of control over their life. Suicide is also common in this age group (Blackburn et al., 2017). Psychological counseling, establishment of social contact and support, and engaging in pleasurable activities on a daily basis help avoid the development of depression. To maintain mental health, the person of advanced old age must be realistic, use strengths and coping strategies to handle physiological changes, and set new goals that are positive and attainable.

Environmental Controls

Reducing the risk of falls and fractures can be achieved by providing a safe environment. For a list of recommended environmental controls to contribute to safe residency, see Placement Alternatives section.

Elder Abuse

Although the exact definition of elder abuse and exploitation varies somewhat depending on state statutes (USDOJ, n.d.), elder abuse is the intentional infliction of mental, sexual, emotional, or physical pain or the failure to provide the care necessary for optimal survival (i.e., neglect). Abuse may also be financial, misappropriating the elder person's income and savings. Dependency, frailty, illness, and metal disability may make the geriatric adult more vulnerable to abuse. When the caregiver is a family member, the combined effect of fatigue and overwhelming responsibilities to spouse,

(Continued)

Lifespan Considerations (*Cont.*)

children, job, and care of a geriatric adult may cause caregiver strain, which may result in some type of elder abuse (Pillemer et al., 2016). Health-care workers can intervene by offering resources for caregiver support, such as respite care, support groups, education, money management programs, stress management, and access to emergency shelters (Pillemer et al., 2016).

Signs of abuse may include depression, social isolation, clusters of bruises, unexplained burns, contractures, undernutrition, dehydration, and missed follow-up health-care appointments. All caregivers should be alert to elder abuse, because it may go unreported by the geriatric adult (USDHHS, 2016). Referral to adult protective services may be necessary, or placement in another environment may be advisable.

Polypharmacy and Medication Errors

Polypharmacy is the use of many medications prescribed for different chronic illnesses. The medications taken may interact with one another and may produce unwanted side effects. Complex medication schedules may contribute to the geriatric person having difficulty taking prescribed medications appropriately. Missing a dose or taking a double dose can result in toxicity and illness. Monitoring of medications is a priority in elder care and is an objective in *Healthy People 2030*. The decreased organ function found in advanced old age contributes to a delay in excretion of the drug from the body, and toxicity can also develop (Halli-Tierney et al., 2019). Drug dosages and effects need to be carefully monitored and explained to patients and their caregivers, and health-care workers should evaluate medication lists to consider discontinuing certain medications if the risks outweigh the benefits.

Placement Alternatives

When polled, 90% of people over the age of 65 would prefer to stay in their own homes as they age and avoid moving into a nursing home or assisted-living facility. "Aging in place" is a growing movement as the elderly population increases in America. Aging in place is the ability to live in one's own home and community safely, independently, and comfortably, regardless of age, income, or ability level (USDHHS, 2020). Converting a home to provide necessary adjustments may be expensive, but as the population of older people grows, innovative opportunities to allow them to remain living in their own home safely increase. Doorways should be widened to allow mobility aids such as walkers or wheelchairs to pass and doorknobs should be replaced with door levers; ramps on exterior stairs and indoor threshold ramps should be installed for smooth transitions; sinks, counter heights, and microwaves should be lowered to be used in a seated position; a bathtub with walk-in shower or bathtub transfer bench or bath chair is necessary as well as safety bars, elevated toilet, and bathroom doors should open outward to allow someone to gain access to the bathroom if a fall occurs; flooring consisting of short-knap carpet is best for walkers or wheelchairs since slippery surfaces may lead to falls and people tend to place throw rugs on cold flooring, which can be a trip hazard; lighting should be bright but not cast shadows or glare, nightlights are useful, and switches should be rocker-type; medical alert systems provide monitoring and assistance when needed; and smart home devices can be set for medication reminders and a plethora of other automated functions (AssistedLivingToday, 2020; Dengarden, 2019; TCPI, 2020; The Helping Home, 2019). Long-term care insurance, if purchased before it is needed, can provide in-home care and assistance. In some communities, visiting health-care workers can attend the homebound geriatric person and can provide supervision, care, and education.

Some facilities offer assisted living in a residential setting for the geriatric adult who needs minimal or moderate supervision and care. Cognitive impairments such as Alzheimer disease, which involves loss of memory, disorientation, and loss of the ability to communicate and function in social situations, and other chronic diseases may lead to the complete dependence on others for activities of daily living (ADLs) such as bathing, tooth-brushing, dressing, and eating may lead to the need for placement in a nursing home or long-term care facility (Box 14.3).

Some nursing homes offer basic nursing care; others offer physical and recreational activities as well. Entering a nursing home often requires relinquishing independence and control over one's life, and many geriatric patients decline rapidly in this type of less personal environment. Selection of a nursing home should include factors such as cost, insurance coverage, accessibility to medical services, philosophy of care, staffing, social services, and availability of occupational, physical, and speech therapy (USDHHS, 2017). Some facilities offer pet therapy, which is the use of pets as friends and dependents. Providing a clean homelike setting with open visiting hours, spiritual care, and pleasant visual surroundings is important (Box 14.4).

BOX 14.3   Activities of Daily Living

Assisted-living facilities can help with cleaning, laundry, meals, and recreational activities. The ability to manage the following activities of daily living (ADLs) is essential for independent living:
- Eating
- Toileting, bathing, and grooming
- Cooking
- Shopping
- Taking medications

BOX 14.4   Concerns Related to Living Arrangements

- Access to health care and assessment
- Individual's perception of move as "dumping" or as assistance
- Control of patient's finances
- Personal space allowed
- Accommodation of special needs
- Privacy or shared room
- Providing pet care, allowing plants in room
- Peer-group activity
- Rehabilitation and therapies available

ROLE OF THE HEALTH-CARE WORKER

Most geriatric adults develop coping strategies to handle the gradual aging process. Often, minor changes in the environment can enhance their ability to function. For example, the

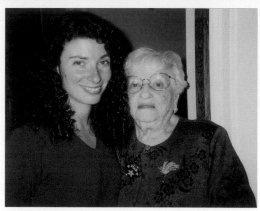

Figure 14.3 A relative visits a woman who has just celebrated her 100th birthday. Adults in the geriatric age group can benefit from assisted-living facilities that enable the older adults to maintain personal independence. Friends, family, and visitors to their homes receive the benefits of the experience, the wisdom, and the expertise of geriatric adults.

geriatric person with decreased lung capacity and high blood pressure may manage well in a ground-floor apartment but may have difficulty if climbing stairs is a required daily activity.

It is important to observe family interaction. Restraining the geriatric person in a wheelchair or in a bed because of the fear of falling will foster dependency that can result in dysfunction and psychological decline. Changes in aging include physiological, psychological, social, economic, and cultural factors that influence the way one ages and the rate of the aging process.

There are many positive aspects of aging. Geriatric adults offer others a wealth of experience, expertise, and wisdom. They provide a grandchild with a relationship that cannot be equaled and that contributes to the development of the child and the well-being of the geriatric adult (Figure 14.3). Understanding the developmental tasks of advanced old age, knowing the physiological and psychological changes and challenges that geriatric persons face, and empowering those in advanced old age to maintain autonomy or control over their lives is the focus of geriatric care (Box 14.5).

BOX 14.5   Principles of Elder Care

- Encourage confidence
- Raise self-image
- Provide empowerment
- Demonstrate kind, caring manner
- Identify and include family and social-support systems
- Actively listen
- Integrate spirituality, hope, and faith
- Assist in setting personal goals
- Monitor exercise and nutrition
- Follow-up on health concerns

KEY POINTS

- Senescence is categorized as including the early-old, middle-old, and late-old.
- The physiological changes in advanced old age affect all body systems, but the degree is dependent on genetics, lifestyle, dietary practices, and social support.
- Immortality versus extinction is the major task or challenge that the advanced old age population must face.
- Some health-promotion activities in which the geriatric adult can participate are physical exercise, balanced nutrition, preventive health maintenance (such as receiving the flu vaccine), and controlling the safety of his or her environment.
- The need for a sense of being loved and valued continues throughout the lifespan and includes fulfilling the sexual needs of the geriatric adult.

- Lifestyle adjustments, including a healthful diet, exercise, and stress management, can aid modern medicine in extending the lifespan.
- Elder abuse is the physical, mental, social, or financial neglect or mistreatment of the geriatric adult.
- A variety of living options are available to geriatric adults, including living in their own homes, with other family members, living in assisted-living apartments, or living in skilled/long-term care facilities.
- Activities of daily living involve the ability to independently eat, dress, wash, toilet, and communicate.
- The health-care worker can provide education and guidance in meeting the life tasks of the geriatric adult.

Clinical Judgment Case Study

Mr. J. is a 77-year-old man who lives in a single-family home with his 84-year-old wife. Mr. J. is in relatively good health and still quite active and fit. Mrs. J. has been declining recently and has been having trouble with hearing and visual limitations, balance, memory, and her nutritional status. Given the fitness and activity levels are so different between them, what are some things that could be done to assist them with continuing to age in place safely?

REVIEW QUESTIONS

1. Match the theories of the aging process with their summary.

Theory	Summary
Free radicals	
Biological clock	
Immune	
Wear and tear	

A. Cells have a programmed lifespan. They break down and are phagocytized at the end of their lifespan.

B. Cells wear out or break down with use over time.

C. Ions within molecules break free more frequently with age and bond with other molecules leading to oxidative stress.

D. An aged immune system is unable to distinguish between healthy and defective cells so therefore destroys both types.

2. Fill in the blanks with the words in the word bank: (words may be used more than once)

harder	less	larger	easier	reduced
gains	increased	smaller	more	loses

The ribs and cartilage become 1._____ _____ rigid, and thus the respiratory muscles work 2._____ _____. Age-related osteoporosis and 3._____ _____ height of the vertebrae results in a 4._____ _____ chest cavity. Lung tissue 5._____ _____ elasticity, which adds to 6._____ _____ lung volume. Surface area within the lung is also 7._____ _____, which impairs oxygen exchange.

3. Match the terms with their definition:

Term	Definition
Ageism	
Glaucoma	
Atrophy	
Senescence	
Apoptosis	
Disengagement	

A. Prejudicial attitudes and discriminatory practices against older people.

B. Decrease in size.

C. Period in which the body begins to age and weaken.

D. Atrophy of the optic nerve and increased intraocular pressure.

E. Process of withdrawing from social contacts and giving up independence.

F. Breaking down of the cell membrane leading to cell death.

4. Age-related changes in the kidneys and bladder can result in: (select all that apply)

A. decreased filtration rate and accumulation of toxins in the bloodstream.

B. increased bladder capacity leading to infrequent urination.

C. urinary retention in men who have enlarged prostates.

D. incontinence or urine leakage with activity.

5. Ms. P. is an 82-year-old woman. She has been losing weight recently and when she had a conversation with her doctor regarding the weight loss, she says, "food just doesn't taste as enticing as it used to." What are some age-related changes that might be contributing to Ms. P's statement? (select all that apply)

A. Taste buds are increased on the surface of the tongue with aging but their sensitivities change.

B. Quantities of saliva increase with aging, which dilutes flavors.

C. Taste buds change to be more sensitive to the taste of bitter with aging.

D. Sense of smell declines with aging contributing to loss of appetite.

E. Taste buds change to be more sensitive to the perception of salt with aging.

F. Digestive enzymes decrease resulting in poor appetite and digestive disturbances.

Planning for the End of Life

OUTLINE

OBJECTIVES

1. Describe the grieving process for the patient who is facing death.
2. List the stages of the dying process.
3. Discuss behaviors related to the dying process.
4. Describe the philosophy of hospice and palliative care.
5. Define quality of life from a child's point of view.
6. Summarize the statements in the Dying Person's Bill of Rights.
7. Discuss the response and needs of the family of the dying patient.
8. Review ethical and legal issues involved in end-of-life care.
9. State the role of the health-care worker in end-of-life care.
10. State three cultural practices related to end-of-life care.
11. Describe the development of the concept of death and dying in young children.
12. Discuss similarities and differences in end-of-life care for adults and children.
13. List signs of impending death.

DEATH AS PART OF THE LIFE CYCLE

Death is a normal part of the life cycle. Many older people prepare for death by writing a last will and testament, documenting in advance directives for health care, or by making advance funeral arrangements, which may include the purchase of a burial plot. Few people, however, are emotionally prepared for the process of dying, which is distinctly different from death itself.

Most people who think about death associate it with the elderly, but death is not unique to the aged. The sudden, unexpected death of a young person causes different emotions and behaviors in the survivors. The process of death can occur in the acute-care hospital surrounded by the unfamiliar, or it can occur in the home or nursing home environment in a room with family and familiar caregivers surrounding the bed.

Cultural Considerations

The care of a dying person, called end-of-life (EOL) care, involves ethical and legal issues and religious and cultural responsibilities that need to be addressed by the health-care team.

No specific technique or procedure can describe exactly what to do for a patient who is dying or for the family who is in anguish. A flexible approach is needed to meet the needs of the patient and family. Often the mere presence of a health-care worker provides the support that is needed. Remaining near the patient and family, or simply holding a hand, provides strength while facilitating the expression of emotions and grief. This is known as therapeutic presence.

Lifespan Considerations

Understanding the patient's and the family's wishes, religious and cultural needs, and legal and ethical protocols is essential for the health-care worker (see Chapter 3 for cultural considerations related to death). The spiritual and psychological needs of the family as a unit are equally as important as physical and social needs. Studies have shown that life satisfaction and spirituality are associated with reduced death anxiety (Renz et al., 2018; Taghiabadi et al., 2017). Most care plans focus on a positive outcome from the care provided, but that is not the goal for EOL care. Providing death with dignity is a quality process in the closure of a life. Helping to decrease pain, promote comfort, and reduce stress are considered positive outcomes in the care of dying patients and the care of their families.

BOX 15.1 Common Signs of Impending Death

- Increasing weakness, immobility
- Weight loss
- Decreased appetite
- Loss of bowel and bladder control
- Decreased awareness of surroundings*
- Diaphoresis (sweating)
- Lung congestion (loose gurgling sound, referred to as the death rattle)
- Altered breathing patterns (periods of apnea, often called Cheyne-Stokes respirations)
- Decreased urine output
- Slowed pulse
- Cold and mottled extremities
- Relaxed and open jaw

*Even though the person may appear to be asleep or in a coma, hearing is the last sense to be lost. Family and caregivers should continue to talk to the dying person.

SIGNS AND SYMPTOMS OF DEATH

The family should be prepared for the symptoms that accompany death (Box 15.1), and the information should be communicated with sensitivity. Even when the death of a person is expected, the finality of the actual death still will come as a shock to most family members. For a list of resources for EOL issues, access the American Psychological Association (2020) End of Life Issues and Care webpage at https://www.apa.org/pi/aging/programs/eol.

THE PROCESS OF DYING

The process of dying is psychological and physiological. *Psychological* death begins when a person is told that he or she has a terminal illness. Sometimes the death of a spouse or a peer causes a person to believe that his or her own death is near. For example, when an older person realizes he is the last of his generation living, he begins to face his own future death. *Physiological* death starts when the body processes decline in function.

Psychological Responses of the Dying Patient

As part of the life cycle, death is accompanied by tasks and responses. Most people who realize they are facing death go through a grieving process (Table 15.1). The process may start with disbelief (e.g., "This can't be happening to me"). This stage is often accompanied by periods of crying and mourning for what will be left behind, future events that will be missed, and unfulfilled opportunities in relationships and activities. This grief process may or may not proceed to clinical depression. The normal sadness of grieving the end of life may occur in spurts as assistance in the activities of daily living (ADLs) is increasingly required, and the deterioration resulting from a condition becomes real. This kind of decrease in independence may trigger a period of sadness.

TABLE 15.1   Behaviors and Stages of Dying

Stages	Behaviors
Denial: "This can't be real"	Shock, numbness
Anger: "Why me?"	Disruptive behaviors, turmoil
Bargaining: Making deals with a god	Anxiety, conflict, confusion
Depression: Feeling of loss	Withdrawal, guilt, grief
Acceptance: "My time has come"	Vulnerability

Data from Kübler-Ross, E. (1969). *On death and dying.* Macmillan; Kinney, M., et al. (1996). *AACN's clinical reference for critical care nursing* (4th ed.). Mosby; Stroebe, H., Hansson, R., Stroebe, W., & Schut, H. (2001). *Handbook of bereavement research: consequences, coping and care.* American Psychological Association.

Disability and increasing dependence on others may cause the patient to lose self-esteem and to be concerned with body image.

The grief process should be supported through the efforts of palliative care and hospice team. The response to the phases of death and dying is different for each person and health-care providers must provide care and support that respects the patient's dignity and personal wishes (Oates & Maani, 2020).

A good social support system can assist the dying patient through the preparatory grief process. The health-care worker can help the person prepare for death by understanding and accepting the stages of grieving, mobilizing support systems, and using coping strategies. *Therapeutic presence* involves simply being present to provide support and comfort for the patient and the family unit. Therapeutic communication involves being understanding of the patient's emotional outbursts or expressions of anger and encouraging venting or verbalization. It is also helpful to have the ability to offer calming words of encouragement. The health-care worker should maintain communication with the family and should explain the stages of grief and the related behaviors. Talking with the patient about family, past achievements, and legacies can also be helpful (Coyle et al., 2015).

Clinical depression can often be avoided by identifying common fears of patients who are facing death and making efforts to alleviate those fears. Therapeutic presence of family and staff can alleviate the fear of abandonment, and fear of the unknown can be reduced by educating the family and patient and by offering support to them. Simple relaxation techniques are often helpful. A spiritual history obtained as part of the care plan can enable assessment of spiritual or cultural needs and practices that would be helpful when providing individualized care. The multidisciplinary health-care team, working closely with the patient and family, can help provide a death with peace and dignity.

Some patients do not progress through the stages as outlined by Kübler-Ross and may never pass beyond the stage of denial (see Table 15.1). Some people regress to previous stages from time to time during their journey toward death. Hope need not be abandoned during any stage. Some people faced with the diagnosis of a terminal illness lose the will to live, whereas others decide to live life to the fullest as long as they are able to. There is no norm for the process of dying.

Family Behaviors Related to the Dying Process

Family members may show a variety of responses when a loved one is dying. In many ways these behaviors are similar to the dying person's responses and must be recognized and acknowledged. Health-care workers are able to help the family most by assessing their needs. Preparation and education are the keys to helping the family cope with whatever lies ahead.

Two specific behaviors, *helplessness* and *guilt*, should be quickly recognized, and appropriate interventions should be implemented as soon as possible. To minimize the sense of helplessness, the health-care worker needs to educate and inform family members about the dying process and allow the family to assist in providing care, which can include washing the patient's face, adjusting a pillow, or simply being present so that they may hold hands with their loved one.

Guilt is a much more difficult behavior for the health-care worker to manage. The setting often determines the level of guilt a family member may experience. For example, if in an intensive-care unit, the family may feel not only overwhelmed with all the machinery but may also feel additional secondary guilt related to the different types of invasive procedures that may be required to support the patient physiologically. In many cases the guilt experience may cause the family member to insist on exhaustive comprehensive care regardless of the outcome or level of suffering the dying person may have to endure. Therefore, it is imperative to help the family member to resolve feelings of guilt, so that a more individualized and appropriate approach can be undertaken in the treatment and plan of care for the dying patient (American Cancer Society, n.d.).

Pain related to dying appears to be a common fear that most people experience. Many state that they "hope it's quick and painless." A variety of pain-relieving techniques can be used to help make the dying person as comfortable as possible. These techniques range from massage, positioning and supports, scented oils or candles, acupressure, acupuncture, herbs, and nonnarcotic or opioid pain relievers. The goal is to ensure that the pain is relieved as much as possible while also allowing the dying person to complete any unfinished tasks (Zeng et al., 2018).

Family, friends, and sometimes even health-care workers may seek advice concerning what to say to a person who is dying. The fear of saying the wrong thing often keeps people away from the bedside of a person who is dying, which often means that the needs of the patient (as well as the needs of others related to or involved with the patient) may remain unmet. Table 15.2 offers some suggestions for what to say and what not to say, often referred to as *therapeutic communication.*

TABLE 15.2 Therapeutic Communication

What to Say (Therapeutic Comments)	What Not to Say (Nontherapeutic Comments)
"Tell me how you are feeling."	"You need to be strong for your family."
"It's okay to cry."	"Don't cry."
"It sounds as if you are dealing with painful memories."	"It is God's will."
"I'm here if you want to talk."	"You will be out of pain soon."

Cultural Considerations

The behaviors of the family related to the care of a terminally ill relative may be influenced in part by the family's cultural and religious beliefs and practices. Health-care workers must be **culturally competent**, that is, they must be aware of the cultural practices of others and accept their practices in a nonjudgmental way. Cultural competence is developed through cultural awareness, knowledge of various cultural practices, skill in incorporating cultural beliefs into a patient care plan, and experience with persons from diverse cultures. Part of health-care education includes encounters with patients and coworkers from diverse settings. Understanding that culture influences thoughts, language, symbolic artifacts (such as bracelets or amulets), and actions that reflect specific traditions, customs, and rituals, helps the health-care worker understand behaviors and practices common to specific cultural groups (Giger & Haddad, 2020).

Culture and health care are interrelated. Culture influences an individual's attitude toward illness, nutrition, health care, and health-care providers. A cultural assessment and history are important parts of a patient's care plan. A family care plan facilitates a more comprehensive cultural assessment, especially when related to EOL care. Interpreters should be provided whenever necessary to ensure accurate communication.

Acute Care of the Dying Patient

Over the past several decades, the medical field has seen a number of positive changes in its ability to care for the sick, injured, or dying. With the advent of new technology, health-care workers are now able to support premature infants of extremely short gestational ages. A gravely ill patient may be kept alive for an indefinite amount of time. However, there are times when modern technology cannot keep vital organ deterioration from occurring. It is usually at this time when the physician speaks to the family to discuss the options and possible outcomes. These options can include continuation of full life support, such as a ventilator (breathing machine), intravenous medications to keep the heart beating and the blood pressure high enough to circulate blood throughout the body, and full cardiopulmonary resuscitation (CPR). The options can also include removing all life support or life-sustaining equipment and stopping all drugs except those that can provide sedation and relief of pain. This time period can be very stressful, especially when conversations surrounding death and dying have not previously occurred among family members. Discussing these topics before a serious event is a gift to yourself and your family (USDHHS, 2020). The Dying Person's Bill of Rights is outlined in Box 15.2.

Palliative Care and Hospice

It is well accepted that death is a part of the human condition but dying can be rife with inequalities. Surveys have shown that the two most common fears associated with the process of dying are the fear of pain and the fear of being a burden to the family (Timm, 2020). Providing compassionate and competent care to dying patients and families is a challenge. Palliative care is defined by the World Health Organization (WHO) as "an approach that improves the quality of life of patients and their families facing the problems associated with life-threatening illness, through the prevention and relief of suffering by means of

---

BOX 15.2   The Dying Person's Bill of Rights

I have the right to be treated as a living human being until I die.

I have the right to maintain a sense of hopefulness, however its focus may change.

I have the right to be cared for by those who can maintain a sense of hopefulness, however its focus may change.

I have the right to express my feelings and emotions about my approaching death in my own way.

I have the right to participate in decisions concerning my care.

I have the right to expect continuing medical and nursing attention even if "cure" goals must be changed to "comfort" goals.

I have the right not to die alone.

I have the right to be free from pain.

I have the right to have my questions answered honestly.

I have the right not to be deceived.

I have the right to have help from and for my family in accepting my death.

I have the right to die in peace and with dignity.

I have the right to retain my individuality and not to be judged for my decisions, which may be contrary to the beliefs of others.

I have the right to discuss and enlarge my religious and spiritual experiences, regardless of what they may mean to others.

I have the right to expect that the sanctity of the human body will be respected after death.

I have the right to be cared for by caring, sensitive, knowledgeable people who will try to understand my needs and will be able to gain some satisfaction in helping me face my death.

Created at the workshop "The Terminally Ill Patient and the Helping Person," sponsored by the Southwestern Michigan In-Service Education Council and conducted by Amelia J. Barbus, Associate Professor of Nursing, Wayne State University, 1975.

From Barbus, A. (1975). The dying patient's bill of rights. *American Journal of Nursing, 75*, 99.

---

early identification and impeccable assessment and treatment of pain and other problems, physical, psychological and spiritual" (WHO, 2020). Palliative care addresses the person as a whole with the goal to improve quality of life for those with serious or life-threatening disease. Palliative care may be accessed at any point in a disease process, in any health-care setting, and can be utilized during diagnosis, curative treatment, follow-up, and end of life. It focuses on physical symptoms, emotional and spiritual needs, assistance for caregivers, and any practical needs such as insurance, legal worries, or employment concerns (National Institutes of Health, 2020). The goal is the best possible quality of life for patients and their families (National Institutes of Health, 2020).

Hospice care is a concept of palliative care that offers comfort to patients and families who have limited life expectancy of 6 months or less. Although symptomatic relief is offered, hospice does not have curative goals and it is expected that patients do not seek aggressive curative treatments while enrolled in hospice. Emotional, spiritual, and physical support is given based on the needs of the patient and the belief that death is imminent and a normal process. Hospice workers also help the survivors through the period of bereavement. The program originated in England as a response to the growing awareness of the unmet needs of the dying patient. The hospice plan is based on the philosophy that death is a part of the normal life cycle. The physical, psychological, spiritual, and social needs of the dying patient are addressed. The hospice program of care started in the Eastern United States in 1974 and became a recognized Medicare benefit in 1982.

The varied settings for hospice care can include the home, nursing facilities, or long-term care facilities. Medication is prescribed for relief of pain and discomfort rather than for curative reasons. The hospice palliative-care program provides comprehensive patient-centered care with a physician and nurse as the key links of a multidisciplinary team. Financing sources for hospice care are insurance companies, veteran's benefit services, Medicare/Medicaid, and private payments. The eligibility requirements for hospice care may be restricted by the rules of the funding source used.

ETHICAL AND LEGAL ISSUES

Ethical issues concerning death are influenced by values, culture, and religion, whereas legal issues are rooted in the law. The responsibilities of health-care workers are to be familiar with the laws, recognize the cultural needs of the patient and family, and make the family aware of options available and the consequences of each option. Informed consent is based on respect for the dignity and rights of individuals and their right to make decisions about themselves and their health care.

The Kennedy Institute of Ethics was established in 1971 in Washington, D.C. This group deals with laws (formal rules), ethics (informal rules), and bioethics (health-care regulations and research). The President's Commission for the Study of Ethical Problems in Medicine and Research was established in 1978, which reported on issues in the health-care system. Decisions concerning EOL care, such as terminating life support, consenting to organ donation, and protecting the rights of incompetent patients, were researched. As a result of the research findings, policies were developed that addressed informed consent, advance directives, and durable power of attorney for health care.

Advance Directives

Advance health-care directives (AHCDs) are used to inform health-care providers and family members of the wishes of the patient as related to the level of lifesaving measures or heroics to be used when the patient is near death and is unable to communicate. The U.S. Congress passed, as part of the Omnibus Budget Reconciliation Act of 1990, the Patient Self-Determination Act. This act became law in December 1991 (U.S. Public Law 101-508). The Patient Self-Determination Act mandates that, at the time of admission to an acute-care or long-term care facility, all patients must be asked if they have executed an AHCD. If they have not, they must be given information defining AHCDs and should be told at the time of admission that they have the right to (1) state such directives and (2) accept or refuse any medical treatment.

There is a significant drawback to waiting for an illness or a hospital admission to draw up an AHCD. Many times, patients are admitted to a hospital with an acute illness or in a crisis. These types of situations typically involve a great deal of physical and emotional stress, and medications may dull the senses and prevent rational, clear thinking. Ultimately, AHCDs written and signed by the patient before he or she becomes critically ill will help lessen the burden of decisions that must be made by the family members in a time of crisis. It is also important to communicate the specifics outlined in an AHCD to the health-care team prior to catastrophic illness. Ensuring these forms are on file with family members, primary medical providers, and local hospitals, as well as posting them in a prominent place in the home so emergency medical personnel has access to them is important in the chain of communication (Scholten et al., 2018).

Durable Power of Attorney for Health Care

The durable power of attorney for health care (DPOH) is a type of advance directive that transfers the health-care decision-making power to a person designated by the patient. It is used when the patient cannot communicate, and it must be set up and signed before the person becomes incapacitated. The DPOH may legally sign consents for treatment. This is not to be confused with a general durable power of attorney that transfers financial transactional decisions to the designated agent. Responsibilities of both types of powers of attorney end with the person's death (Legalzoom, 2020).

Living Will

A living will is usually drawn up before a patient is terminally ill or incapacitated. It describes the wishes of the person concerning EOL care. State laws vary concerning the recognition of living wills, but such documents are more valid as expressions of a person's wishes than casual statements made during family discussions, and the living will is usually respected and upheld by the courts (Legalzoom, 2020).

Do Not Resuscitate Order

A do not resuscitate (DNR) order can be written only by a physician on the basis of the patient's living will or DPOH. DNR means that if a patient stops breathing or the heartbeat is incompatible with life (e.g., asystole or "flat line"), aggressive methods of resuscitation such as CPR will not be attempted (AAFP, 2020).

Physician's Order for Life-Sustaining Treatment (POLST)

A POLST is a document written by a health-care provider during a conversation with the patient that equates to a physician order outlining specific medical treatments that the patient wishes to have immediately based on their diagnosis, prognosis, and goals of care. This document is appropriate for persons with medical conditions that are likely to result in frequent hospitalizations and possibly life-threatening clinical events. It is more detailed and specific than a DNR order, and the instructions must be followed regardless of where the patient is being treated. Specific details within a POLST vary by state (Everplans, 2020).

Assisted Suicide and Euthanasia

Suicide is the taking of one's own life. Assisted suicide is the facilitation of suicide where the person knowingly takes lethal drugs provided by a doctor for this purpose. The word euthanasia comes from the Greek eu ("good") and thanatos ("death"). Euthanasia is an intentional act (such as the lethal injection of a drug), with the purpose of causing death. Both assisted suicide and euthanasia involve legal, moral, and ethical issues that have been tested in the courts through the years and remain controversial. Currently, nine states have legalized physician-assisted suicide: California, Colorado, Hawaii, Maine, New Jersey, Oregon, Vermont, Washington, and District of Colombia. Montana has legal physician-assisted suicide via a court ruling (ProCon, 2019). The Netherlands, Germany,

Switzerland, Belgium, Finland, Canada, and Luxembourg permit physician-assisted suicide, and some permit active euthanasia (ProCon, 2020).

Health-care professionals are often asked by the patient or family to participate in hastening the end of life. The core of the debate against assisted suicide and euthanasia is the premise that providing effective palliative, pain-free EOL care will eliminate the need for people to request such an action.

ROLE OF THE HEALTH-CARE WORKER IN END-OF-LIFE CARE

The health-care worker must understand the process of dying, offer support and empathy to the patient and family, and assist the family to recognize and manage options and supportive resources. Standards of professional practice in nursing have been developed jointly by the Hospice and Palliative Nurses Association, the American Nurses Association, and the National Hospice and Palliative Care Organization. The role of the nurse and health-care worker in EOL care is to perform the following:

- Ensure education of the patient and family concerning the diagnosis.
- Ensure that informed consent is provided with a clear offer of all available options of care.
- Ensure that the patient's and family's cultural and personal wishes are respected.
- Communicate with the multidisciplinary health-care team when death is imminent or has occurred.

CHILDREN'S CONCEPT OF DYING AND DEATH

An understanding of death is often first taught to children as they learn about the life cycle of plants and animals in school. Students in sociology classes discuss cultural and religious customs of funerals and burials. The media review the life and death of celebrities. High school students may receive an assignment to write an opinion paper concerning the right to die or the final destiny of death.

Health-care workers often help parents guide children in developing a positive attitude toward and a fuller understanding of dying and death. Discussion of experiences with loss in everyday life using a plant, pet, or movie character creates opportunities to discuss dying and death in a nonthreatening manner. Many children's books are available to introduce the concepts at age-appropriate levels. A list of books to help children understand death and grief may be found on Scholastic Books' website: https://www.scholastic.com/parents/books-and-reading/raise-a-reader-blog/7-touching-books-to-help-kids-understand-death-and-grief.html.

Discussion of life and death should be a normal part of the growth and development experience to prepare a child to understand and manage death whenever it occurs. The concept of death is often influenced by exposure and discussion at home, in school, or at church, although the understanding of death is closely related to Piaget's stages of cognitive development (see Chapter 5). A child's first experience with death usually occurs when a pet dies. Telling a child that a pet is being put to sleep does not add to the understanding of death and in fact may cause the child to be afraid to go to sleep. Often the child's first experience with the death of a person occurs when a grandparent dies. The occurrence of death should not be hidden but should be openly discussed to enable effective coping strategies to be developed.

The Dying Child

Children who have a terminal illness typically progress through specific stages as they prepare for death, and they are often more aware of their condition than their parents realize. Children as young as age 2 respond to their parents' emotions and nonverbal behavior. Truthfulness, using age-appropriate terms in a supportive, nonthreatening manner, is the optimal approach in the care of a terminally ill child (APA, 2020). Efforts at minimizing or denying the terminal nature of the condition merely obstruct vital communication between the parent and child, and communication could be more useful than false cheer.

The initial stage of awareness (Bluebond-Langner, 1996) involves the child adapting to an identity or niche in the family as being the sick child. Special privileges or attention may be given to the child, and siblings often do not understand the favored status. The dying child soon learns that there is a relationship among medications, treatments, and recovery and adapts to the need for daily medication. Eventually, as the condition deteriorates, the child begins to realize he or she is different from peers. As the illness progresses, the child sees the illness as a lifelong challenge and feels he or she will always be sick. In the final stage, the child develops an awareness of the terminal nature of the illness, often asks direct questions about death, and may express inner fears and fantasies. The focus of care may initially be on educating the child and family about the disease. Later, specific fears expressed by the child or family are an appropriate focus of care. Studies show lasting detrimental effects on surviving siblings in terms of educational success and family formation during adulthood (Fletcher et al., 2013). Siblings should be included in the plan of care, so they do not feel abandoned or punished or do not develop an overwhelming sense of sibling rivalry and, later, feelings of guilt.

The role of the health-care worker is to provide support for the patient, parents, siblings, family, and school contacts. The death of a child is not normally a part of the natural life cycle, and so the emotional impact on the family is often devastating. The dying child should be provided with age-appropriate routines and activities for as long as possible. Contact with all family members should be encouraged. Questions should be answered truthfully, and the health-care worker should attempt to empower the child as much as possible (Bates & Kearney, 2015). The adolescent is most aware of the loss of expected life experiences when facing death. Outbursts of anger are common and should be expected and understood. Caregivers also need a support system of peers to cope with the death of a child. Parents will need help with coping strategies and assistance with the care of other children and family members during the grief process. Community resources should be used to help the family through the difficult times.

Developmental Concepts of Death and Dying

Death and dying are understood in different ways by children of different ages and developmental stages (Table 15.3). It is important to recognize the ability of the child to understand what is happening and to help the family communicate with the dying child or the child who has lost a family member. In infants and young children, a separation anxiety disorder may occur that is evidenced by the stages of *protest* (crying), *despair* (sadness), and eventual *disengagement* with the deceased person.

TABLE 15.3   Developmental Concepts of Death and Dying*

Age	Concept	Response	Interventions
Infants	Not applicable.	React to separation and alteration of routine or stress behavior of caregiver.	Maintain a familiar daily routine if possible.
Toddlers	Perceive anxiety of those around them. Do not understand permanence of death or that they can die.	Take on the anxiety and emotions of those around them.	Maintain a familiar routine. Explain in simple terms what is happening.
Preschool-age children	Understand that death is feared by adults. View death as reversible and may see it as being similar to sleep. *Magical thinking* may distort reality of death.	Often ask why and how questions about death. May feel their thoughts or actions caused the death or caused their own illness as a punishment. May cling or withdraw.	Avoid explaining death as a type of sleep. Accept temporary regression. Reassure that they are not the cause of the death. Help facilitate the grieving process through play.
School-age children	Begin to understand death as permanent and inevitable but often feel it occurs in others or in the remote future. May believe in continuation of life in another form.	Curious about details of death. May fear separation from family or friends. May romanticize death according to TV experiences.	Emotional restraint of caregiver makes it more difficult for child to express emotions. Encourage active participation in grieving process. Encourage the asking of questions and the expression of feelings. Answer questions truthfully.
Adolescents	Understand death is permanent and inevitable. May begin to question the meaning of life.	Can relate death to cultural or religious beliefs or practices. Most feel immortal and may become defiant and rebellious when facing their own deaths. Faith can help adolescents cope.	Extra effort is needed to help parent maintain communication with adolescent. Listen to adolescents' thoughts and fears and answer questions truthfully. Include adolescents in family discussions and decisions.

*The ability of the child to understand the nature and consequences of death varies according to culture, experiences, cognitive development, and family stability. The child's external behavior often does not reflect the internal intensity of his or her feelings.

Toddler

The toddler views separation as temporary, because he or she is just learning to separate from the parent and to understand object permanence. The toddler's behavior may reflect a response to changes in caregivers and routines, or reflect anxiety and fear seen in those around them (Stanford Children's Health, 2020).

Preschooler

The thinking of a preschooler is not logical in the way that an adult's is. The preschool-age child thinks of death as reversible. The preschooler employs magical thinking and may believe his or her own negative thoughts caused the ill sibling to go away and be laden with guilt and shame. Death should never be described as "sleep." He or she may also fear abandonment. Serious illness in a preschooler may be misunderstood as punishment, or inability of parents to protect him or her (Stanford Children's Health, 2020).

School-Age Child

Concrete thinking enables the school-age child to realize death is permanent and the deceased sibling will be absent from family activities. During this developmental stage, thanatophobia, or fear of death, is common, seeing death as a terrifying state of nothingness without understanding the cause or what happens to them after death (Fritscher, 2020). The school-age child should attend the funeral or memorial service. The school-age child may not yet understand his or her own mortality.

Adolescent

Adolescents can think abstractly and understand the permanence of death. The adolescent mourns and understands the effect of death on others and their own religious or cultural rituals will be followed. A dying teen usually resents his or her dependence on others. Comfort and pain relief are critical, and the adolescent should be involved in decision-making. Adolescents may have difficulty coping with their own death and will often deny their own mortality by engaging in risky activities (Stanford Children's Health, 2020).

It is important to understand that quality of life for a child means participating in age-appropriate activities as normal, healthy children do. Visits from friends and attending school even part time help the child and the family to cope with the dying process.

PHYSICAL CARE AFTER DEATH

The physical care of the patient is performed according to the culture of the patient and the protocols of the institution. The health-care worker should communicate with the family concerning policies and routines related to care and transport of the body, because cultural or religious practices may require flexibility in the procedure. The time of death may be the last opportunity for some family members to see or touch their loved one, so they may appreciate some private time with the deceased to help with closure. Often when a child dies the parents may wish to hold the child snugly wrapped in a blanket for a time.

Family members may need assistance in notifying extended family or friends and helping to facilitate phone calls is valuable. Talking about the death is part of the healing process. Providing referral for the funeral arrangements and for the planning of the memorial service may also be helpful. The use of community resources for bereavement support groups helps survivors realize that they are not alone. See Chapter 16 concerning the bereavement process. The American Association for Retired Persons (2020) has many resources to assist patients and family members during this period. For a list of what to do when a loved one dies, access their website at https://www.aarp.org/home-family/friends-family/info-2020/when-loved-one-dies-checklist.html.

KEY POINTS

- The grieving process of a patient facing death includes the stages of denial, anger, bargaining, depression, and acceptance.

- Hospice care is based on the philosophy that death is a normal part of the life cycle. The physical, psychological, spiritual, and social needs of the dying person are addressed in hospice care without the use of aggressive curative efforts.

- Palliative care is the total care of patients. Comfort is the core of this type of care.

- Some ethical and legal issues involved in end-of-life care include understanding of advanced directives, living wills, and DNR orders.

- Assisted suicide or euthanasia is the action of a person other than the patient to facilitate suicide. It is not legal in most states and remains a controversial legal, moral, and ethical issue.

- Cultural practices of the family should be respected during end-of-life care.

- Family and friends should continue to talk to the dying person, because hearing is the last sense to be lost.

- An understanding of death is taught to children as they study the life cycle of plants and animals in school. Students and teachers in sociology classes discuss customs and cultures. The death of a family pet may be a common experience that children share concerning death.

- Death and dying are understood in different ways by children of different ages and developmental stages. Communication with children at their level of understanding is important.

- Quality of life for ill children involves inclusion in age-appropriate routines and activities for as long as possible.

- Some signs of impending death include weakness, immobility, altered breathing patterns, cold and mottled extremities, and decreased awareness of surroundings.

- The role of the health-care worker in end-of-life care is to educate the family and patient concerning options and resources, to provide support, and to maintain communication with the health-care team. The health-care worker can provide the family with strategies and resources to cope with end-of-life care.

Clinical Judgment Case Study

Mrs. M is a 78-year-old female previously diagnosed with stage 4 colon cancer. She had been treated with surgical resection and chemotherapy. Her cancer did not respond to chemotherapy and she currently is in liver failure. Mrs. M. states she no longer wishes aggressive treatment and her adult children are in agreement with her wishes. Discuss the next steps in Mrs. M's plan of care.

REVIEW QUESTIONS

1. Categorize each goal as consistent with palliative care, hospice, or both.

Goal	Palliative Care	Hospice	Both
Reduction of pain			
May include aggressive, curative treatments			
Improving psychological and spiritual states			
Offers support specifically for patients with a 6-month life expectancy or less			
Includes early identification, assessment, and treatment of life-threatening illnesses			
Helps survivors through a period of bereavement			

2. Match the document to its definition.

Document	Definition
Advanced Health Care Directive	
Durable Power of Attorney for Health Care	
Do Not Resuscitate Order	
Physicians' Order for Life-Sustaining Treatment	

   A. Portable medical order form recording detailed and specific patient wishes in the event of a medical emergency.
   B. Legal document that appoints someone to make medical decisions on a person's behalf and only is active if the person becomes incapacitated.
   C. Legal document defining what actions should be taken if the patient is no longer able to make decisions for themselves because of illness or incapacity.
   D. Also known as "No Code" or "Allow Natural Death" indicating the person does not want physical or chemical resuscitation at the moment the heart stops beating and/or the person stops breathing.

3. Which of the following statements are included in the Dying Person's Bill of Rights? (Select all that apply)
   A. I have the right to be cared for by those who can maintain a sense of hopefulness, however its focus may change.
   B. I have the right to expect daily visits from family and friends in an effort to maintain my mental health.
   C. I have the right to be free from pain.
   D. I have the right to expect that the sanctity of my body will be respected after death.
   E. I have the right to be buried in the location of my choice, regardless of cost or convenience.
   F. I have the right to not be deceived.

4. Complete each sentence by circling the correct term from the options given in parentheses.
   A. The school-aged child believes death is (permanent, reversible). B. (Fear, acceptance) of death is common. C. They (should not, should) attend the funeral. D. They (may, may not) understand their own mortality.
   1. A. permanent; B. reversible
   2. A. fear; B. acceptance

3. A. should not; B. should

4. A. may; B. may not

5. Mark the column to appropriately define the intervention.

Intervention	Comfort Care	Assisted Suicide	Euthanasia
Sleeping pills in a large dose (Seconal 9000 mg) prescribed by a physician for the patient to take voluntarily			
Morphine within normal dosing parameters as ordered by the physician to relieve pain			
Large dose of morphine (300 mg) injected by a caregiver into comatose patient			

Loss, Grief, and Bereavement

http://evolve.elsevier.com/Leifer/growth

OUTLINE

OBJECTIVES

1. List the normal losses that occur during the stages of the life cycle.
2. State how the response to normal losses influences responses to loss of life.
3. List the stages and tasks of the grieving process.
4. Explain the difference between grief, mourning, and bereavement.
5. State the importance of understanding cultural practices related to death.
6. Describe an emotional, cognitive, and behavioral response to grief.
7. List two components of an abnormal grief response.
8. State the response to loss and grief at different development stages within the lifespan.
9. Discuss the achievement of the letting-go phase of the grief process.
10. State four ways condolences can be expressed.

KEY TERMS

anticipatory grief
bereavement
compassion
complicated grief
condolence
culture

delayed grief
empathy
eulogy
funeral
grief

legacy
maturational loss
mourning
situational loss
sympathy

THE CONCEPT OF LOSS

Loss is a natural part of life, but it is often painful and requires difficult adjustments. The experience of loss occurs at almost every stage of life, not just at life's end.

NORMAL LOSSES DURING THE LIFE CYCLE

Situational loss occurs when an unexpected and traumatic life experience takes place such as a loss of a source of income, or loss from a serious illness. Maturational loss is an occurrence as one passes through the life cycle (Vasquez, 2020). Perhaps the first experience of maturational loss is the newborn's loss of the security of the womb. When the newborn later develops an attachment to the mother, the goal of the newborn is to prevent the loss of the mother, who is needed for survival. The act of attachment of the infant to his or her mother or the husband to his wife makes the person vulnerable to the experience of loss.

The toddler endures the loss of being the exclusive focus of his or her parents when a sibling arrives who can be viewed as a rival in sharing the love of the parents. Puberty often involves loss when the body image of adulthood they had in their mind does not come to be.

When the teen leaves home for college, the teen loses the securities of home and family, and the parents lose control over their child. We lose our dreams of what might be when we settle for more realistic life goals. As we age, we lose our youth, our beauty, our energy, our sight, and our health, and we must learn to cope with all these losses.

The normal losses of each stage of the life cycle involve some form of letting go and adapting. How a person responds to the various losses during life contributes to the development of that person's personality and how bereavement is managed when loss of life occurs.

ABNORMAL OR ATYPICAL LOSSES

Families across the nation suffered a loss of national security when Pearl Harbor was bombed on December 7, 1941. Confidence in the safety and security of our country was again lost when the World Trade Center towers and the Pentagon were attacked on September 11, 2001. Families in the United States had felt protected by the moat-like surroundings of the oceans that seemed impenetrable, and the loss of that feeling of security affected everyone in the country. Profound multifaceted loss occurred during the COVID-19 pandemic in 2020. By August 2020, 155,204 people died of COVID-19 in the United States (CDC, 2020), and loss of many aspects of "normal life" during times of quarantine affected every person in the nation and beyond (Zhai & Du, 2020).

RESPONSES TO LOSS

To adapt to the various normal losses in life, the individual must learn how to cope with disappointments, and this learning usually results in maturity and personal growth. The response to normal losses during each phase of the life cycle determines how losses in old age are perceived and managed. The attitude toward death and loss often determines the quality of life that is maintained (Renz et al., 2018). When past losses are not resolved, the losses involved in later life stages may reactivate old, unresolved sorrows (Gesi et al., 2020). Passing successfully through Erikson's stages of the life cycle determines whether the older person will enjoy life to its end with new strengths and goals or just spend time waiting to be claimed by death.

TASKS ASSOCIATED WITH DEATH

Death is the ultimate loss – the loss of life. It is important to establish communication with those who are dying, but many people avoid discussions of death. The experience of death is a stage in life with its own tasks. Some people wish not to be conscious of death as it occurs. They opt for sedation and yearn for death during sleep. The hospice movement has enabled the terminally ill to experience the task of dying with dignity (Rodriguez-Prat et al., 2016) (also see Chapter 15). Being satisfied with the legacy or the family one has left to the world may give the person a feeling of immortality. The legacy can be a grandchild, property, a culture, an organization, or writings. Establishing a spiritual connection and belief that there is an afterlife, a final reunion of all, also can be a meaningful task to pursue during the death process.

Grief

Grief is the emotional response to a loss of anyone or anything an individual is attached to deeply. It may be a loved one, but it also may be a pet, a job, a spouse, one's health, or many other cherished items (Meyers, 2016). Grief can occur before the actual loss, when a terminal illness is diagnosed, or it may be initiated upon the actual death of the loved one. Mourning is the outward expression of grief. Mourning is often based on cultural practices and traditions. Delayed grief occurs when emotions in response to the loss are postponed, often triggered by another major life event. Grief that occurs before the loss is known as anticipatory grief (St. Elizabeth Health Care, 2020). Complicated grief is grief that may be prolonged and debilitating, complicated by a sense of disbelief regarding the death, anger and bitterness, painful emotions with intense yearning, and intrusive and distressing thoughts of the deceased, all of which remain severe and impairing (Hamilton, 2016). Bereavement involves grief and mourning. It involves the time survivors first react to the reality of the loss, the adjustment to the loss, and the entering of a period where they can move on and continue with the fabric of life (Figure 16.1). Understanding the dynamics of loss, dying, and grief is essential to help the patient and family go through the process of bereavement (Centre for the Grief Journey, 2018). Verbal and nonverbal communication, therapeutic presence, and collaboration with the multidisciplinary health-care team are the core responsibilities of the health-care professional.

Culture, Religion, and Death

How individuals grieve is often directed by cultural and religious traditions and practices. Some may process loss through verbal or physical expressions, while some may process loss through introspection (Meyers, 2016). Culture is a pattern of behavior, language, and practices that are transmitted through the generations (see Chapter 3). Within each culture, these practices may vary. Understanding common religious and cultural practices enables health-care workers to individualize their approach to the grieving survivor and family following the death of a loved one.

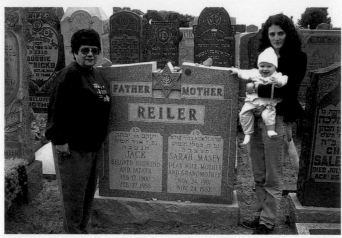

Figure 16.1 Most cultures include a ritual of memorializing family members who have died. Periodic visits to the cemetery to reflect, to offer respect, and to say prayers are healthy adaptations during the grieving process.

Normal Grief Responses

The grief process involves a series of stages, but travel through these stages is rarely orderly. Normal grief reactions often involve *physical symptoms* (e.g., lack of energy, weight gain, weight loss, or insomnia), *emotional symptoms* (e.g., anger, anxiety, relief, or despair), *cognitive reactions* (e.g., disbelief, confusion, or inability to concentrate), and *behavioral symptoms* (e.g., crying, impaired functioning, withdrawal, or changing of relationships) (Smith et al., 2019).

Several theorists outlined stages of grief that are widely accepted today.

Sigmund Freud developed the "Grief Work" theory in which the survivor breaks ties with the deceased, readjusts to a new life, and builds new relationships (Freud, 1917).

Elisabeth Kübler-Ross (1969) proposed the "Stage Theory" where grief follows a series of predictable stages of:

1. shock, denial, and isolation;
2. anger;
3. bargaining, resentment and guilt;
4. depression; and
5. acceptance (Axelrod, 2020).

Schulz (1978) and Bowlby (1980) outlined three stages of grief that involve

1. initial shock and disbelief;
2. numbness and overwhelming sadness, with yearning and protest; and
3. reflection in search of meaning and possibly eventual acceptance.

Current concepts are that life proceeds in a nonlinear timetable, with passage through or regressing to former stages influenced by sudden and unpredicted events (disruptors) that reshape the course of life. Transition into a new stage after a disruptor may take an average of five years, and thus, normal grief reactions after a loss may not progress in an orderly fashion, nor be resolved quickly (Feiler, 2020).

See Table 16.1 for a description of the tasks of the grieving process and suggested interventions.

TABLE 16.1 Tasks of the Grief Process

Stage	Task	Interventions
Notification of death	Share event with extended family and friends	Assist with initial coping or refer to community resources as needed. Assess support system.
Recognition of reality of death	Share the response by expressing grief	Understand anger may be directed toward health-care professional. Survivors may need help with feelings of guilt.
Adjustment or reintegration	Reorganize family structure and life goals	Survivor may need help setting up memory book and also planning for future and reintegrating into society.

Modified from Kübler-Ross, E. (1969). *On death and dying.* Macmillan.

The health-care worker should maintain a pleasant and nonjudgmental attitude while providing therapeutic presence and should help survivors identify and mobilize a strong support system. Referral to support groups or bereavement counselors for needed guidance is important. Hospice agencies can assist with accessing these resources.

Dysfunctional Grieving

Dysfunctional grieving is the failure to follow a predictable course of a normal grieving process to a resolution, resulting in the person resorting to abnormal or maladaptive coping strategies. Dysfunctional grieving involves the expression of unresolved issues and symptoms that result in interference with life's functioning (St. Elizabeth Health Care, 2020). In some instances, the signs and symptoms appear similar to a major depressive episode. These signs and symptoms include insomnia, emotional lability, changes in appetite, and withdrawal from friends or social support systems (Box 16.1). Support groups, therapists, or grief counselors can be beneficial.

BOX 16.1 Signs and Symptoms of Dysfunctional Grief

- Profound continuous sadness
- Pessimistic expressions about life in general
- Irritability, anger, or bitterness
- Sleep disturbances including being unable to sleep or sleeping all the time
- Declining attention to personal appearance
- Withdrawal from social interactions and activities
- Denial and defensiveness
- Distracted job performance
- Worsening of any preexisting mental health conditions
- Obsessing over or avoiding mementos of the deceased
- Inability to manage necessary daily affairs
- Reckless, impulsive, or potentially self-destructive behavior
- Talk of suicide, or actual suicide attempts

Modified from Bridges to Recovery (2020). *What are the signs of complicated grief disorder?* https://www.bridgestorecovery.com/complicated-grief/signs-complicated-grief-disorder/.

BOX 16.2   Special Aspects of Grief Following a Suicide

- Event involves social stigma
- Blaming often occurs
- Police investigation increases guilt
- Survivors feel death could have been prevented
- Survivors may feel decreased self-esteem
- Survivors feel rejected and deserted
- Family may worry about inherited predisposition

It is important to note that some of the signs and symptoms may be normal for the first few months after the death of a loved one. Typically, bereaved individuals slowly begin to resume normal activities of daily living (ADLs), maintain contact with family and friends, and accept other forms of support. It is not normal, however, to continue to remain isolated or removed from the real world for prolonged periods. Some form of intervention, whether medical, psychological, or both, may be necessary if the bereavement process is prolonged (Linde et al., 2017). Suicidal ideas may occur when the survivor begins to feel that life is not worth living without the deceased person. Professional intervention may be necessary. The death of a loved one by suicide also affects the grief process of the survivors. Box 16.2 describes the typical grief response following a death by suicide.

Role of the Health-Care Worker

The responsibility of the health-care worker does not end at the death of the patient. Preparing the family for the grief process and referring the family to community resources for counseling and other assistance are important. The focus of care is on the patient and the family unit, as described in Chapter 4. Cultural competence is the key to successful communication and support (see Chapter 3). See Table 16.2 (and Chapter 15) for some suggestions of what to say and not to say.

TABLE 16.2   Communicating With the Bereaved*

What to Say (Therapeutic Comments)	What Not to Say (Nontherapeutic Comments)
"I am sorry for your loss."	"I know how you feel."
"It is okay to be angry."	"You must not blame God. You should not feel like that."
"Grieving takes time. Take your time. Don't feel pushed to do anything."	"You will be okay in a week or so."
"It is not easy for you. Tell me about the person you lost."	"He lived a long and full life."
"Would you like to talk? I will listen."	"Tell me what happened."
"You did the best you could. It is okay to cry."	"Do not feel guilty. Do not cry."

*The most important thing to do is to listen.

GRIEF EARLY IN THE LIFE CYCLE

Pregnant Women

Perinatal loss is common, with estimations of up to 20% of recognized pregnancies ending in miscarriage and 1% ending in stillbirth of fetuses after 20 weeks of gestation. It is a profound grief experience (Weir, 2018). Because pregnant women experience movement of the fetus by the second trimester of pregnancy, an attachment between the mother and fetus begins to evolve. Typically, the parents join together in planning their future and the future of their unborn infant. When a stillbirth occurs, both parents respond, but often the mother suffers a more intense grief reaction, which may spark interpersonal problems. The health-care team must take the time to provide much needed support during this difficult time.

Clear information should be provided about the cause of death and any implications for future pregnancies. Women who become pregnant after experiencing a loss in a previous pregnancy need to be guided through the milestones of the subsequent pregnancy to promote a positive attitude and to anticipate a joyful outcome (Wojcieszek et al., 2018).

If the mother experiencing a pregnancy loss is an adolescent, the responses may be complicated by the thinking process of that level of development and the attitudes of the adults around her. If the adolescent who experiences this loss is not given permission to grieve, they are at great risk for developing depression, anger, or feelings of guilt that will affect their own growth and development process (NIH, n.d.). Health-care workers need to offer to the adolescent information about the grief process, referral for counseling, and general empathy and support.

In the case of the loss of an infant, acknowledging the existence of the baby as a separate person is important and may include taking careful pictures or footprints or cutting and preserving a curl of hair as a memento (Mayo Clinic, 2020). A "memory kit" may be assembled to include items of importance to the parents (Figure 16.2).

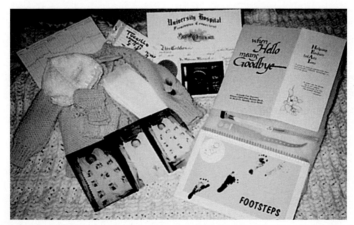

Figure 16.2 After pregnancy loss, the parents may take home a "memory kit." The kit can include pictures of the infant, the death certificate, footprints, identification bands, an ultrasound picture, or the first set of clothing, among other individual items that are important to the parents. These memory kits can be designed for persons of any age to give meaningful memories to the family.

Some parents wish to hold their infants, take photographs, and dress the baby in cherished garments to say good-bye. Parents should be taught about the grieving process, so each will understand what behaviors to expect. Options for funeral arrangements should be offered, and parents should be referred to support groups that may be beneficial in the weeks and months following their loss. Providing empathetic listening, therapeutic touch, and nonverbal support to the parents is most helpful. Attention to siblings and extended family is also important because other family members may not verbalize their feelings as readily as the parents.

Infants

By the age of 10 months, when they have established an attachment, infants are capable of responding to loss. This response to loss may resurface in adulthood and may manifest as an inability to form attachments or as a more intense response to normal loss experiences. See Table 15.3 for the developmental concepts of death and dying and suggested interventions for infants and children.

Children

Young children may react to death in a manner reflecting their developmental stage. By age 6, children realize death is not reversible. Children may show anger at the person who left them, guilt because they blame themselves for the loved one's leaving, and fear that they will not be cared for and loved. Their immaturity prevents them from coping with these feelings and often prevents them from expressing these feelings (Schonfeld & Demaria, 2016). Young children need the support and guidance of understanding adults to help them through this stressful experience (Box 16.3).

Adolescents

Loss due to death is common for adolescents and 71% have experienced a loss by the time they graduate from high school (Zakeri, 2020). Adolescents who lose a parent are usually at the point of moving into the adult role and may mourn the adult-to-adult relationship they had anticipated. The adolescent is establishing a sense of identity and may mourn the loss of

---

BOX 16.3 Children Coping With Loss

- Remember children are concrete thinkers. Avoid expressions such as "passed," or "went to sleep." Answer questions simply and honestly but only offer details they can understand.
- Allow them to talk about their fears and express their sorrow.
- Play activities are a way children express grief. They can be physical in their grief.
- Expect their grief to reawaken during strong reminders of the loss.
- Allow children to remember, reminisce, and talk about the deceased, but allow them to make choices for a sense of control.
- Maintain regular routines as much as possible.

Modified from Mental Health America (2020). *Helping children cope with loss*. https://www.mhanational.org/helping-children-cope-loss.

sharing accomplishments with the parent who died. Adolescents may feel the need to take on the role of the deceased parent to help the surviving parent and family members, or they may grieve in less productive ways through academic withdrawal, reverting to earlier developmental behaviors, or physical complaints such as headaches or abdominal pain (MHA, 2020).

Young Adults

Grief is thought of as sadness, but young adults may respond with rage at lost opportunities, anxiety about the future, resentment, guilt, irritation, or even relief. All emotions are normal and all timelines for coping are acceptable. Young adults may not only grieve the loss of the person who died, but the loss of the life they had before the death, how the death changed relationships with others, and how future events will change (The Dougy Center, 2020). Helping the survivor through the grief process toward integration of the loss and associated emotions into their daily life is both challenging and rewarding.

THE HEALING PROCESS

Reintegration and Adjustment

Many people remain in emotional pain years after the loss of a loved one. Complicated grief, as previously defined, was formerly termed unresolved grief. The smooth integration back into a "new normal" is blocked and successful adaptation does not occur (Zisook & Reynolds, 2017). Grief is considered to be a private emotion, and others may not reach out because they do not know what to say or do. Some people say, "Don't feel bad," or "Don't cry." This type of response implies that the person who is grieving should not show the grief.

When a child loses a pet dog, parents may avoid having the child cope with grief by saying, "Don't worry – we will get you another dog." This implies that the loss can be easily replaced. Not showing the grief that is felt and trying to replace what is lost are not appropriate responses to grief, because they do not allow recovery to occur. Encouraging the cover-up of grief forces the person to act as if he or she has successfully managed the loss to ensure acceptance back into his or her social group. Isolation from social contacts who may feel uncomfortable when he or she shows grief adds to emotional pain, and sleeplessness, confusion, and changes in behavior. Complicated grief is also more likely to occur when the death is sudden or violent, when the deceased had a particularly close relationship with the grieving person, or when the grieving person had mental health issues or poor support systems in place prior to the death (Zisook & Reynolds, 2017). Unresolved issues in the grieving process can lead to physical and mental illness. The health-care worker should try to help the grieving survivor master tasks that lead toward the healthy healing of grief. Exercises such as grief journaling, storytelling, letter writing, or art therapy may be helpful (Art Therapy Resources, 2020; Raab, 2019).

Mastering Tasks Leading Toward Grief Healing

The health-care worker can help survivors in the task of grief healing by offering the following suggestions:
1. Talk about the death of the loved one with friends, fellow survivors, or grief recovery groups. Avoidance can lead to isolation.

2. Accept your feelings. A wide range of emotional response is normal.
3. Take care of yourself and your family by eating a healthy diet, exercising, and getting adequate sleep to improve physical and emotional health.
4. Find ways to help others dealing with the same loss. Feeling you are assisting someone else gives you purpose and makes you feel better as well.
5. Remember and celebrate the life of your loved one. Honor your loved one during special dates such as birthdays and anniversaries, but also in little things every day. Enjoying things such as favorite foods, activities, music, or art can kindle remembrance (APA, 2020).

HELPING GRIEVING SURVIVORS
Condolence

The word condolence means to express sympathy or to grieve together especially on the occasion of a death. Sympathy, in its pure form, however, has negative meanings of unwanted, pity-based response with a lack of understanding on the part of the person offering it. Empathy is an emotional response that acknowledges and attempts to understand the suffering of the other person. Compassion is motivated by love and kindness and uses the insights provided by empathy (Sinclair et al., 2016). To offer condolence to someone experiencing grief, one must elect to approach the grieving person, which can be emotionally challenging. As one offers comfort and understanding to the survivor, profound perceptions about life and loss are sparked. Disturbing questions arise, such as "What would I do if I was in this situation?" Often the person offering condolence does not know what to say and is concerned about saying the wrong thing. A feeling of helplessness follows, and the challenge of offering condolence may become overwhelming.

The health-care worker may offer condolences to the family after the death of a patient by sending a letter to the survivor or family. Friends of the deceased patient often look to the health-care worker for advice on how to offer condolences to the grieving survivors.

The grief experience is life-changing. The goal is to integrate successfully into a new life. Supporting the bereaved means helping them preserve their dignity and understand the process they must journey through. The outcome of condolence is not meant to cure grieving persons of their feelings of loss. It is not meant to cheer them up. However, condolence may ease the emotional pain, allow the grieving person to feel supported rather than abandoned, and help facilitate a healthy passage through the grieving process. A person providing condolence may receive the reward of strengthening his or her own coping strategies.

Some ways to offer condolence include:

1. *Writing a letter:* A personal letter of condolence is more meaningful to a grieving survivor than a preprinted card from a store. Comments concerning the deceased person will be treasured, and sincere words of condolence will be a tribute to the deceased and will bring comfort to the grieving survivor. A favorite memory and a sincere offer to help when needed would be appropriate. The letter should not diminish the intensity of the grieving person's feelings with phrases such as, "I know exactly how you feel." It should not offer advice to bury the feelings by saying, "Don't cry." It should offer compassion and support, reminiscence of a memory, and assistance.

2. *Visiting the survivor*: A spoken word of comfort, a supporting hand on the shoulder, and face-to-face encounters are very meaningful to the grieving person. Touch breaks through the numbness stage of grief and may bring the grieving person out of isolation.

3. *Helping with phone calls and arrangements for the funeral and receptions*: Try to help with hotel accommodations for family members who must travel to attend the funeral.

4. *Selecting a gift or service to provide*: Cook a meal, babysit for younger children, or perform any other activity that will relieve the responsibilities of the grieving survivor.

5. *Helping the adjustment of the household*: Offer to assist with disposition of clothes or help to list the legal responsibilities and to set a list of priorities.

6. *Including the survivor in occasional positive activities*, especially during holiday times.

7. *Remembering the anniversary* of the death, offering support, and reinforcing coping strategies during any remembrance services.

8. *Offering resources for coping*: A book, website, or a community support group may help the grieving survivor to move through the grieving process.

The health-care worker has an important role in helping grieving survivors through the bereavement process. The end of a life is part of the life cycle and coping with loss can be a developmental task in any stage. For a list of options to assist with sympathy and condolence, visit Legacy.com (2019) website at https://www.legacy.com/news/sympathy-and-condolence-advice/.

Funerals and Tasks of the Family

Preparing for a funeral is often the first task facing the family of the deceased. A funeral is an activity shortly after death involving a meaningful ceremony to remember the life of the deceased. It may or may not involve religious rituals. For the deceased, it serves the purpose of respectful recognition and disposition of the remains. For the family, it serves the purpose of confirming the reality and finality of the death, providing a climate to express grief, and an opportunity for the community to pay respects. The funeral typically recognizes, remembers, and honors the life of the one who has died.

Funerals are held in a variety of locations and for varied time periods. In some cultures, the family prepares a eulogy, a speech usually presented at the funeral ceremony intended to memorialize the deceased by including a condensed life history, details of interests and achievements at home and at work, family memories, and a summary of what the deceased enjoyed in life. It can contain humorous moments to remember as well as serious comments that honor the life of the deceased. Green burials, military honors, and New Orleans Jazz processions are all options for the endless variety in ceremony (Funeralwise, 2020).

Family tasks related to loss of a family member may also include the reorganization of roles. Decisions need to be made regarding who will do the laundry, cook, care for the young or disabled, or earn money to pay the bills. Often children are required to fill adult roles. Parents who suffer a loss of a loved one may not be able to respond to the needs of young children. The resources of the family need to be assessed and used appropriately (Potts, 2020). In the weeks, months, and years after the death, however, overt support wanes, especially if family members live many miles apart. Professional help may be needed if financial issues spark animosity among survivors. Survivors who have had the opportunity to anticipate the death of a loved one may be better prepared for the changes and challenges they will face. However, when the actual event occurs, the typical stages of the grief process are set into motion.

Death and Funeral Rituals Around the World

Every culture and religion has well-documented traditional customs and practices related to the death and funeral of a person (Giger & Haddad, 2021). Practices may revolve around religious traditions and offer guidance to the grieving family. Most all death and funeral rituals have a similar purpose: to bring people together to mourn the loss, prevent isolation, offer respectful care of the dead, and remember the deceased in a meaningful way (Meyers, 2016). Mourning rituals may include a dress code for the deceased and the mourners, reciting specific prayers or incantations, certain treatments of the deceased's body, or holding special ceremonies (Everplans, 2020). Some practices involve a simple remembrance, ceremony, and funeral, others have more elaborate practices. The community and family are often invited to share the grief. Almost all religions remember the dead and celebrate their life. Many celebrate an afterlife. Mourning and funeral practices change over time and vary between cultures, but grief itself has not. What rituals remain must be respected, as it offers a sense of control over a situation in which there is none and gives meaning to a difficult but natural time in our lives.

In times of prolonged forced isolation such as during the global coronavirus pandemic of 2020, grief and funeral rituals were difficult to carry out as many were unable to come in close contact with those who died, and group gatherings were not permitted. Traditions such as preparing the body and performing a ceremony were rarely possible and alterations to usual traditions had to be created (CDC, 2020). Family members learn their cultural and religious traditions as they experience them growing up, and documents such as personal Wills, and Living Trusts often outline these final wishes of the deceased. But it is best when active family discussions regarding final wishes take place prior to serious illness or death.

KEY POINTS

- Loss is a part of life. Normal loss occurs in every stage of life, and coping strategies are developed in response to these losses.
- Understanding common religious and cultural rituals related to death (cultural competence) enables the health-care worker to meet the individual needs of the grieving survivor and family.
- Grief is the emotional response to loss.
- Anticipatory grief occurs before the death of a loved one, when death appears imminent. Some preparation for the grief process may occur, but the stages of the grief process remain the same.
- Mourning is the outward experience of grief.
- Bereavement involves grief and mourning.
- Stages of grieving generally involve shock, disbelief, and numbness; overwhelming sadness with yearning and protest; and reflection and search for meaning.

- The tasks of the grieving process include sharing the event, recognition of the reality of the loss, sharing the expression of grief, and reorganizing and reintegrating life goals.
- Alterations of the grieving process may occur in the case of sudden deaths, in unanticipated deaths, and in deaths involving children.
- When past losses are not resolved, handling the losses involved in retirement, aging, and the death of a spouse may be dysfunctional.
- Hiding the expression of grief or attempting to replace what is lost does not allow for healthy adaptation and recovery.
- Expressing grief, accepting changes, and establishing positive and negative memories help a person progress through the grieving process.
- The ability to express positive and negative memories of the deceased without suffering severe anguish may indicate that the survivor has successfully achieved the letting-go phase of the grieving process.
- Condolence is the sharing of grief with the survivors. There are many ways condolences can be expressed.

Clinical Judgment Case Study

A family consisting of two parents, a newborn infant, a 2-year-old child, an adolescent, and a grandparent reside together in a small single-family home along with their much loved 14-year-old pet dog. The family acquired the dog as a puppy when their first child was born, but since the grandparent is home the majority of the day, the dog has become their close companion. When the dog passes away from old age, discuss how each of the family members might grieve in relation to the loss based on their stage of development.

REVIEW QUESTIONS

1. Referring to the above case study, place the below grief reactions of the parents, adolescent, and grandparent in the appropriate columns:

Normal Grief Response   **Response Indicating Dysfunctional Grief**

A. Having a memory plaque placed in the garden where the pet's ashes are buried.
B. Avoiding all contact with friends and neighbors who also have a dog for a prolonged period.
C. Tearing up when looking at photos of the dog.
D. Pretending the death did not occur for a prolonged period.
E. Holding a funeral ceremony for the dog.
F. Placing all photos or reminders of the dog in the garbage.

2. Place the developmental stage in the row that corresponds to the *most common* grief responses for that developmental stage.

Developmental Stage	Grief Responses
	Taking on a parental role or declining academic performance.
	Inconsolable crying, calling out for missing loved one.
	Having anxiety about what the long-term future will be without the person who died.
	Fear of not being cared for, or anger at the person who died.

A. Infants.

B. Young children.

C. Adolescents.

D. Young adults.

3. Match the type of response with its definition.

Type of Response	Definition
Grief	
Mourning	
Delayed grief	
Anticipatory grief	
Complicated grief	
Bereavement	

A. Emotions in response to grief are postponed and often triggered later.

B. Emotional response to the loss of anything an individual is deeply attached to.

C. Debilitating, painful, and intrusive thoughts and feelings.

D. The outward expression of grief.

E. The process of reacting, adjusting, and moving on from loss.

F. Grief that occurs before the loss.

4. Put the stages of grief in the proper order:

A. depression.

B. bargaining.

C. anger.

D. acceptance.

E. shock, denial, and isolation.

5. A 36-year-old woman recently gave birth to a stillborn full-term infant. Which of the following responses are signs of *normal* grief reactions? (Select all that apply)

A. Planning a funeral for her baby.

B. Donating the furniture in the nursery to a charity.

C. Neglecting her personal hygiene for an extended period of time.

D. Having a memory kit made that includes the layette her sister purchased for the baby.

Multilingual Glossary of Symptoms

glossary of Symptoms

Symptom	Definition	
Abnormal Bleeding	Unusual loss of blood from stools, urine, bleeding gums, internal organs.	
Chills	A feeling of being cold and shivering, usually with pale skin and a high temperature.	
Cough	Rapid expulsion of air from the lungs in order to clear fluid, mucous, or phlegm.	
Diarrhea	Having loose and watery stools (bowel movements) often.	
Disorientation	To lose a sense of time, place, and one's personal identity.	
Dizziness	A feeling of unsteadiness.	
Dyspnea	Shortness of breath or difficulty breathing.	
Fever	A rise in the temperature of the body above normal, usually when the body has an infection. (A temperature taken by mouth greater than 100.4° Fahrenheit means you have a fever.)	
Headache	A pain located in the head, as over the eyes, at the temples, or at the bottom of the skull.	
Hemoptysis	Coughing up blood (or bloody mucous).	
Jaundice	Yellowing of eyes, skin.	
Loss of Appetite	No desire to eat.	
Loss of Consciousness (Unconscious)	Not responsive, not aware, not feeling, not thinking (sometimes as a result of fainting).	
Malaise	Feeling generally weak and tired, and bodily discomfort.	
Nausea	An unpleasant feeling in the stomach, with an urge to vomit (throw up).	
Pain	An unpleasant feeling in the body that can range from being mild to extremely painful. The pain can be physical or emotional. Body pain is physical pain, usually due to tissue damage.	
Rash	Red bumps (or flaky patches) on the body that are sometimes itchy.	
Sore Throat	Pain or discomfort in swallowing.	
Tremor	An uncontrollable trembling, shaking, or quivering from physical weakness, emotional stress, or disease.	
Vomiting	To throw up what is inside the stomach through the mouth.	

Division of Communicable Disease Control

IMM-835 (3/05)

Reproduced with permission from the California Department of Public Health, Immunization Branch

glossary of Symptoms

Symptom	Spanish	Chinese	Korean	
Abnormal Bleeding	Sangrado anormal	異常出血	비정상 출혈	
Chills	Escalofrío	寒顫	오한	
Cough	Tos	咳嗽	기침	
Diarrhea	Diarrea, excrementos líquidos	腹瀉	설사	
Disorientation	Desorientación, confusión mental	定向障礙	방향 감각 상실	
Dizziness	Sentirese desmayado	頭暈	현기증	
Dyspnea	Dificultad de respirar	呼吸困難	호흡 곤란	
Fever	Fiebre	發燒	열	
Headache	Dolor de cabeza intenso	頭痛	두통	
Hemoptysis	Tos con sangre	咯血	객혈	
Jaundice	Piel y ojos de color amarillo (ictericia)	黃疸	황달	
Loss of Appetite	Pérdida del apetito	食欲不振	식욕 부진	
Loss of Consciousness (Unconscious)	Desmayarse	失去知覺	무의식	
Malaise	Indisposción o malestar	不舒服	권태감	
Nausea	Ganas de vomitar o náuseas	噁心	메스꺼움	
Pain	Dolor	疼痛	통증	
Rash	Erupción o sarpullido	皮疹	발진	
Sore Throat	Dolor de garganta	喉嚨痛	목앓이	
Tremor	Temblor continuo	震顫	떨림	
Vomiting	Vómito	嘔吐	구토	

Division of Communicable Disease Control   IMM-835 (3/05)

Reproduced with permission from the California Department of Public Health, Immunization Branch

glossary of **Symptoms**

Symptom	Japanese	Tagalog	Cambodian	
Abnormal Bleeding	異常出血	Di-normal na Pagdugo	ឈាមហូរខុសធម្មតា	
Chills	悪寒	Ginaw	ព្រឺដង្ហ័រ	
Cough	咳	Ubo	ក្អក	
Diarrhea	下痢	Pagtatae	ជម្ងឺរាគ	
Disorientation	方向感覚の喪失	Pagkalito	វង្វេងស្មារតី	
Dizziness	めまい	Pagkahilo	វិលមុខ	
Dyspnea	呼吸困難	Pangangapos ng Hininga	ពិបាកដកដង្ហើម	
Fever	発熱	Lagnat	ក្ដៅ	
Headache	頭痛	Sakit ng Ulo	ឈឺក្បាល	
Hemoptysis	血を吐く	Pag-ubo ng Dugo	ក្អកផ្លាក់ឈាម	
Jaundice	黄疸	Paninilaw ng Mata at Balat	ជម្ងឺខាន់លឿង	
Loss of Appetite	食欲不振	Pagkawala ng Ganang Kumain	មិនឃ្លានអាហារ	
Loss of Consciousness (Unconscious)	意識不明	Pagkawala ng Malay	៥គដឹងខ្លួន	
Malaise	倦怠感	Panlulupaypay	ធ្ងឹកឆ្លេ	
Nausea	吐き気	Nasusuka	ចង់ក្អួត	
Pain	痛み	Masakit	ឈឺ	
Rash	発疹	Singaw sa Balat	កន្ទួលលើស្បែក	
Sore Throat	喉の痛み	Masakit na Lalamunan	ឈឺបំពង់ក	
Tremor	震え	Pangangatal	ញ័រញ្យាក់	
Vomiting	嘔吐	Pagsusuka	ក្អួត	

Division of Communicable Disease Control   IMM-835 (3/05)

Reproduced with permission from the California Department of Public Health, Immunization Branch

glossary of Symptoms

Symptom	Hmong	Laotian	Vietnamese	
Abnormal Bleeding	Los ntshav	ເລືອດອອກຜິດປົກກະຕິ	Chảy Máu Bất Thường	
Chills	No	ຫນາວໄຂ້ສັ່ນ	Ớn Lạnh	
Cough	Hnoos	ອາການໄອ/ໄອ	Ho	
Diarrhea	Thoj plab	ຖອກທ້ອງ	Tiêu Chảy	
Disorientation	Feeb tsis meej	ສັບສົນ	Bối Rối Mất Định Hướng	
Dizziness	Kiv taubhau	ສີກວິນວຽນຫົວ	Chóng mặt	
Dyspnea	Txog Siav	ຫາຍໃຈຝືດ	Hụt Hơi Khó Thở	
Fever	Kub cev	ເປັນໄຂ້	Sốt	
Headache	Mob taubhau	ເຈັບຫົວ	Nhức Đầu	
Hemoptysis	Hnoos tau ntshav	ໄອອອກເລືອດ	Ho Khạc Ra Máu	
Jaundice	Daj ntseg	ເປັນຂີ້ຫມາກເຫລືອງ	Vàng Da	
Loss of Appetite	Tsis qab los	ກິນເຂົ້າບໍ່ແຊບ	Biếng ăn	
Loss of Consciousness (Unconscious)	Looj lawm	ຫມົດສະຕິ (ສະຫລົບ)	Bất Tỉnh	
Malaise	Nkees	ອາການບໍ່ສະບາຍ	Mệt Mỏi Uể Oải	
Nausea	Xeev siab	ປວດຮາກ	Buồn Nôn	
Pain	Mob	ເຈັບ/ປວດ	Đau Nhức	
Rash	Ua xua	ຕຸ່ມແດງ	Da nổi mụn đỏ	
Sore Throat	Mob cajpas	ເຈັບຄໍ	Đau Cổ Họng	
Tremor	Tshee	ສັ່ນ	Run Rẩy	
Vomiting	Ntuav	ຮາກ	Ói Mửa	

Division of Communicable Disease Control   IMM-835 (3/05)

Reproduced with permission from the California Department of Public Health, Immunization Branch

glossary of Symptoms

Symptom	Arabic	Farsi	Armenian	
Abnormal Bleeding	نزيف شديد غبر طبيعي	خونريزى غيرعادى (اَب نُرمال بليدينگ)	Արտասովոր Արյունահոսություն	
Chills	قشعريرة	لرز (چيلز)	Սարսուռություն	
Cough	سعال / كحة	سرفه (كاف)	Հազ	
Diarrhea	إسهال	اسهال (دايريا)	Լուծ	
Disorientation	توهان	اختلال درجهت يابى (ديس اُرينتيشن)	Ապակողմնորոշում	
Dizziness	دوخة/دوار	سرگيجه	Գլխապտույտ	
Dyspnea	ضيقة نفس / صعوبة في التنفس	تنگى نفس (ديسپينيا)	Ապավարար Շնչառություն	
Fever	سخونة شديدة	تب (فيور)	Ջերմություն	
Headache	صداع	سردرد (هد إك)	Գլխացավ	
Hemoptysis	سعال مع بصق الدم / كحة مع بصق الدم	خلط خونى (هِمّتا يسپس)	ԱրյունախերՀազ	
Jaundice	الصفراء	يرقان . زردى (جانديس)	Դեղնախտ	
Loss of Appetite	فقدان الشهية/عدم الرغبة في الطعام	بى اشتهايى	Ախորժակի Կորուստ	
Loss of Consciousness (Unconscious)	فقدان الوعي (فاقد الوعي)	ناهوشيارى (آنكانشيس نس)	Ուշաթափություն (ուշակորույս լինել)	
Malaise	تعب في الجسم كله	احساس بيحالى و ناخوشى. كوفتگى (مَليز)	Թուլություն	
Nausea	ميل للتقيؤ / غثيان	حال بهم خوردگى. تهوع (نازيا)	Սրտախառնություն	
Pain	ألم	درد (پين)	Ցավ	
Rash	طفح	جوش و دانه هاى قرمز روى پوست (رَش)	Ցան	
Sore Throat	ألم في الزور	گلو درد (سُرتُرت)	Կոկորդի Բորբոքում	
Tremor	رعشة	لرزش و تكان غير ارادى (ترمُر)	Դող	
Vomiting	تقيؤ	استفراغ (واميتينگ)	Փսխումներ	

Division of Communicable Disease Control

IMM-835 (3/05)

Reproduced with permission from the California Department of Public Health, Immunization Branch

glossary of Symptoms

Symptom	Russian	Punjabi	
Abnormal Bleeding	Кровотечение в брюшную полость	ਬਹੁਤ ਖੂਨ ਪੈਣਾ	
Chills	Озноб	ਪਾਲਾ	
Cough	Кашель	ਖੰਘ	
Diarrhea	Понос	ਟੱਟੀਆਂ ਲੱਗਣਾ	
Disorientation	Дезориентация	ਬੌਂਦਲਣਾ	
Dizziness	Головокружение	ਚੱਕਰ ਆਉਣੇ	
Dyspnea	Одышка	ਸਾਹ ਲੈਣ ਵਿਚ ਮੁਸ਼ਕਲ	
Fever	Жар	ਬੁਖਾਰ	
Headache	Головная боль	ਸਿਰਦਰਦ	
Hemoptysis	Кровохарканье	ਖੰਘ ਨਾਲ ਖੂਨ ਆਉਣਾ	
Jaundice	Желтуха	ਪੀਲੀਆ	
Loss of Appetite	Потеря аппетита	ਭੁੱਖ ਨਾ ਲੱਗਣਾ	
Loss of Consciousness (Unconscious)	Потеря сознания	ਬੇਹੋਸ਼ੀ	
Malaise	Недомогание	ਕਮਜ਼ੋਰੀ	
Nausea	Тошнота	ਜੀਅ ਕੱਚਾ ਹੋਣਾ	
Pain	Боль	ਦਰਦ	
Rash	Сыпь	ਧੱਫੜ	
Sore Throat	Больное горло	ਗਲਾ ਦੁਖਣਾ	
Tremor	Дрожь	ਕੰਬਣਾ	
Vomiting	Рвота	ਉਲਟੀਆਂ	

This glossary includes only the most common signs and symptoms of most communicable diseases. Disease investigators can use this as a supplement when interviewing non-English speaking clients. Languages included are the most common ones in California. A phonetic pronunciation supplement is available online for download at **www.cdlhn.com**.

Division of Communicable Disease Control   IMM-835 (3/05)

Reproduced with permission from the California Department of Public Health, Immunization Branch

Glossary

Abstinence: Voluntarily refraining from indulging in practices such as sexual intercourse.

Accreditation: The process by which an institution is recognized as meeting specific predetermined standards of care.

Acculturation: The adjustment to a new culture.

Activities of daily living (ADL): Tasks that enable a person to meet his or her own basic needs, such as toileting, eating, and dressing.

Adolescence: The period between childhood and adulthood, which can be considered as between the ages of 10 and 20.

Advance health-care directive (AHCD): A legal document that guides health-care personnel concerning a patient's wishes when that patient is no longer capable of making decisions.

Age-appropriate toys: Toys that are safe and promote the cognitive and motor development of a specific age group.

Ageism: Discrimination or avoidance because of a person's age.

Aging in place: The ability of a person to remain in their own home for the duration of their lifespan while maintaining their safety and independence.

Allele: A pairing of genes that contain specific inheritable characteristics.

Alternative medicine: Therapies used *instead* of Western medical care.

Alzheimer disease: A progressive decline in mental function related to degeneration of the brain.

Anticipatory grief: Grief that occurs before a loss.

Apgar score: A scoring system to evaluate the newborn at 1 and 5 minutes after birth.

Apoptosis: The programmed death of cells. Referred to as the biological clock, it leads to menopause and senescence.

Assisted suicide: An action of a person other than the patient to facilitate suicide.

Assistive devices: Items such as canes, walkers, and hearing aids that help a person maintain independent living.

Asynchronous: Not synchronous; exhibiting asynchrony; not occurring at the same time, as when different parts of the body mature at different times causing an awkward appearance (e.g., during adolescence).

Atrophy: A decrease in the size of an organ or tissue.

Attachment: An affectionate bond that occurs over time as a result of interaction.

Autonomy: Freedom from external control or influence; independence.

Behavioral theories: Theories designed to explain the development of specific behaviors and suggest their relationships to other developing social skills.

Behaviorist theory: A theory that describes how and why behavioral learning alters behavior.

Behaviors: Individual responses or reactions to internal stimuli and external conditions.

Beliefs: Cultural teachings of practices and values handed down for generations that determine how one behaves and responds to daily life and health-care practices.

Bereavement: A period of sadness and adjustment after the loss of a loved one.

Biological clock: A programmed cell death that leads to menopause and deterioration associated with senescence.

Biology: An individual's genetic makeup (those factors with which he or she is born), family history (which may suggest risk for disease), and the physical and mental health problems acquired during life.

Blended family: One or both parents may bring children from a previous marriage or relationship to form a new, blended family.

Bonding: The development of a strong emotional attachment between individuals, such as a mother and her infant.

Cephalocaudal: The progression of the growth pattern that proceeds from head to toe.

Chromosome: A thread of protein and DNA contained in the nucleus of every cell.

Classical conditioning: Relates a positive or negative event to a specific behavior to promote or prevent that behavior from recurring.

Climacteric: The change of life in which hormonal shifts result in cessation of the reproductive ability in women and a corresponding decrease in sexual drive in men.

Clique: A social group with a fixed exclusive membership that shares similar interests, values, and tastes.

Cognitive style: A pattern of thought and reasoning.

Cognitive theories: Theories that focus on advancement of the development of thinking.

Coitus: Sexual intercourse.

Compassion: Reactions to others that are motivated by love and kindness.

Competence: Effective interactions; ability.

Complementary and Alternative Medicine (CAM): Non-Western medicinal practices such as essential oils, acupressure, acupuncture, Qi gong, herbal supplements, or meditation.

Complementary medicine: Therapies used *together with* Western therapies.

Complicated grief: Prolonged and debilitating grief.

Conception: The union of the male sperm and female ovum; fertilization.

Condolence: The expression of sympathy or grieving together.

Cooperative play: A group of two or more children who cooperate by playing together.

Coping skill: A behavior that helps an individual adapt to or manage a stressful situation.

Corporal punishment: Spanking; focuses on the pain of the punishment and can role model aggression, in which case it will not accomplish the true goal of discipline.

Cultural assimilation: A process by which members of a specific cultural group lose some of the characteristics of that group and adapt to the practices of another group.

Cultural awareness: Recognizing the history of patients' ancestry or culture and how their customs influence the handling of problems, issues, or teachings.

Cultural care: Health-promotion activities initiated by a culturally competent health-care worker who enables a patient to modify health behaviors toward beneficial outcomes while respecting the patient's cultural values, beliefs, and practices.

Cultural competence: Involves cultural awareness, acceptance, and respect toward behaviors and practices that are different from one's own.

Cultural interventions: Interventions achieved when health-care information is presented in a way that includes specific cultural styles, colors, pictures, symbols, and so forth, that add credibility to the content by reflecting cultural values.

Cultural relativism: The concept that normalcy comes from the standard social practices of a specific culture.

Cultural sensitivity: Observing, using, and showing knowledge of culturally appropriate verbal language, body language, use of personal space, and gestures of respect toward family members while providing health care or teaching.

Cultural stereotyping: The assumption that all the people of one culture behave the same way and believe the same thing.

Culture: A set of learned values, beliefs, customs, and behaviors that is shared by interacting individuals, such as a family.

Culture shock: The effect of a sudden, drastic change in the cultural environment of an individual or family.

Defense mechanism: A reaction that is protective to the individual or helps conceal conflicts or anxieties.

Delayed grief: Postponed emotions in response to a loss, triggered by another stressful event.

Dental caries: Tooth decay.

Determinants of health: Genetic makeup, lifestyle behaviors, social and physical environment, and general policies and interventions that affect the health of the population.

Development: Indicates an increase in function and mastery of tasks for the specific phase in the lifespan.

Developmental stage: Patterns of development related to perception and response to environment.

Developmental task: A competency or skill that helps a person cope with the environment or advance personal development.

Discipline: A technique used to guide, teach, or correct behavior; it may include consequences but is not punishment.

Disengagement: Implies removing of emotional attachments to people, places, and objects.

Dizygotic: A type of twin that occurs when two ova are released at ovulation and each ovum is fertilized by a separate sperm.

Dominant gene: A gene that overpowers other genes so that its characteristics will be inherited.

Durable power of attorney for health care: A type of advance directive that gives decision-making power concerning health care to a person designated by the patient, to be used when the patient cannot speak for himself or herself.

Dysbiosis: A shifting or impairment of microbiomes that allows inflammation or chronic disorders to develop.

Dysfunctional family: A family unit that does not offer consistency of membership or rules, may exhibit poor interpersonal relationships among its members, handles conflicts and problems poorly, and often cannot reach out to the community for help.

Early childhood: A period that includes children between the ages of 1 and 6. Early childhood is typically separated into two phases; ages 1–2 is the toddler phase, and ages 2–6 is the preschool phase.

Ectopic pregnancy: A pregnancy that occurs outside the uterus, usually in the fallopian tube.

Ejaculation: Release of semen and sperm during orgasm.

Elder abuse: The infliction of harm or neglect through actions or acts of omission on an older person. The abuse can be physical, emotional, or financial and can include neglect or obstruction of personal rights.

Electra anxiety: Occurs when little girls compete with their mothers for love and attention from their fathers.

Empathy: Acknowledgment of emotions of another person and an attempt at understanding how others feel.

Empowerment: Providing tools and knowledge to the family to enable informed participation in decision making.

Empty nest syndrome: When grown children start to leave home for the first time, causing parents to feel lonely or isolated.

En face: Face to face.

Engrossment: When fathers or significant others develop an intense focus on a newborn.

Ethnicity: A cultural pattern shared by people with the same cultural heritage. Language, preferred diet, specific customs, family roles, and religious beliefs are often shared among those with the same ethnicity.

Ethnocentrism: The belief that one's own culture is the standard of behavior and is better than other cultures.

Eulogy: A speech usually presented at the funeral ceremony intended to memorialize the deceased.

Euthanasia: An intentional act that causes death for the purpose of relieving pain and suffering.

Exercise: Specifically planned and structured repetitive activities designed for a level of calorie burning that increases endurance, balance, strength, or flexibility.

Expressive language: The ability to express thoughts in the words of a language.

Extrovert: An outgoing person who focuses on others in the environment.

Facebook depression: Depression that affects one who overuses social networking to the point of altering sleep and eating habits and isolating himself from peers and family, eventually succumbing to general depression.

Family: A basic human social system that involves commitment and interaction among its members.

Family systems theory: Theories that explain interconnected family functions and responses.

Federal Register: Federal legislation concerning health care is recorded and published in this document.

Fetal alcohol syndrome: A group of symptoms present in a newborn infant resulting from maternal ingestion of alcohol during pregnancy.

Fetus: An unborn infant from the ninth week of conception to birth.

Food insecurity: The state of being without reliable access to a sufficient quantity of affordable, nutritious food.

Free radicals: When one ion of a molecule breaks off and is no longer paired. Free radicals produce a harmful effect on body tissues.

Funeral: An activity shortly after death involving a meaningful ceremony to remember the life of the deceased.

Gamification: Electronic media activities that apply gaming elements to real world activity.

Gender dysphoria: Involves conflict between assigned sex and gender identity.

Gender identity: Refers to a feeling of how a person identifies themselves as feminine, masculine, or some combination of the two (nonbinary).

Gender nonconformity: The situation in which a person identifies as their assigned gender but behaves in a nonstereotypical gender manner.

Gene therapy: Involves placing a therapeutic gene on the back of a virus vector, which will then carry the new gene into the cell that has a missing or defective gene.

Generativity: Contributing in a positive way to family or community. This contribution improves self-image and promotes subjective well-being.

Genetic code: The code contained in the genes of living cells that will determine what characteristics will be inherited.

Genetic counseling: The communication between a geneticist (a specialist in inherited conditions) and the parents regarding the risk of their infant inheriting genes that can result in an abnormality.

Genome: A complete set of chromosomes and DNA that contain all the genetic information in the human cell.

Geriatrics: The study of old age, including the biological, psychological, physiological, and sociological aspects of aging.

Gestation: The period between conception and birth.

Gestational diabetes: Diabetes that occurs during pregnancy.

Gingivitis: Gum irritation or infection.

Grief: The emotional response to a loss and is a process through which a survivor accepts the loss.

Growth: Indicates an increase in size.

Gonads: A term used to refer to ovaries in females and testicles in males.

Health indicators: The public health issues and concerns linked to the objectives of *Healthy People 2030.*

Health maintenance organization (HMO): A group medical practice that offers prepaid care for members.

Health status: Details concerning illness and other factors that affect health, which are measured by factors such as birth and death rates, life expectancy, and accessibility to health care.

Healthy People 2030: An evidence-based 10-year report card describing health-care accomplishments within the United States from the years 2010 to 2020 and a prescription for what needs to be done between now and the year 2030.

Homeopathy: The use of minute portions of chemicals for their healing power.

Hormone replacement therapy (HRT): Hormone supplementation to relieve discomforts associated with perimenopause and menopause.

Hospice: A plan of noncurative terminal care that is based on the philosophy that death is a normal part of the life cycle. Hospice involves palliative care that meets the physical, psychological, spiritual, and social needs of the dying patient.

Hot flashes: A sensation caused by blood rushing to the surface of the skin as a result of dilation of capillaries.

Humanist theories: Theories that describe the influence of human experiences such as love and attachment on behavior and personality development.

Hydrotherapy: Therapy using water.

Hysterectomy: Removal of the uterus.

Identity accommodation: Changing the concept of one's own identity to fit what is real, rather than what was dreamed or imagined.

Immune theory: A theory of aging that involves the concept that as one ages, the body finds it more difficult to tell the difference between healthy and defective cells.

Immunity: The body's resistance to disease-causing organisms.

Infant: The period between ages 4 weeks and 1 year.

Infant mortality rate: The number of deaths that occur before age 1 per 1000 live births.

Information processing: An input of information followed by a thought mechanism resulting in an output of judgment or decision-making.

Information processing theory: Theory based on the idea that information is input, is processed mentally, and is then followed by an output of judgment and decision-making. This processing matures in a continuous pattern of development as opposed to maturation in stages.

Informed consent: Providing the patient with information, in a language that the patient can understand, regarding the risks of, advantages to, and possible alternatives available for a medical or surgical procedure.

Initiative: The ability to take the first step or the leading movement.

Intimacy: Not only involving sexuality, intimacy involves developing a warm, trusting, honest relationship with another person with whom it is safe to be open and to express and share private thoughts.

Intimate partner violence: A term related to domestic violence, which can include psychological, physical, sexual, financial, and social abuses between intimate partners.

Introvert: A quiet person who focuses inwardly on himself or herself.

Latchkey children: Children who are allowed to remain without direct supervision, usually during the hours after school, because both parents work and extended family are not available to care for the children.

Late adulthood: The ages between 65 and 74 years.

Leading Health Indicators: Selected high-priority issues within *Healthy People 2030* for the current 10-year period.

Legacy: What one leaves to the world that may give a person a feeling of immortality; can be a child, grandchild, property, a culture, an organization, or writings.

Length: Referring to measurement of height of an infant while the infant is lying down.

Life expectancy: The average number of years a person born in a particular year is expected to live.

Looking-glass self: The development of a self-image by combining the way we portray ourselves to others and the way others evaluate us.

Managed care organization: An organization that standardizes medical practice guidelines to maintain the quality of care provided at the same time as it controls the costs of health care.

Maturational loss: Losses experienced during passage through the life cycle, such as decreased physical strength or perceived beauty.

Medicaid: A type of federal welfare program in which benefits are provided on a basis of need or level of poverty.

Medicare: A type of a government-provided insurance program in which benefits are received after contributions are made through payroll deductions.

Menarche: The very first menstrual period.

Menopause: The cessation of the menstrual period as a result of hormonal changes in the body.

Menstrual cycle: Consists of (1) maturing of the egg in the ovary, (2) formation of blood and mucus in the lining of the uterus, (3) ovulation, and (4) expulsion of the unfertilized egg with the blood and mucous lining from the uterus. This cycle lasts approximately 28 days and repeats until menopause.

Microbiome: Micro (tiny) and biome (organism) are large communities of trillions of tiny organisms that live in our body.

Middle adulthood: The ages between 40 and 65 years.

Middle childhood: The ages of children between 6 and 12 years.

Midlife crisis: A stressful period when an adult tries to make up for lost opportunities of the past or challenge the inevitability of the future.

Midlife transition: The process of aging in which one is able to realign themselves with the next stage of life in a healthy way.

Mnemonic technique: The use of rhymes for remembering certain things, such as the number of days in each month.

Monozygotic: A type of twin that develops when one single fertilized ovum separates into two separate embryos.

Moral behavior: Actions based on moral reasoning.

Moral reasoning: A capacity that develops in a child as he or she learns to understand rules and determine if an action is right or wrong.

Mourning: The outward expression of grief.

Multifetal: More than one fetus – that is, twins, triplets, quadruplets, septuplets.

Mutated: Malformed.

Neonatal: The first 30 days of life after birth.

Nocturnal emission: Ejaculation of semen during sleep.

Nonverbal language: The language of the motions, postures, and gestures of the body that is learned as part of communication.

Norms: Averages that can be used as guidelines for comparison concerning, for example, the age that specific abilities or skills are achieved or disappear.

Nurse practice acts: The scope of practice for each level of professional practice in nursing.

Nursing caries: Tooth decay that occurs when the infant is put to bed while sucking on a bottle of milk or juice. The milk or juice pools in the mouth, allowing bacterial organisms to grow.

Nursing Licensure Compact: A multistate licensing arrangement that enables traveling nurses to function in multiple states.

Object permanence: Knowing an object is there even though it is not within sight.

Occupational Health and Safety Act (OSHA): Standards of safety that must be maintained by employers to protect the health and safety of employees; mandates reporting of injuries sustained by workers.

Oedipus complex: Arises during the phallic stage of development. Freud suggested that little boys compete with their father for the mother's love and attention.

Operant conditioning: Involves behavioral consequences such as reward or punishment.

Ordinal position: Birth order; whether the infant is an only child, older child, youngest child, or middle child may influence the age and rapidity of mastering developmental tasks.

Oropharynx: The part of the anatomy that includes the mouth and throat.

Osteoporosis: The loss of bone mass.

Ovulation: Release of a matured egg from the ovary into the fallopian tube that leads to the uterus.

Palliative care: Care interventions with the primary focus of improving quality of life rather than length of life of patients and families during life-threatening illnesses.

Parallel play: When a young child plays next to a friend but does not interact with the friend during play.

Pelvic inflammatory disease: A serious complication of some sexually transmitted infections (STIs), especially chlamydia and gonorrhea, that infects the uterus, fallopian tubes, and other reproductive organs.

Personality: A unique combination of characteristics that results in the individual's recurrent pattern of behavior.

Physical activity: Daily actions that use energy, such as dog walking or gardening.

Physical environment: Things that can be seen, touched, heard, smelled, and tasted and less tangible elements, such as radiation and ozone.

Physician's Orders for Life Sustaining Treatment (POLST): Physician order drawn up in partnership with the patient that specifically states what is to be done and not to be done during a life-threatening illness.

Pincer action or grasp: The ability to pick up small objects with the thumb and forefinger.

Plan of care: A tool for communication among multidisciplinary health-care team members.

Plaque: A sticky, transparent mass of bacteria that grows on the surface and spreads to the roots of teeth.

Political action committees (PACs): Groups that influence governmental legislation by offering monetary contributions to legislators who support their needs and that provide lobbying efforts to create an awareness of needed legislation.

Polypharmacy: The ingestion of multiple medications in one day.

Postformal operational thought: The process of integrating various points of view to develop knowledge and understanding.

Posttraumatic stress disorder (PTSD): The development of characteristic symptoms following an extreme traumatic stressor.

Preferred provider organization (PPO): An organization that contracts with professionals in the medical field to provide care to a specific group of patients at an agreed-on fee-for-service rate.

Preschool phase: Age between 2 and 6 years.

Preverbal: Body language before the ability to speak.

Psychodynamic theories: Theories that focus on personality trait development and psychological challenges at different ages.

Proximodistal: From the midline of the body to the periphery.

Puberty: The age at which sexual maturity occurs; having the functional ability to reproduce. Puberty involves physical and psychological changes.

Receptive language: Ability to understand words.

Relatedness: A sense of belonging.

Reproductive health: A term used to describe the health of the reproductive organs in males and females.

Sandwich generation: A period in middle adulthood when persons must deal with increased financial and emotional responsibilities related to their children and increased demands placed on them by their older and possibly dependent parents.

Scope of practice: "The identification of and legal limitations to the usual and customary skill practices of a professional. The usual and customary practices are determined by the educational preparation for that profession" (From Nurse Practice Act, Business and Professional Code).

Secondary sex characteristics: The development of pubic, facial, and body hair; also, in boys the enlargement and darkening of the scrotum and an increase in penis size; in girls the enlargement of breasts and darkening around the areola.

Senescence: A period in an adult's life in which the body begins to age and weaken more noticeably.

Separation anxiety: When an infant cries or protests when the parent leaves the room or when approached by a stranger. Separation anxiety usually emerges after 6 months of age.

Sexual orientation: Refers to sexual attractions and preference for a sexual partner.

Sexuality: Beliefs and behaviors that surround physiological responses, emotions, and sociocultural values. Involves communication, a sense of closeness, and mutual comfort.

Sexually transmitted infection (STI): Illness that is transmitted through sexual intercourse and in some cases through oral copulation (oral sex).

Sexting: The sending or receiving of sexually explicit text messages and pictures.

Sibling rivalry: The competition between brothers and sisters, usually for parental attention and love.

SIDS: Sudden infant death syndrome.

Situational loss: Unexpected loss as a result of an encountered situation such as loss of a job, loss of living arrangements, etc.

Social cognition: An awareness and understanding of how a person's actions may affect other people. When children begin to understand social cognition, it enables them to cooperate better with peers, and it can enhance the child's self-concept.

Social environment: Interactions with family, friends, coworkers, and others in the community and social institutions, such as law enforcement, the workplace, places of worship, and schools.

Social learning theory: Involves exposure to and imitation of a behavior.

Sociocultural theories: Theories that describe how culture influences behavior.

Somatic: Pertaining to the body.

Spermatogenesis: The production of sperm.

Stagnation: The failure to achieve generativity.

Standards of practice: Guidelines used to determine type and quality of care provided to patients.

Stereotyping: Assuming that all people from a specific cultural or ethnic group behave or believe the same way.

Structure: Referring to Levinson's four seasons of life, each with a structure during which significant choices are made, separated by transitional periods during which those choices are evaluated.

Sympathy: A pity-based response to grief.

Syndrome: A group of symptoms or signs of an abnormal condition.

Teaching moment: The point at which the learner is most receptive to change or growth within a situation.

Testicular self-examination (TSE): Self-examination of the testicles.

Thanatophobia: Fear of death.

Theory: A group of concepts that form the basis for understanding observations. An accepted theory is logical, consistent, and integrates past and current research.

Therapeutic communication: A form of communication that involves accepting the patient's emotional outbursts and expressions and encouraging venting and verbalization.

Therapeutic presence: Remaining near the patient and family, or simply holding a hand, thus providing strength while facilitating emotional expressions in patients and families during times of grief or stress.

Time-out: A form of discipline implemented as a response to unacceptable behavior. Effective discipline technique for children between the ages of 1 and 6 years.

Toddler phase: Period between the ages of 1 and 2 years.

Transitional phase: A period of young adulthood during which life choices are reviewed and reevaluated, and changes may be made.

Trial of labor after cesarean (TOLAC): Females who previously gave birth via cesarean are allowed to labor in an attempt to facilitate vaginal birth as opposed to scheduling cesarean before natural labor begins.

Vaginal birth after cesarean (VBAC): A controversial practice in which a woman who previously had a cesarean section attempts to deliver a subsequent baby vaginally.

Values: Deep feelings about what is right or wrong, good or bad.

Viable: Able to survive outside the uterus.

Vigorous exercise: At least 20 minutes of exercise that causes sweating or breathing hard.

Virus vector: A virus that has the ability to enter specific cells in the body and act as a vehicle to carry substances to that cell.

Wear-and-tear theory: Like machinery, parts of the human body begin to wear out or break down over time.

Young adult: Person between the ages of 20 and 39 years.

Bibliography and Online Resources

CHAPTER 1 *HEALTHY PEOPLE 2030*

Centers for Disease Control (2019). National vital statistics report, 68(7), 1-66. Retrieved April 26, 2020 from https://www.cdc.gov/nchs/data/nvsr/nvsr68/nvsr68_07-508.pdf.

Centers for Disease Control and Prevention (2017). Healthy People 2020 midcourse review. Retrieved August 16, 2020 from https://www.cdc.gov/nchs/healthy_people/hp2020/hp2020_midcourse_review.htm.

Centers for Disease Control and Prevention (2017). National Center for Health Statistics adolescent health. Retrieved April 26, 2020 from https://www.cdc.gov/nchs/fastats/adolescent-health.htm.

Centers for Disease Control and Prevention (2018). Health, United States. Retrieved August 16, 2020 from https://www.cdc.gov/nchs/hus/index.htm.

Centers for Disease Control and Prevention (2019). Reproductive health, infant mortality. Retrieved April 26, 2020 from https://www.cdc.gov/reproductivehealth/maternalinfanthealth/infantmortality.htm.

Central Intelligence Agency (2020). Country comparison: Life expectancy at birth. The world factbook. Retrieved April 26, 2020, from https://www.cia.gov/library/publications/the-world-factbook/fields/355rank.html.

Central Intelligence Agency (2020). The world factbook country comparison infant mortality rate. Retrieved April 26, 2020 from https://www.cia.gov/library/publications/the-world-factbook/rankorder/2091rank.html.

Dietary Guidelines Advisory Committee (2020). Scientific report of the 2020 Dietary Guidelines Advisory Committee: Advisory report to the Secretary of Agriculture and the Secretary of Health and Human Services. US Department of Agriculture, Agricultural Research Service.

National Academies of Sciences, Engineering, and Medicine (2020). *The leading health indicators 2030: Advancing health, equity, and well-being.* The National Academies Press. https://doi.org/10.17226/25682.

National Vital Statistics System, National Center for Health Statistics, Center for Disease Control and Prevention (2017). 10 leading causes of death by age group United States 2017. Retrieved April 26, 2020, from https://www.cdc.gov/injury/wisqars/pdf/leading_causes_of_death_by_age_group_2017-508.pdf.

Office of Disease Prevention and Health Promotion (2020). Healthy People 2030 Framework. Retrieved April 26, 2020 from https://www.healthypeople.gov/2020/About-Healthy-People/Development-Healthy-People-2030/Framework.

Office of Disease Prevention and Health Promotion (2020). Secretary's advisory committee on national health promotion and disease prevention objectives for 2030: Recommendations for an approach to Healthy People 2030. Retrieved April 26, 2020 from https://www.healthypeople.gov/sites/default/files/Full%20Committee%20Report%20to%20Secretary%205-9-2017_1.pdf.

U.S. Department of Health and Human Services (2000). *Healthy People 2010.* International Publishing, Inc.

United Nations (2020). Millennium development goals. Retrieved April 26, 2020 from https://www.undp.org/content/undp/en/home/sdgoverview/mdg_goals.html.

United States Department of Health and Human Services (2014). Healthy People 2020 leading health indicators: Progress update. Retrieved April 26, 2020 from https://www.healthypeople.gov/sites/default/files/LHI-ProgressReport-ExecSum_0.pdf.

United States Department of Health and Human Services (2020). Healthy People 2030. Retrieved from https://health.gov/healthypeople.

United States Department of Health and Human Services (2020). Proposed objectives for inclusion in healthy people 2030. Retrieved April 26, 2020 from https://www.healthypeople.gov/sites/default/files/ObjectivesPublicComment508.pdf.

United States Department of Health and Human Services (2020). Secretary's advisory committee on national health promotion and disease prevention objectives for 2030. Report #7 assessment and recommendations for proposed objectives for Healthy People 2030. Retrieved April 26, 2020 from https://www.healthypeople.gov/sites/default/files/Report%207_Reviewing%20Assessing%20Set%20of%20HP2030%20Objectives_Formatted%20EO_508_05.21.pdf.

United States Environmental Protection Agency (2018). *EPA's environmental quality index supports public health*. Retrieved from https://www.epa.gov/healthresearch/epas-environmental-quality-index-supports-public-health.

Weiss, H., & Ferrand, R. (2019). Improving adolescent health: an evidence-based call to action. *The Lancet*, *393*(10176), 1073–1075.

Online Resources

https://health.gov/healthypeople
https://www.cdc.gov/
https://www.healthypeople.gov/2020/About-Healthy-People/Development-Healthy-People-2030/Framework
https://www.hhs.gov/
https://www.who.int/

CHAPTER 2 GOVERNMENT INFLUENCES ON HEALTH CARE

American Hospital Association (2003). The patient care partnership understanding expectations, rights, and responsibilities. Retrieved May 1, 2020 from https://www.aha.org/system/files/2018-01/aha-patient-care-partnership.pdf.

American Medical Association (2017). American health care act. Retrieved May 1, 2020 from https://www.ama-assn.org/sites/ama-assn.org/files/corp/media-browser/public/government/advocacy/ahca-top-line-summary.pdf.

Centers for Disease Control and Prevention (2015). State school immunization requirements and vaccine exemption laws. Retrieved May 1, 2020 from https://www.cdc.gov/phlp/docs/school-vaccinations.pdf.

Centers for Medicare & Medicaid Services (2010). The affordable care act's new patient's bill of rights. Retrieved May 1, 2020 from https://www.cms.gov/CCIIO/Resources/Fact-Sheets-and-FAQs/aca-new-patients-bill-of-rights.

Chen, I., Richter, P., & Miner, L. (2011). FDA's new role in tobacco control. *Contemporary Pediatrics*, *28*(11), 39–45.

Mason, D., Perez, A., McLemore, R., & Dickson, E. (2020). *Policy and politics in nursing and health care* (8th ed.). Elsevier.

National Council of State Boards of Nursing, Inc. (2020). NLC member states. Retrieved May 1, 2020 from https://www.ncsbn.org/nlcmemberstates.pdf.

National Council of State Boards of Nursing, Inc. (2020). Nurse licensure compact. Retrieved May 1, 2020 from https://www.ncsbn.org/nurse-licensure-compact.htm.

Schiff, E., Attias, S., Matter, I., Sroka, G., Nae, B., Arnon, Z., Samuels, N., Grinberg, O., & Ben-Arye, E. (2019). Complementary and alternative medicine interventions for perioperative symptoms: A comparative effectiveness study. *Complementary Therapies in Medicine*, 44, 51–55. Retrieved May 1, 2020 from https://www.sciencedirect.com/science/article/abs/pii/S0965229919301190#!.

Social Security Agency (2020). Retirement benefits. Retrieved May 1, 2020 from https://www.ssa.gov/planners/retire/agereduction.html.

The Joint Commission (2013). Accreditation guide for hospitals. Retrieved May 9, 2020, from https://www.jointcommission.org/-/media/deprecated-unorganized/imported-assets/tjc/system-folders/assetmanager/accreditation_guide_hospitals_2011pdf.pdf?db=web&hash=350D19DE3CEF201A9C270B07B7D0FBCD.

Online Resources

https://www.aha.org/
https://www.cdc.gov/phlp/index.html
https://www.ncsl.org/
https://www.fda.gov/tobacco-products
https://smokefree.gov/
https://teens.drugabuse.gov/

CHAPTER 3 CULTURAL CONSIDERATIONS ACROSS THE LIFESPAN AND IN HEALTH AND ILLNESS

Banwell, C., Ulijaslek, S., & Dixon, J. (2013). *When culture impacts health*. Elsevier.

Cherry, B., & Jacob, S. (2019). *Contemporary nursing issues, trends, & management* (8th ed.). Elsevier.

Giger, J., & Davidhizar, R. (2002). Transcultural nursing assessment. *International Nursing Review*, 37(1), 199–203.

Giger, T., & Haddad, L. (2020). *Transcultural nursing: assessment and intervention* (8th ed.). Elsevier.

Kaiser Family Foundation (2013). Race/ethnicity. Retrieved May 1, 2020 from https://www.kff.org/medicaid/state-indicator/medicaid-enrollment-by-raceethnicity/?currentTimeframe=0&sortModel=%7B%22colId%22:%22Location%22,%22sort%22:%22asc%22%7D.

Micozzi, M. (2018). *Fundamentals of complimentary, alternative, and integrative medicine* (6th ed.). Elsevier.

Pew Research Center (2016). 10 demographic trends shaping the U.S. and the world in 2016. Retrieved July 25, 2020 from https://www.pewresearch.org/fact-tank/2016/03/31/10-demographic-trends-that-are-shaping-the-u-s-and-the-world/.

Riley, J. (2019). *Communication in Nursing* (9th ed.). Elsevier.

The Church of Jesus Christ of Latter-Day Saints (n.d.). Word of wisdom. Retrieved July 25, 2020 from https://www.churchofjesuschrist.org/study/manual/gospel-topics/word-of-wisdom?lang=eng.

United Nations World Population Prospects (2019). United States population 2020 (live). Retrieved July 25, 2020 from https://worldpopulationreview.com/countries/united-states-population.

United States Census Bureau (2017). American community survey. Retrieved May 1, 2020 from https://www.census.gov/acs/www/data/data-tables-and-tools/data-profiles/2017/.

United States Census Bureau (n.d.). Quick facts United States. Retrieved May 1, 2020 from https://www.census.gov/quickfacts/fact/table/US/PST045219.

Wold, G. (2008). *Basic geriatric care* (4th ed.). Mosby/Elsevier.

Online Resources

https://minorityhealth.hhs.gov/omh/browse.aspx?lvl=2&lvlid=53

https://www.ahrq.gov/

https://www.ausmed.com/cpd/articles/cultural-assessment

https://www.hhs.gov/ash/oah/resources-and-training/tpp-and-paf-resources/cultural-competence/index.html

https://www.hrsa.gov/

https://www.nccih.nih.gov/

https://www.NCCIH.NIH.gov/health/complimentary

https://www.nih.gov/institutes-nih/nih-office-director/office-communications-pub-lic-liaison/clear-communication/cultural-respect#:~:text=Cultural%20respect%20benefits%20consumers%2C%20stakeholders%2C%20and%20communities%20and,also%20critical%20for%20achieving%20accuracy%20in%20medical%20research.

CHAPTER 4 THE INFLUENCE OF FAMILY ON DEVELOPING A LIFESTYLE

American Academy of Child and Adolescent Psychiatry (2018). Social media and teens. Retrieved May 7, 2020 from https://www.aacap.org/AACAP/Families_and_Youth/Facts_for_Families/FFF-Guide/Social-Media-and-Teens-100.aspx.

American Psychiatric Association (2015). *Cognitive and behavioral intervention for PTSD Nov 2015 Position Statement*. Retrieved from https://www.apa.org/ptsd-guideline/treatments.

American Psychiatric Association (2019). *AAP guidelines for treatment of depression*. Retrieved from www.ARA.org.

Baronowski, T., & Nader, P. (1985). Family health behavior. In D. Turk, & R. Kerns (Eds.), *Health, illness and family*. Wiley [classic].

Bowlby, J. (1951). *Maternal care and mental health*. Columbia University Press [classic].

Chartrand, M., Frank, D., White, L., & Shope, T. (2008). Effects of parents' wartime deployment on behavior of young children in military families. *Archives of Pediatrics and Adolescent Medicine, 162*(11), 1009–1114.

Chen, W., & Adler, J. (2019). Assessment of screen exposure in young children, 1997 to 2014. *Journal of American Medical Association Pediatrics, 173*(4), 391–393.

Child Welfare Information Gateway (2019). Foster care statistics 2017. U.S. Department of Health and Human Services, Children's Bureau. Retrieved May 7, 2020 from https://www.childwelfare.gov/pubPDFs/foster.pdf.

Child Welfare Information Gateway (2020). *Reasonable efforts to preserve or reunify families and achieve permanency for children*. U.S. Department of Health and Human Services, Administration for Children and Families, Children's Bureau. https://www.childwelfare.gov/pubPDFs/reunify.pdf.

Duvall, E., & Miller, B. (1985). *Marriage and family development* (6th ed.). Harper and Row [classic].

Eth, S., & Pynoos, R. (Eds.). (1985). *PTSD in children*. American Psychiatric Press [classic].

Federal Trade Commission. (2013). Children's online privacy protection rule, final rule. *Federal register*, 78(12). Retrieved May 7, 2020 from https://www.ftc.gov/enforcement/rules/rulemaking-regulatory-reform-proceedings/childrens-online-privacy-protection-rule.

Firth, J., Torous, J., Stubbs, B., Firth, J., Steiner, G., Smith, L., Alvarez-Jimenez, M., Gleeson, J., Vancampfort, D., Armitage, C., & Sarris, J. (2019). The "online brain": How the internet may be changing our cognition. *World Psychiatry*, 18(2), 119–129. https://10.1002/wps. 20617.

Garfield, C. (2009). Variations in family composition. In W. Carey, A. Crocker, W. Coleman, E. Elias, & H. Feldman (Eds.), *Developmental-behavioral pediatrics* (4th ed.). Saunders.

Graham, J., & Forstadt, L. (2010). *Child development and screen time: bulletin #4100*. University of Maine Cooperative Extension Publications. Retrieved from www.HTTP://UofMaine.EDU/publications/4100e.

Havighurst, R. (1974). *Developmental tasks and education*. David McKay [classic].

JAMARDA Resources (2020). Cultural diversity training and educational products for health care providers. Retrieved July 11, 2020 from http://www.jamardaresources.com/.

Kaiser Family Foundation (2010). *Generation M2: media in the lives of 8-18 year olds*. Retrieved November 2011 from www.KFF.org/entmedia.

Kaiser Permanente (2019). Screen time and kids: Setting limits for better health. Retrieved May 4, 2020 from https://thrive.kaiserpermanente.org/thrive-together/live-well/screen-time-kids-setting-limits-better-health.

Kim, H. (2011). Children of divorced parents often fall behind classmates in math and social skills. *American Sociological Review*, 78(3), 487–511.

Kleigman, R., Stanton, B., St Geme, J., III, Schor, N., & Behrman, R. (Eds.). (2016). *Nelson textbook of pediatrics* (20th ed.). Elsevier.

Landry, G. (2016). Sports medicine. In R. Kleigman, B. Stanton, J. St Geme, III, N. Schor, & R. Behrman (Eds.), *Nelson textbook of pediatrics* (20th ed.). Elsevier.

Leifer, G. (2019). *Introduction to maternity & pediatric nursing* (8th ed.). Elsevier.

Pagani, L., Fitzpatrick, C., Barnett, T., & Dubow, E. (2010). Prospective association between early childhood TV exposure and academic, psychosocial, and physical well-being by middle childhood. *Archives of Pediatrics and Adolescent Medicine*, 64(5), 425–431.

Pew Research Center (2019). Social media fact sheet. Retrieved May 7, 2020 from https://www.pewresearch.org/internet/fact-sheet/social-media/.

Popenoe, D. (1989). The family transformed. *Family Affairs*, 2(2–3), 1–5. [classic].

Population Reference Bureau (2020). U.S. household composition shifts as the population grows older; more young adults live with parents. Retrieved May 7, 2020 from https://www.prb.org/u-s-household-composition-shifts-as-the-population-grows-older-more-young-adults-live-with-parents/.

Rocha, S. (2019). Talking with teens and families about digital media use. The Brown University Child and Adolescent Behavior Letter. Retrieved May 4, 2020 from https://onlinelibrary.wiley.com/doi/full/10.1002/cbl.30361.

Smilkstein, G. (1978). The family Apgar: a proposal for a family function test and its use by physicians. *Journal of Family Practice, (6)*, 1231–1238.

Tanner, J. L. (2009). Separation, divorce and remarriage. In W. Carey, A. Crocker, W. Coleman, E. Elias, & H. Feldman (Eds.), *Developmental-behavioral pediatrics* (4th ed.). Saunders.

Teng, Z., Nie, Q., Guo, C., Zhang, Q., Liu, Y., & Bushman, B. J. (2019). A longitudinal study of link between exposure to violent video games and aggression in Chinese adolescents: The mediating role of moral disengagement. *Developmental Psychology, 55*(1), 184–195. https://doi.org/10.1037/dev0000624.

Thyen, U., & Perrin, J. (2009). Chronic health conditions. In W. Carey, A. Crocker, W. Coleman, E. Elias, & H. Feldman (Eds.), *Developmental-behavioral pediatrics* (4th ed.). Saunders.

Torres, F. (2020). *What is post traumatic stress disorder*? American Psychiatric Association. Retrieved from www.psychiatry.org/patients-families/PTSD/What-is-PTSD.

U.S. Bureau of Labor Statistics (2020). Employment characteristics of families summary. Retrieved May 7, 2020 from https://www.bls.gov/news.release/famee.nr0.htm.

U.S. Department of Health and Human Services (2019). Characteristics of families served by the child care and development fund (CCDF) based on preliminary FY2018 data. Retrieved May 7, 2020 from https://www.acf.hhs.gov/occ/resource/characteristics-of-families-served-by-child-care-and-development-fund-ccdf.

U.S. Department of Labor (2017). 12 stats about working women. Retrieved May 7, 2020 from https://blog.dol.gov/2017/03/01/12-stats-about-working-women.

Online Resources

https://www.mhanational.org/
https://www.urban.org/
https://thebowencenter.org/theory/

CHAPTER 5 THEORIES OF DEVELOPMENT

Alligood, M. (2016). *Nursing theorists and their work* (9th ed.). Elsevier.

Arlin, P. (1975). Cognitive development in adulthood: a 5th stage? *Developmental Psychology, 11*, 602. [classic].

Bandura, A. (1977). *Social learning theory.* Prentice-Hall [classic].

Brofenbrenner, U. (1979). *The ecology of human development.* Harvard University Press [classic].

Carey, W., Crocker, A., Coleman, W., Elias, E., & Feldman, H. (Eds.). (2009). *Developmental-behavioral pediatrics* (4th ed.). Saunders.

DuVall, E. (1977). *Marriage and family development.* JB Lippincott [classic].

Erikson, E. (1994). *The life cycle completed: a review.* WW Norton.

Gopnik, A. (2016). Cognitive development: Domains and theories. In R. Kleigman, B. Stanton, J. St Geme, III, N. Schor, & R. Behrman (Eds.), *Nelson textbook of pediatrics* (20th ed.). Elsevier.

Gormly, A., & Brodzinsky, D. (1989). *Lifespan human development*. Harcourt Brace [classic].

Haggerty, R., & Friedman, S. (2003). History of developmental and behavioral pediatrics. *Journal of Developmental and Behavioral Pediatrics, 24*, 215.

Haith, M., & Benson, J. (2008). *Encyclopedia of infant and early childhood development*. Elsevier.

Havighurst, R. (1974). *Developmental tasks and education*. D. McKay [classic].

Hoover, W. (2006). White House Conference on Child Health: Address to the White House on Child Health and Protection, 1930. In J. Wooley, & E. Peters (Eds.), *The American Presidency Project*. Santa Barbara California University. Gerhard Peters Database on-line https://oac.cdlib.org/findaid/ark:/13030/kt6j49r12c/.

Kegan, R. (1982). *The evolving of self: a theory of human development*. Howard Press [classic].

Kleigman, R., Stanton, B., St Geme, J., III, Schor, N., & Behrman, R. (Eds.). (2016). *Nelson textbook of pediatrics* (20th ed.). Elsevier.

Kohlberg, L. (1964). Development of moral character and moral ideology. In H. Hoffman, & L. Hoffman (Eds.), *Review of child development research*. Russell Sage [classic].

Leifer, G. (2019). *Introduction to maternity and pediatric nursing* (8th ed.). Elsevier.

Levinson, D. J., Darrow, C. N., & Klein, E. B. (1978). *The seasons of a man's life*. Knopf [classic].

Loevinger, J. (1979). *Scientific ways in the study of ego development*. Clark University Press [classic].

Piaget, J. (1926). *The language of the child*. Harcourt Brace [classic].

Reider, P., Wisiniewski, P., Alderman, B., & Campbell, S. (2017). Microbes and mental health: A review. *Brain, Behavior, and Immunity, 66*(1), 1–17.

Reitzes, D., & Mutran, E. (2004). Transition to retirement: stages and factors that influence retirement adjustment. *International Journal of Aging and Human Development, 59*(1), 63–84.

Skinner, B. (1987). *Verbal behavior*. Appleton-Century-Croft [classic].

Stambuk, A., Rusac, S., & Sucic, A. (2013). Process of retirement: an attempt at checking Atchley's model of adjustment. *Periodicum Biologorum, 115*(4), 567–574.

Vygotsky, L. (1962). *Thoughts and language*. MIT Press [classic].

Watkins, O. (2016). Development of the authentic self: An exploration of gender neutral parenting. *Journal of Undergraduate Research School of Education and Childhood, 2016*(1), 21–30. Leeds Beckett University. Retrieved June 5, 2020 from https://www.leedsbeckett.ac.uk/-/media/files/riches/spotlight-volume-1-2016.pdf#page=22.

CHAPTER 6 PRENATAL INFLUENCES ON HEALTHY DEVELOPMENT

Bentley, A., Collier, S., & Rotimi, C. (2017). Diversity and inclusion in genomic research: Why the uneven progress? *Journal of Community Genetics, 8*(4), 255–266. https://doi.org/10.1007/s12687-017-0316-6.

Brazelton, T. (1973). *The neonatal behavioral assessment scale*. JB Lippincott [classic].

Dunlop, A., Muller, J., Ferrante, E., Edwards, S., Dunn, A., & Corwin, E. (2015). Maternal microbiome and pregnancy outcomes that impact infant health: a review. *Advances in Neonatal Care, 15*(6), 377–385.

Flynn, J. (1987). Massive IQ gains in 14 nations: what IQ tests really measure. *Psychological Bulletin, 101*, 171. [classic].

Giger, J. (2016). *Transcultural nursing.* Elsevier.

Halvatsiotis, P., Panagiotou, O., Koulouvaris, P., Raptis, A., Bamias, A., Kalantaridou, S., & Valsamakis, G. (2020). Benefits of exercise in pregnancies with gestational diabetes [published online ahead of print, 2020 Jul 7]. *Journal of Maternal-Fetal & Neonatal Medicine.* https://doi.org/10.1080/14767058.2020.1786515.

Kim, H., Sitarik, A., Woodcroft, K., Johnson, C., & Joratte, E. (2019). Birth mode, breast feeding, pet exposure and antibiotic use associated with gut microbiome and sensitization. *Current Allergy and Asthma Reports, 19*(4), 22. https://doi.org/10.1007/s11882-019-0851-9.

Leifer, G. (2012). *Maternity nursing, an introductory text* (11th ed.). Saunders.

Lundstrom, K. (2019). Gene therapy today and tomorrow. *Diseases, 7*(2), 37. https://doi.org/10.3390/diseases7020037.

Moore, K. L., & Persaud, T. V. N. (2008). *The developing human: clinically oriented embryology* (8th ed.). Saunders.

Murray, S. S., McKinney, E. S., & Gorrie, T. M. (2001). *Foundations of maternal-newborn nursing* (3rd ed.). Saunders.

Mutic, A., Jordan, S., Edwards, S., Ferrante, E., Taylor, A., & Yang, I. (2019). The postpartum maternal and newborn microbiomes. *American Journal of Maternal Child Nursing, 42*(6), 326–331.

National Institutes of Health (2020). What are genome editing and CRISPR-Cas9? Retrieved May 24, 2020 from https://ghr.nlm.nih.gov/primer/genomicresearch/genomeediting.

Neu, J. (2013). The pre- and early microbiome: Relevance to subsequent health and development. *Journal of Neurology, 13*(2), e592–e599.

Nio Leon, R. (2005). *Are IQ tests biased?* Retrieved November 2001 from www.Psychpage.com.

Poyatos-León, R., García-Hermoso, A., Sanabria-Martínez, G., Álvarez-Bueno, C., Cavero-Redondo, I., & Martínez-Vizcaíno, V. (2017). Effects of exercise-based interventions on postpartum depression: A meta-analysis of randomized controlled trials. *Birth, 44*(3), 200–208. https://doi.org/10.1111/birt.12294.

Ross, M., & Ervin, H. (2016). Fetal development and physiology. In S. Gabbe, J. Niebyl, J. Simpson et al. (Eds.), *Obstetrics: Normal and problem pregnancies.* Elsevier.

Ross, M., & DeSal, M. (2017). Developmental origins of adult health and disease. In S. Gabbe, J. Niebyl, J. Simpson, M. Landon et al. (Eds.), *Obstetrics: Normal and problem pregnancies.* Elsevier.

Rubin, R. (1961). Maternal behavior. *Nursing Outlook,* (9), 692.

Rubin, R. (1961). Puerperal change. *Nursing Outlook, 9*(12), 743–755.

Rubin, R. (1963). Maternal touch at first contact with the newborn infant. *Nursing Outlook, 11*, 828. [classic].

Rubin, R. (1967). Attainment of the maternal role: part 1 processes. *Nursing Research,* (16), 237–245.

Rubin, R. (1975). Maternal tasks in pregnancy. *American Journal of Maternal-Child Nursing, 4*(3), 143.

Rubin, R. (1977). Binding-in in the postpartum period. *American Journal of Maternal-Child Nursing, 6*(1), 65–75.

Rubin, R. (1984). *Maternal identity and the maternal experience.* Springer.

Valentine, G., Prince, A., & Aagaard, K. (2019). The neonatal microbiome and metagenomics: What do we know now and what is the future? *NeoReviews*, *20*(5), e258–e271.

Vargas-Terrones, M., Nagpal, T. S., & Barakat, R. (2019). Impact of exercise during pregnancy on gestational weight gain and birth weight: an overview. *Brazilian Journal of Physical Therapy*, *23*(2), 164–169. https://doi.org/10.1016/j.bjpt.2018.11.012.

Wu, W., Kong, Q., Tian, P., Zhai, Q., Wang, G., Liu, X., Zhao, J., Zhang, H., Lee, Y., & Chen, W. (2019). Targeting gut microbiota dysbiosis: potential interventional strategies for neurological disorders. *Engineering*, *6*(4), 415–423. https://doi.org/10.1016/j.eng.2019.07.026.

Online Resources

https://thinkculturalhealth.hhs.gov/

https://www.genome.gov/human-genome-project

https://www.hhs.gov/surgeongeneral/reports-and-publications/physical-activity-nutrition/index.html

https://www.hmpdacc.org/overview/

CHAPTER 7 THE INFANT

Erikson, E. (1994). *The life cycle completed: a review.* WW Norton.

Carey, W., Crocker, A., Elias, E., Feldman, H., & Coleman, W. (Eds.) (2009). *Developmental-behavioral pediatrics* (4th ed.). Saunders.

Czaenabay, D., Dalmago, J., Martins, A., & Quaeroz, A. (2019). Repeated three-hour maternal deprivation as model of early life stress alters maternal behavior, olfactory learning and neural development. *Journal of Neurobiology of Learning and Memory*, *163*(9), 107040. https://doi.org/10.1016/J.NLM.2019.107040.

Feigelman, S. (2016). Development of behavior: overview and assessment of variability. In R. Kleigman, B. Stanton, J. St Geme, III, N. Schor, & R. Behrman (Eds.), *Nelson textbook of pediatrics* (20th ed.). Elsevier.

Gaensbauer, T. (2002). Representation of trauma in infancy: clinical and theoretical implications for understanding early memory. *Journal of Infant Mental Health*, *23*(3), 259–277.

Hoecker, J. (2016). *What is the best way to predict a child's height?* Mayo Clinic Children's Health.

Kleigman, R., Stanton, B., St Geme, J., III, Schor, N., & Behrman, R. (Eds.). (2016). *Nelson textbook of pediatrics* (20th ed.). Elsevier.

Leifer, G. (2019). *Introduction to maternity & pediatric nursing* (8th ed.). Elsevier.

National Association for Sport and Physical Education (2009). Active start: A statement of physical activity guidelines for children birth to age 5 (2nd ed.). Accessed June 29, 2020 from www.aahperd.org.

Parks, E., Shaikhkhalil, A., Groleau, V., & Wendell, D. (2016). Feeding healthy infants, children and adolescents. In R. Kleigman, B. Stanton, J. St Geme, III, N. Schor, & R. Behrman (Eds.), *Nelson textbook of pediatrics* (20th ed.). Elsevier.

Virgilio, S., & Clements, R. (2020). Active start: A statement of physical activity guidelines for children birth to Age 5 (3rd ed.). Accessed December 18, 2020 from www.ShapeAmerica.org/standards/guidelines/activestart.aspx.

Online Resources

https://heal.nih.gov/research/infants-and-children/healthy-brain
https://www.hhs.gov/surgeongeneral/reports-and-publications/physical-activity-nutrition/index.html
https://www.nidcd.nih.gov/health/speech-and-language
www.brightfutures.org/mentalhealth/index.html

CHAPTER 8 EARLY CHILDHOOD

Burr, H. (1933). Modern theories of development. *Yale Journal of Biologic Development,* *6*(2), 201–203. [classic].

Douglass, J., & Clark, M. (2015). Integrating oral health to overall health care to prevent early childhood caries: Need, evidence and solutions. *Pediatric Dentistry, 37*(3), 266–274.

Feigelman, S. (2016). The preschool years. In R. Kleigman, B. Stanton, J. St Geme, III, N. Schor, & R. Behrman (Eds.), *Nelson textbook of pediatrics* (20th ed.). Elsevier.

Feldman, H., & Messick, C. (2009). Language and speech disorders. In W. Carey, A. Crocker, W. Coleman, E. Elias, & H. Feldman (Eds.), *Developmental-behavioral pediatrics* (4th ed.). Saunders.

Gottfried, A., & Bathurst, L. (1983). Hand preference across time is related to intelligence in young girls, not boys. *Science, 221,* 1074. [classic].

Greenbaum, L. (2016). Micronutrient mineral deficiencies. In R. Kleigman, B. Stanton, J. St Geme, III, N. Schor, & R. Behrman (Eds.), *Nelson textbook of pediatrics* (20th ed.). Elsevier.

Hillman, J., & Spigarelli, M. (2009). Sexuality development and direction. In W. Carey, A. Crocker, E. Elias, H. Feldman, & W. Coleman (Eds.), *Developmental-behavioral pediatrics* (4th ed.). Saunders.

Kinsey, A., Pomeroy, W., & Martin, C. (1948). *Sexual behavior in the human male.* Saunders [classic].

Leifer, G. (2019). *Introduction to maternity & pediatric nursing* (8th ed.). Elsevier.

Marcdante, K., & Kleigman, R. (2019). *Nelson essentials of pediatrics.* Elsevier.

Parks, E., Shaikhkhalil, A., Groleau, V., & Wendell, G. (2016). Feeding healthy infants, children and adolescents. In R. Kleigman, B. Stanton, J. St Geme, III, N. Schor, & R. Behrman (Eds.), *Nelson textbook of pediatrics* (20th ed.). Elsevier.

Shaywitz, E., & Shaywitz, B. (2016). Dyslexia. In R. Kleigman, B. Stanton, J. St Geme, III, N. Schor, & R. Behrman (Eds.), *Nelson textbook of pediatrics* (20th ed.). Elsevier.

Simms, M. (2016). Language development and communication disorders. In R. Kleigman, B. Stanton, J. St Geme, III, N. Schor, & R. Behrman (Eds.), *Nelson textbook of pediatrics* (20th ed.). Elsevier.

Turk, M. (2016). Health and wellness for children with disabilities. In R. Kleigman, B. Stanton, J. St Geme, III, N. Schor, & R. Behrman (Eds.), *Nelson textbook of pediatrics* (20th ed.). Elsevier.

USDA (2020). *Dietary guidelines for Americans* (9th ed.). Retrieved from https://www.dietaryguidelines.gov/.

Weiss, C. E., & Lillywhite, H. E. (1976). *Communication disorders: a handbook for prevention and early detection.* Mosby.

Online Resources

https://www.medic8.com/healthguide/sports-medicine/prevention/equipment.html
https://www.nhtsa.gov/equipment/car-seats-and-booster-seats
https://www.nhtsa.gov/road-safety/child-safety
www.aap.org
www.AAP.org/periodicityschedule.
www.allergicchild.com
www.CDC.gov/vaccines

CHAPTER 9 MIDDLE CHILDHOOD

Airton, L. (2019). *Gender: your guide. Adams Media*. Simon & Schuster.

American Academy of Child and Adolescent Psychiatry (2017). *Bulletin Facts for Families # 46 Home Alone Children*

American Academy of Pediatrics (2019). *Reference manual of pediatric dentistry* (pp. 341-353, 220-224).

Betz, C., Hunsberger, M., & Wright, S. (1994). *Family centered nursing care of children* (2nd ed.). Saunders.

Bus, A., Takas, Z., & Kegal, C. (2015). Affordance and limitation of electronic storybooks for young children's emerging literacy. *Developmental Review, 35*(1), 79–97.

Carey, W., Crocker, A., Coleman, W., Elias, E., & Feldman, H. (Eds.). (2009). *Developmental-behavioral pediatrics* (4th ed.). Saunders.

Feigelman, S. (2016). Middle childhood. In R. Kleigman, B. Stanton, J. St Geme, III, N. Schor, & R. Behrman (Eds.), *Nelson textbook of pediatrics* (20th ed.). Elsevier.

Felt, L., & Robb, M. (2016). *Technology addiction: Concern, controversy, and finding a balance*. Retrieved from https://www.commonsensemedia.org/sites/default/files/uploads/research/csm_2016_technology_addiction_research_brief_1.pdf.

Guernsey, L., & Levine, M. (2015). *Tap, click, and read: Growing readers in a world of screens*. Jossey-Bass.

Kabali, H., Irigoyen, M., & Nunez-Davis, R. (2016). Exposure and use of mobile media devices by young children. *Pediatrics, 136*(6), 644–650.

Kim, B. (2015). The popularity of gamification in the mobile and social era. *Library Technology Reports, 51*(2), 5–9.

Kleigman, R., Stanton, B., St. Geme, J., Schor, N., & Behrmann, R. (Eds.). (2016). *Nelson textbook of pediatrics* (20th ed.). Elsevier.

Kollmayer, M., Schober, B., & Spiel, C. (2018). Gender stereotypes in education: Development, consequences, and interventions. *European Journal of Developmental Psychology, 15*(4), 361–377. https://doi.org/10.1080/17405629.2016.1193483.

Kollmayer, M., Schultes, M., Schober, B., Hadosi, T., & Spiel, C. (2018). Parent's judgement about desirability of toys for their children: Association with gender role attitude, gender typing of toys, and demographics. *Journal of Sex Roles, 791*, 329–341. https://doi.org/10.1007/s11199-017.

Leifer, G. (2019). *Introduction to maternity & pediatric nursing* (8th ed.). Elsevier Saunders.

McClellan, M. (1984). On their own: Latchkey children. *Pediatric Nursing, 10*(2000), 198–202.

Naglieri, J. (2020). 100 Years of intelligence testing: We can do better. Traditional intelligence tests are outdated and should be replaced by those based on brain function. *APA Newsletter.*

Olitsky, S., Hug, D., Plummer, L., Stahl, E., Ariss, M., & Lindquist, T. (2016). Growth and development of the eye. In R. Kleigman, B. Stanton, J. St Geme, III, N. Schor, & R. Behrman (Eds.), *Nelson textbook of pediatrics* (20th ed.). Elsevier.

Rappley, M., & Kallman, G. (2009). Middle childhood. In W. Carey, A. Crocker, E. Elias, H. Feldman, & W. Coleman (Eds.), *Developmental-behavioral pediatrics* (4th ed.). Saunders.

Reed, J., Hirsch-Pasek, K., & Golinoff, R. (2017). Learning on hold: Cellphones side-track parent-child interactions. *Developmental Psychology, 53*(8), 1428–1436.

Rodesky, J., Christakis, D., Moreno, M., & Cross, C. (2016). Council on communication and media. *Pediatrics, 138*(5), e2162593. https://doi.org/10.1542/peds.2016-2593.

Sege, R., & Siegel, B. (2018). Council on child abuse and neglect and committee on social aspects of child and family health, effective discipline to raise healthy children. *Pediatrics, 142*(6), e20183112. https://doi.org/10.1542/peds.2018-3112.

SIECUS (2020). *The future of sex education initiative 2020: National sex education standard: Core content and skills K-12.* SIECUS Publications.

Sturner, R. (2009). General principles of psychological testing. In W. Carey, A. Crocker, E. Elias, H. Feldman, & W. Coleman (Eds.), *Developmental-behavioral pediatrics* (4th ed.). Saunders.

Substance Abuse and Mental Health Services Administration (2020). Why you should talk with your child about alcohol and other drugs. Retrieved June 14, 2020 from https://www.samhsa.gov/underage-drinking/parent-resources/why-you-should-talk-your-child.

Watkins, O. (2016). Development of the authentic self: An exploration of gender neutral parenting. *Journal of Undergraduate Research School of Education and Childhood, 1,* 21–30. Leeds Beckett University. Retrieved June 15, 2020 from https://www.leedsbeckett.ac.uk/-/media/files/riches/spotlight-volume-1-2016.pdf#page=22.

World Health Organization (2018). *Physical activity.* Retrieved from https://www.who.int/news-room/fact-sheets/detail/physical-activity.

Online Resources

www.SIECUS.org
www.CDC.gov/vaccines/index.HTML
www.Healthychildren.org

CHAPTER 10 ADOLESCENCE

ACOG (2016). Committee opinion #653 concerns regarding social media and health issues in adolescents and young adults. Retrieved from https://pubmed.ncbi.nlm.nih.gov/26942388/.

Adelson, S., & Schuster, M. (2016). Gay, lesbian and bisexual behavior. In R. Kleigman, B. Stanton, J. St Geme, III, N. Schor, & R. Behrman (Eds.), *Nelson textbook of pediatrics* (20th ed.). Elsevier.

American Psychiatric Association (2016). What is gender dysphoria? Retrieved July 3, 2020 from https://www.psychiatry.org/patients-families/gender-dysphoria/what-is-gender-dysphoria.

Aoyama, B., & McGrath-Morrow, S. (2020). Vaping: Poisoning a new generation of kids: Vaping and electronic cigarette use in the pediatric population. *Contemporary Pediatrics, 37*(4), 20–25.

Bockting, W. (2016). Sexual identity development. In R. Kleigman, B. Stanton, J. St Geme, III, N. Schor, & R. Behrman (Eds.), *Nelson textbook of pediatrics* (20th ed.). Elsevier.

Burstein, R. (2016). The epidemiology of adolescent health problems. In R. Kleigman, B. Stanton, J. St Geme, III, N. Schor, & R. Behrman (Eds.), *Nelson textbook of pediatrics* (20th ed.). Elsevier.

Centers for Disease Control and Prevention (2020). Physical activity. Retrieved from https://www.cdc.gov/physicalactivity/index.html.

Cherian, S., Kumar, A., Estrada, Y., & Martin, R. (2020). E cigarette and vaping products associated with lung injury: A review. *American Journal of Medicine, 133*(6), 657–663. https://pubmed.ncbi.nlm.nih.gov/32179055/.

Cullen, K., Gentzke, A., Sawdey, M., Chang, J., Anic, G., Wang, T., Creamer, M., Jamal, A., Ambrose, B., & King, B. (2019). E cigarette use among youth in US. *JAMA, 332,* 2095–2103. https://pubmed.ncbi.nlm.nih.gov/31688912/.

Evans-Polce, R., Velez, P., Boyd, C., McCabe, W., & McCabe, C. (2020). Trends in e-cigarette, cigarette, cigar and smokeless tobacco among US adolescents 2014-2018. *American Journal of Public Health, 110*(2), 163–165.

Holland-Hall, C., & Burstein, G. (2016). The adolescent physical and social development. In R. Kleigman, B. Stanton, J. St Geme, III, N. Schor, & R. Behrman (Eds.), *Nelson textbook of pediatrics* (20th ed.). Elsevier.

Kaljee, L. (2016). Cultural issues in pediatric care. In R. Kleigman, B. Stanton, J. St Geme, III, N. Schor, & R. Behrman (Eds.), *Nelson textbook of pediatrics* (20th ed.). Elsevier.

Kleigman, R., Stanton, B., St. Geme, J., Schor, N., & Behrmann, R. (Eds.). (2016). *Nelson textbook of pediatrics* (20th ed.). Elsevier.

Leifer, G. (2019). *Introduction to maternity & pediatric nursing* (8th ed.). Elsevier.

Lindsey, L. (2020). *Gender roles: A sociological perspective* (6th ed.). Prentice Hall.

Spinks-Franklyn, A. (2019). Teens gone wild: Helping parents navigate adolescent challenges. Presentation October 22, 2019 to AAP Annual Conference & Exhibition, New Orleans, LA. Retrieved from https://www.aappublications.org/news/2019/08/19/nce19wildteensvideo081919.

Stager, R. (2016). Substance abuse. In R. Kleigman, B. Stanton, J. St Geme, III, N. Schor, & R. Behrman (Eds.), *Nelson textbook of pediatrics* (20th ed.). Elsevier.

WHO (2020). Economic and financing considerations of self-care interventions for sexual and reproductive health and rights summary report. Retrieved from https://www.who.int/reproductivehealth/publications/economic-financing-considerations-self-care-interventions-srhr/en/.

Zimlich, R. (2019). How to help teen parents navigate adolescence. AAP Conference and Exhibition in New Orleans LA. Contemporary Pediatrics News Media October 2019.

Online Resources

www.aap.org/
www.plannedparenthood.org
www.seventeen.com/sexsmarts
www.siecus.org

https://www.contemporarypediatrics.com/

http://teenmentalhealth.org/wp-content/uploads/2019/10/teening-your-parent-LATEST-min-2.pdf

CHAPTER 11 YOUNG ADULTHOOD

Ainsworth, B., Haskell, W., Whitt, M., Irwin, M., Swartz, A., Strath, S., O'Brien, W., Bassett, D., Schmitz, K., Emplaincourt, D., Jacobs, D., & Leon, A. (2000). Compendium of physical activities: An update of activity codes and MET intensities. *Medicine and Science in Sports and Exercise*, *32*(Suppl 9), S498–S504. https://doi.org/10.1097/00005768-200009001-00009.

Augustyn, M., Frank, D., & Zuckerman, B. (2009). Infancy and toddler years. In W. Carey, A. Crocker, E. Elias, H. Feldman, & W. Coleman (Eds.), *Developmental-behavioral pediatrics* (4th ed.). Saunders.

Barbieri, R. (2017). The American College of Obstetricians and Gynecologists. Practice bulletin no. 184: Vaginal birth after cesarean delivery. *Obstetric Gynecology*, *130*, 1167. https://doi.org/10.1097/AOG.0000000000002398.

Berger, K. S. (2020). *The developing person through the lifespan* (8th ed). Worth Publishers.

Centers for Disease Control and Prevention (2016). Mean age of mothers is on the rise: United States, 2000-2014. Retrieved from https://www.cdc.gov/nchs/products/databriefs/db232.htm.

Centers for Disease Control and Prevention (2020). *HPV vaccine safety*. Retrieved from https://www.cdc.gov/vaccines/vpd/hpv/hcp/safety-effectiveness.html.

Central Intelligence Agency (2019). *Mother's mean age at first birth*. Retrieved from https://www.cia.gov/the-world-factbook/field/mothers-mean-age-at-first-birth/.

Commons, M., Richards, F., & Armon, C. (1982). *Beyond formal operations: late adolescent and adult cognitive development*. Praeger [classic].

Dong, L., Block, G., & Mandel, S. (2004). Activities contribution to total energy expenditure in US: Results of NHAPS study. *International Journal of Behavioral Nutrition and Physical Activity*, *1*(4), 1–4.

Gilligan, T., Lin, D., Aggarwal, R., Chism, D., Cost, N., Derweesh, I. H., Emamekhoo, H., Feldman, D. R., Geynisman, D. M., Hancock, S. L., LaGrange, C., Levine, E. G., Longo, T., Lowrance, W., McGregor, B., Monk, P., Picus, J., Pierorazio, P., Rais-Bahrami, S., & Pluchino, L. A. (2019). Testicular cancer, version 2.2020, NCCN Clinical Practice Guidelines in Oncology. *Journal of the National Comprehensive Cancer Network*, *17*(12), 1529–1554. https://doi.org/10.6004/jnccn.2019.0058.

Leifer, G. (2019). *Introduction to maternity & pediatric nursing* (8th ed.). Elsevier.

Levinson, D., Darrow, C., & Klein, E. B. (1978). *The seasons of a man's life*. Knopf [classic].

Lowdermilk, D. L., Perry, S. E., & Bobak, I. M. (2000). *Maternity and women's health care* (7th ed.). Mosby.

Martin, S. J., Sherly, M., & McLeod, M. (2018). Adverse effects of sports supplements in men. *Australian Prescriber*, *41*(1), 10–13. https://doi.org/10.18773/austprescr.2018.003.

Murstein, B. (1982). Marital choices. In B. Wolman (Ed.), *Handbook of developmental psychology*. Prentice Hall [classic].

Piercy, K., Troiano, R., & Ballard, R. (2018). Physical activity guidelines for Americans. *JAMA*, *320*(19), 2020–2028.

Rawlins, P., Williams, S., & Beck, C. (1993). *Mental health psychiatric nursing*. Mosby.

Rowe, D., Welsh, G., & Hell, D. (2011). Stride rate recommendations for moderate intensity walking. *Medicine and Science in Sports and Exercise, 43*(2), 312–318.

Seigel, R., Miller, K., & Jemal, A. (2019). Cancer statistics, 2019. *CA, A Cancer Journal for Clinicians, 69*(1), 7–34.

Smock, P., & Schwartz, C. (2020). The demography of family: A review of pattern and change. *Journal of Marriage and Family, 82*(1), 9–34.

Tambo, A., Roshan, A., & Pace, N. (2016). Testosterone and cardiovascular disease. *The Open Cardiovascular Medicine Journal, 10*, 1–10. https://doi.org/10.2174/1874192401610010001.

Troino, R. P., Berrigan, D., Dodd, K. W., Mâsse, L. C., Tilert, T., & McDowell, M. (2008). Physical activity in the US measured by accelerometer. *Medicine and Science in Sports and Exercise, 40*(1), 181–188.

U.S. Preventive Services Task Force (2020). *A and B recommendations.* Retrieved from https://www.uspreventiveservicestaskforce.org/uspstf/recommendation-topics/uspstf-and-b-recommendations.

United States Department of Health and Human Services (2018). Physical guidelines for Americans (2nd ed.). Retrieved from https://health.gov/sites/default/files/2019-09/Physical_Activity_Guidelines_2nd_edition.pdf. U.S. Department of Health and Human Services/U.S. Department of Agriculture, 2015-2020.

Online Resources

https://www.dietaryguidelines.gov/sites/default/files/2020-12/Dietary_Guidelines_for_Americans_2020-2025.pdf

https://oldwayspt.org/traditional-diets/latin-american-diet/latin-american-diet-pyramid

https://www.uspreventiveservicestaskforce.org/uspstf/recommendation-topics/uspstf-and-b-recommendations

www.cancer.org

www.cdc.gov/ncipc/dvp/youpt/datviol.htm

CHAPTER 12 MIDDLE ADULTHOOD

Adlin, E. V. (2020). Age-related low testosterone. *Annals of Internal Medicine, 172*(2), 151–152. https://doi.org/10.7326/M19-3815.

American Psychological Association (2020). Sandwich generation moms feeling the squeeze. Retrieved June 16, 2020 from https://www.apa.org/helpcenter/sandwich-generation.

Brickwood, K. J., Watson, G., O'Brien, J., & Williams, A. D. (2019). Consumer-based wearable activity trackers increase physical activity participation: Systematic review and meta-analysis. *Journal of Medical Internet Research mHealth and uHealth, 7*(4), e11819. https://doi.org/10.2196/11819.

Crimmins, E., Shim, H., Zhang, Y., & Kim, J. (2019). Differences between men and women in mortality and the health dimensions of the morbidity process. *Clinical Chemistry, 65*(1), 135–145. https://doi.org/10.1373/clinchem.2018.288332.

Erikson, E. (1994). *The life cycle completed: a review.* WW Norton.

Harvard Men's Health Watch (2019). Mars vs. Venus: The gender gap in health. Retrieved June 16, 2020 from https://www.health.harvard.edu/newsletter_article/mars-vs-venus-the-gender-gap-in-health.

Levinson, D., Darrow, C., & Klein, E. (1978). *The seasons of a man's life*. Knopf.

Malone, J. C., Liu, S. R., Vaillant, G. E., Rentz, D. M., & Waldinger, R. J. (2016). Midlife Eriksonian psychosocial development: setting the stage for late-life cognitive and emotional health. *Developmental Psychology, 52*(3), 496–508. https://doi.org/10.1037/a0039875.

Masters, W., Johnson, V., & Kolodny, R. (1986). *Masters and Johnson on sex and human loving*. Little Brown [classic].

Mukhalalati, B., & Taylor, A. (2019). Adult learning theories in context: A quick guide for healthcare professional educators. *Journal of Medical Education and Curricular Development, 6*. https://doi.org/10.1177/2382120519840332.

National Cancer Institute (2018). Menopausal hormone therapy and cancer. Retrieved June 16, 2020 from https://www.cancer.gov/about-cancer/causes-prevention/risk/hormones/mht-fact-sheet.

Newton, N., Vandewater, E., & Stewart, A. (2016). Stagnation: is it the dark side of generativity? *The Gerontologist, 56*(3), 243.

Thomas, H. N., Hamm, M., Hess, R., & Thurston, R. (2015). Correlates of sexual activity and satisfaction in midlife and older women. *Annals of Family Medicine, 13*(4), 336–342. https://doi.org/10.1370/afm.1820.

Thomas, H. N., Hamm, M., Hess, R., & Thurston, R. (2018). Changes in sexual function among midlife women: "I'm older and I'm wiser.". *Menopause, 25*(3), 286–292. https://doi.org/10.1097/GME.0000000000000988.

U.S. Preventive Services Task Force (2020). Screening recommendations. Retrieved June 16, 2020 from https://www.uspreventiveservicestaskforce.org/uspstf/topic_search_results?category%5B%5D=All&searchterm=screening.

World Health Organization (2020). Sexual and reproductive health. Retrieved June 16, 2020 from https://www.who.int/reproductivehealth/topics/sexual_health/sh_definitions/en/.

Online Resources

https://www.cdc.gov/cancer/breast/basic_info/risk_factors.htm

https://www.mayoclinic.org/healthy-lifestyle/mens-health/basics/mens-health/hlv-20049438

www.nlm.nih.gov/medlineplus/hormonereplacementtherapy.html

CHAPTER 13 LATE ADULTHOOD

Administration for Community Living (2018). 2017 profile of older Americans. Retrieved July 12, 2020 from https://acl.gov/sites/default/files/Aging%20and%20Disability%20in%20America/2017OlderAmericansProfile.pdf.

American Psychiatric Association. (2013). *Diagnostic and statistical manual of mental disorders* (5th ed.). American Psychiatric Publishing.

American Psychological Association (2020). Memory changes in older adults. Retrieved July 3, 2020 from https://www.apa.org/research/action/memory-changes.

Anderson, M., & Perrin, A. (2017). *Tech adoption climbs among older adults*. Pew Research Center. Retrieved July 24, 2020 from https://www.pewresearch.org/internet/2017/05/17/tech-adoption-climbs-among-older-adults/.

Britannica (2020). Old age. Retrieved July 28, 2020 from https://www.britannica.com/science/old-age.

Burns, E., & Ramakrishna, K. (2018). Deaths from falls among persons aged ≥65 years – United States, 2007-2016. *MMWR Morbidity and Mortality Weekly Report, 67*, 509–514.

Butler-Browne, G., Mouly, V., Bigot, A., & Trollet, C. (2018). *How muscles age, and how exercise can slow it.* The Scientist. Retrieved July 3, 2020 from https://www.the-scientist.com/features/how-muscles-age--and-how-exercise-can-slow-it-64708.

Ewing, J. (1984). Detecting alcoholism: the CAGE questionnaire. *JAMA, 252*, 1905–1907. [classic].

Goldin, A., Weinstein, B. E., & Shiman, N. (2020). How do medical masks degrade speech perception? *Hearing Review, 27*(5), 8–9. Retrieved September 17, 2020 from https://www.hearingreview.com/hearing-loss/health-wellness/how-do-medical-masks-degrade-speech-reception.

Havighurst, R. (1974). *Developmental tasks and education.* David McKay [classic].

Khoury, R., Chakkamparambil, B., Chibnall, J., Rajamanickam, J., Kumar, A., & Grossberg, G. (2020). Diagnostic accuracy of the SLU AMSAD scale for depression in older adults without dementia. *Journal of the American Medical Directors Association, 21*(5), 665–668.

Mandsager, K., Harb, S., & Cremer, P. (2018). Association of cardiorespiratory fitness with long-term mortality among adults undergoing exercise treadmill testing. *JAMA, 1*(6), e183605. https://doi.org/10.1001/jamanetworkopen.2018.3605.

Mather, M., Scommegna, P., & Kilduff, L. (2019). *Fact sheet: aging in the United States.* Population Reference Bureau. Retrieved July 24, 2020 from https://www.prb.org/aging-unitedstates-fact-sheet/.

Merriam-Webster (n.d.). Senior citizen. Retrieved July 28, 2020 from https://www.merriam-webster.com/dictionary/senior%20citizen.

Munsterman, E. (2020). Our aging patients: Are we prepared? *Gastroenterology Nursing, 43*(4), 320–321.

National Council for Aging Care (2020). Alcohol abuse amongst the elderly: a complete guide. Retrieved July 24, 2020 from https://aging.com/alcohol-abuse-amongst-the-elderly-a-complete-guide/.

National Institutes of Health (NIH), National Institute on Aging (2017). Facts about aging and alcohol. Retrieved July 24, 2020 from https://www.nia.nih.gov/health/facts-about-aging-and-alcohol.

National Institutes of Health (NIH), National Institute on Alcohol Abuse and Alcoholism (2014). Harmful interactions, mixing alcohol with medicines. Retrieved July 24, 2020 from https://pubs.niaaa.nih.gov/publications/Medicine/medicine.htm.

Pew Research Center (2020). More older Americans are working and working more, than they used to. Retrieved July 3, 2020 from https://www.pewrescarch.org/fact-tank/2016/06/20/more-oldcr-americans-are-working-and-working-more-than-they-used-to/.

Reas, E., Laughlin, G., Bergstrom, J., Kritz-Silverstein, D., Richard, E., Barrett-Connor, E., & McEvoy, L. (2019). Lifetime physical activity and late-life cognitive function: The Rancho Bernardo study. *Age and Ageing, 48*(2), 241–246. https://doi.org/10.1093/ageing/afy188.

Ryan, C., & Bauman, K. (2016). Educational attainment in the United States: 2015. US Census Bureau. Retrieved July 12, 2020 from https://www.census.gov/content/dam/Census/library/publications/2016/demo/p20-578.pdf.

Thomson Healthcare. (2007). *PDR for herbal medicines* (4th ed.). Thomson Reuters.

United States Department of Health and Human Services (USDHHS) Administration for Community Living (2018). 2017 Profile of older Americans. Retrieved July 3, 2020 from https://acl.gov/sites/default/files/Aging%20and%20Disability%20in%20America/2017 OlderAmericansProfile.pdf.

US Department of Health and Human Services (2011). Evidence-based practices KIT; knowledge information transformation guide to EBPs. Treatment of depression in older adults evidence-based practices (EBP) KIT. Retrieved July 3, 2020 from https://store. samhsa.gov/product/Treatment-Depression-Older-Adults-Evidence-Based-Practices-EBP-Kit/SMA11-4631.

US Preventative Services Task Force (2020). Recommendation topics A and B recommendations. Retrieved July 12, 2020 from https://www.uspreventiveservicestaskforce. org/uspstf/recommendation-topics/uspstf-and-b-recommendations#:~:text=Main%20 navigation,-Home&text=The%20USPSTF%20recommends%201%2Dtime,years%20 who%20have%20ever%20smoked.&text=The%20USPSTF%20recommends%20 screening%20for,who%20are%20overweight%20or%20obese.

USPSTF Grade Definitions. Retrieved July 25, 2020 from https://www.uspreventiveservicestaskforce.org/uspstf/grade-definitions.

Vespa, J. (2019). The graying of America: more older adults than kids by 2035. The U.S. joins other countries with large aging populations. US Census Bureau. Retrieved July 24, 2020 from https://www.census.gov/library/stories/2018/03/graying-america.html.

Vespa, J., Engelberg, J., & He, W. (2020). *Old housing, new needs: are U.S. homes ready for an aging population? P23-217.* U.S. Department of Commerce, U.S. Census Bureau. Retrieved July 24, 2020 from https://www.census.gov/content/dam/Census/library/publications/2020/demo/p23-217.pdf.

Online Resources

https://adaa.org/

https://store.samhsa.gov/product/Treatment-Depression-Older-Adults-Evidence-Based-Practices-EBP-Kit/SMA11-4631.

https://www.abct.org/Home/

https://www.census.gov/library/publications.html

www.aagponline.org/proffacts_mh.asp

www.agingstats.gov

www.DHHS.gov/aging

CHAPTER 14 ADVANCED OLD AGE AND GERIATRICS

Alvis, B., & Hughes, C. (2016). Physiology considerations in the geriatric patient. *Anesthesiology Clinics, 33*(3), 447–456. https://doi.org/10.1016/j.anclin.2015.05.003.

Amarya, S., Singh, K., & Sabharwal, M. (2018). *Aging process and physiological changes.* Intechopen. https://doi.org/10.5772/intechopen.76249. Retrieved July 31, 2020 from https://www.intechopen.com/books/gerontology/ageing-process-and-physiological-changes.

American Psychological Association (2016). Geropsychology: it's your future. Retrieved August 6, 2020 from https://www.apa.org/pi/aging/resources/geropsychology.

American Psychological Association (2020). Older adults health and age-related changes. Retrieved August 2, 2020 from https://www.apa.org/pi/aging/resources/guides/older.

AssistedLivingToday (2020). 5 must-have home modifications for seniors aging in place. Retrieved August 3, 2020 from https://assistedlivingtoday.com/blog/home-modifications-for-seniors-aging-in-place/.

Blackburn, P., Wilkins-Ho, M., & Wiese, B. (2017). Depression in older adults: diagnosis and management. *BC Medical Journal*, *59*(3), 171–177. Retrieved August 2, 2020 from https://bcmj.org/articles/depression-older-adults-diagnosis-and-management.

Butler, R. (1969). Age-ism: Another form of bigotry. *Gerontologist*, *9*(4), 243–246. [classic].

Centers for Disease Control (2020). Recommended adult immunization schedule. Retrieved August 2, 2020 from https://www.cdc.gov/vaccines/schedules/downloads/adult/adult-combined-schedule.pdf.

Chia, C., Egan, J., & Ferrucci, L. (2018). Age-related changes in glucose metabolism, hyperglycemia, and cardiovascular risk. *Circulation Research*, *123*(7), 886–904. https://doi.org/10.1161/CIRCRESAHA.118.312806.

Coxwell, K. (2017). Growing old is optional! More stories of amazing accomplishments by people older than you. Retrieved July 28, 2020 from https://www.newretirement.com/retirement/growing-old-is-optional-more-stories-of-amazing-accomplishments-by-people-older-than-you/.

Crossman, A. (2020). *Disengagement theory*. Retrieved from https://www.thoughtco.com/disengagement-theory-3026258.

Cummings, E., & Henry, W. (1961). *Growing old*. Basic Books [classic].

Dengarden (2019). Elderly care house design for our old age-elderly care home. Retrieved August 3, 2020 from https://dengarden.com/safety/Home-Design-Ideas-for-Our-Old-Age.

Dhingra, I., De Sousa, A., & Sonavane, S. (2016). Sexuality in older adults: clinical and psychological dilemmas. *Journal of Geriatric Mental Health*, *3*(2), 131–139. https://doi.org/10.4103/2348-9995.195629.

Dodig, S., Cepelak, I., & Pavic, I. (2019). Hallmarks of senescence and aging. *Biochemia Medica*, *29*(3), 030501. https://doi.org/10.11613/BM.2019.030501.

Duffin (2020). Population of the United States by sex and age 2019. Statistica. Retrieved August 3, 2020 from https://www.statista.com/statistics/241488/population-of-the-us-by-sex-and-age/#:~:text=Population%20of%20the%20United%20States%20by%20sex%20and,and%2024-years-old%20in%20the%20United%20States%20in%202019.

Fernandez, J., Rodriguez-Vallejo, M., Martinez, J., Tauste, A., & Pinero, D. (2018). From presbyopia to cataracts: a critical review on dysfunctional lens syndrome. *Journal of Ophthalmology*. Article ID 4318405. https://doi.org/10.1155/2018/4318405.

Gladyshev, V. (2014). The free radical theory of aging is dead. Long live the damage theory! *Antioxidants & Redox Signaling*, *20*(4), 727–731. https://doi.org/10.1089/ars.2013.5228.

Halli-Tierney, A., Scarbrough, C., & Carroll, D. (2019). Polypharmacy: evaluating risks and deprescribing. *American Family Physician*, *100*(1), 32–38. Retrieved August 2, 2020 from https://www.aafp.org/afp/2019/0701/p32.html.

Harvard Health (2018). Sexually transmitted disease? At my age? Retrieved July 31, 2020 from https://www.health.harvard.edu/diseases-and-conditions/sexually-transmitted-disease-at-my-age.

Health Research Funding (2020). The activity theory of aging explained. Retrieved August 3, 2020 from https://healthresearchfunding.org/the-activity-theory-of-aging-explained/.

Illiades, C. (2020). *A healthy sex life after angioplasty*. Healthgrades. Retrieved August 6, 2020 from https://www.healthgrades.com/right-care/angioplasty/a-healthy-sex-life-after-angioplasty.

Lee, S., Shih, S., Leu, Y., Chang, W., Lin, H., & Ku, H. (2017). Implications of age-related changes in anatomy for geriatric-focused difficult airways. *International Journal of Gerontology, 11*(3), 130–133.

Leung, E., Wongrakpanich, S., & Munshi, M. (2018). Diabetes management in the elderly. *Diabetes Spectrum, 31*(3), 245–253. https://doi.org/10.2337/ds18-0033.

Levine, H. (2019). How your eyes change with age. Retrieved August 3, 2020 from https://www.aarp.org/health/conditions-treatments/info-2019/eye-changes-with-age.html.

Lohler, J., Cebulla, M., Shehata-Dieler, W., Volkenstein, S., Volter, C., & Walther, L. (2019). Hearing impairment in old age, detection, treatment, and associated risks. *Deutsches Arzteblatt International, 116*(17), 301–310. https://doi.org/10.3238/arztebl.2019.0301.

Mancino, R., Martucci, A., Cesareo, M., Giannini, C., Corasaniti, M., Bagetta, G., & Nucci, C. (2019). Glaucoma and Alzheimer disease: One age-related neurodegenerative disease of the brain. *Current Neuropharmacology, 16*(7), 971–977. https://doi.org/10.2174/1570159X16666171206144045.

Masters, W., & Johnson, V. (1976). *The pleasure bond*. Bantam [classic].

McPhee, J., French, D., Jackson, D., Nazroo, J., Pendleton, N., & Degens, H. (2016). Physical activity in older age: perspectives for healthy ageing and frailty. *Biogerontology, 17*, 567–580. https://doi.org/10.1007/s10522-016-9641-0.

Metzger, E. (2017). Ethics and intimate sexual activity in long-term care. *AMA Journal of Ethics, 19*(7), 640–648. https://doi.org/10.1001/journalofethics.2017.19.7.ecas1-1707.

National Council on Aging (2020). Older Americans Act. Retrieved August 2, 2020 from https://www.ncoa.org/public-policy-action/older-americans-act/.

National Institutes of Health. (2017). *Sexuality in later life*. National Institute on Aging. Retrieved August 3, 2020 from https://www.nia.nih.gov/health/sexuality-later-life.

National Institutes of Health (2019). Diabetic retinopathy. National Eye Institute. Retrieved August 3, 2020 from https://www.nei.nih.gov/learn-about-eye-health/eye-conditions-and-diseases/diabetic-retinopathy.

Patton, K. T. (2018). *Anatomy & physiology* (10th ed.). Mosby.

Pillemer, K., Burnes, D., Riffin, C., & Lachs, M. (2016). Elder abuse: global situation, risk factors, and prevention strategies. *The Gerontologist, 56*(Suppl 2), S194–S205. https://doi.org/10.1093/geront/gnw004.

Queen, N., Hassan, Q., & Cao, L. (2020). Improvements to healthspan through environmental enrichment and lifestyle interventions: where are we now? *Frontiers in Neuroscience, 14*. https://doi.org/10.3389/fnins.2020.00605.

Sanderson, W., Scherbov, S., & Gerland, P. (2017). Probabilistic population aging. *PLoS One, 12*(6), e0179171. https://doi.org/10.1371/journal.pone.0179171.

Shanbhag, S., Nayak, A., Nayayan, R., & Nayak, U. (2019). Anti-aging and sunscreens: Paradigm shift in cosmetics. *Advanced Pharmaceutical Bulletin, 9*(3), 348–359. https://doi.org/10.1571/apb.2019.042.

TCPI (2020). Understanding the lighting needs of the aging eye. Retrieved August 3, 2020 from https://www.tcpi.com/lighting-aging-eye-understanding-lighting-need-growing-population/.

The Helping Home (2019). Alexa for seniors: 21 extremely practical ways older adults can use Amazon Echo devices. Retrieved August 3, 2020 from https://thehelpinghome.

com/alexa-for-seniors-21-extremely-practical-ways-older-adults-can-use-amazon-echo/.

Trzewikoswki de Lima, G., & De Gaspari, E. (2019). Study of the immune response in the elderly: is it necessary to develop a vaccine against *Neisseria meningitidis* for the aged? *Journal of Aging Research, 2019*, 9287121. https://doi.org/10.1155/2019/9287121.

U.S. Census Bureau (2017). American Community Survey. Retrieved August 3, 2020 from https://www.census.gov/acs/www/data/data-tables-and-tools/narrative-profiles/2017/report.php?geotype=nation&usVal=us.

U.S. Department of Health and Human Services National Institute on Aging (2016). Elder abuse. Retrieved August 2, 2020 from https://www.nia.nih.gov/health/elder-abuse.

U.S. Department of Health and Human Services National Institutes of Health, National Institute on Aging (2020). Aging in place: Growing older at home. Retrieved August 6, 2020 from https://www.nia.nih.gov/health/aging-place-growing-older-home.

U.S. Department of Health and Human Services National Institutes of Health, National Institute on Aging (2017). How to choose a nursing home. Retrieved August 3, 2020 from https://www.nia.nih.gov/health/how-choose-nursing-home#:~:text=%20How%20to%20Choose%20a%20Nursing%20Home%20,the%20nursing%20direc-tor.%20The%20Medicare%20Nursing..%20More%20.

United States Department of Health and Human Services (2020). Healthy People 2030. Retrieved from https://health.gov/healthypeople.

United States Department of Justice (n.d.). Elder abuse and elder financial exploitation statutes. Retrieved August 6, 2020 from https://www.justice.gov/elderjustice/prosecu-tors/statutes?page=8.

US Preventative Services Task Force (2020). Recommendation topics A and B recom-mendations. Retrieved July 12, 2020 from https://www.uspreventiveservicestaskforce.org/uspstf/recommendation-topics/uspstf-and-b-recommendations#:~:text=Main%20navigation,-Home&text=The%20USPSTF%20recommends%201%2Dtime,years%20who%20have%20ever%20smoked.&text=The%20USPSTF%20recommends%20screening%20for,who%20are%20overweight%20or%20obese.

Vanhaelen, Q. (2019). Non-programmed (non-adaptive) aging theories. Retrieved July 31, 2020 from https://www.researchgate.net/profile/Quentin_Vanhaelen/publication/333609513_Non-programmed_Nonadaptive_Aging_Theories/links/5cf8ecd0299bf1fb185bca9b/Non-programmed-Nonadaptive-Aging-Theories.pdf.

Westerhof, G., Bohlmeijier, E., & McAdams, D. (2017). The relation of ego integrity and despair to personality traits and mental health. *Journals of Gerontology, 72*(3), 400–407. https://doi.org/10.1093/geronb/gbv062.

World Health Organization (2020). Sexual and reproductive health. Retrieved August 6, 2020 from https://www.who.int/reproductivehealth/topics/sexual_health/conceptual_elements/en/.

Zugich, J. (2018). The twilight of immunity: Emerging concepts of aging of the immune system. *Nature Immunology, 19*, 10–19. https://doi.org/10.1038/s41590-017-0006-x.

Online Resources

https://www.ahrq.gov/prevention/guidelines/index.html
https://www.cdc.gov/violenceprevention/elderabuse/index.html

https://www.guidelinecentral.com/summaries/sexuality-in-the-older-adult-in-evidence-based-geriatric-nursing-protocols-for-best-practice/#section-396

https://www.mhanational.org/preventing-suicide-older-adults

https://www.nimh.nih.gov/about/directors/thomas-insel/blog/2010/the-under-recognized-public-health-crisis-of-suicide.shtml

CHAPTER 15 PLANNING FOR THE END OF LIFE

American Academy of Family Physicians (2020). Advance directives and do not resuscitate orders. Retrieved August 4, 2020 from https://familydoctor.org/advance-directives-and-do-not-resuscitate-orders/.

American Cancer Society (n.d.). Coping with the loss of a loved one. Retrieved August 2, 2020 from https://www.cancer.org/content/dam/CRC/PDF/Public/6036.00.pdf.

American Psychological Association (2020). When your child is diagnosed with chronic illness. Retrieved August 2, 2020 from https://www.apa.org/topics/chronic-illness-child.

American Association for Retired Persons (2020). https://www.aarp.org/home-family/friends-family/info-2020/when-loved-one-dies-checklist.html.

Barbus, A. (1975). The dying patient's bill of rights. *American Journal of Nursing, 75,* 99.

Bates, A., & Kearney, J. (2015). Understanding death with limited experience in life: dying children's and adolescents' understanding of their own terminal illness and death. *Current Opinion in Supportive and Palliative Care, 9*(1), 40–45. https://doi.org/10.1097/SPC.0000000000000118.

Bluebond-Langner, M. (1996). *In the shadow of illness: Parents of siblings of the chronically ill child.* Princeton University Press.

Coyle, N., Manna, R., Johnson Shen, M., Banerjee, S., Penn, S., Pehrson, C., Krueger, C., Maloney, E., Zaider, T., & Bylund, C. (2015). Discussing death, dying, and end-of-life goals of care: A communication skills training module for Oncology nurses. *Clinical Journal of Oncology Nursing, 19*(6), 697–702. https://doi.org/10.1188/15.CJON.697-702.

Everplans (2020). What's a POLST (Physicians Orders for Life Sustaining Treatment)? Retrieved August 2, 2020 from https://www.everplans.com/articles/whats-a-polst-physicians-orders-for-life-sustaining-treatment.

Feifel, F. (1977). *The meaning of death to children: new meanings of death.* McGraw-Hill [classic].

Fletcher, J., Mailick, M., Song, J., & Wolfe, B. (2013). A sibling death in the family: common and consequential. *Demography, 50*(3), 803–826. https://doi.org/10.1007/s13524-012-0162-4.

Fritscher, L. (2020). *Helping your child with the fear of death. What parents should know about thanatophobia.* VeryWellMind. Retrieved August 4, 2020 from https://www.verywellmind.com/fear-of-death-in-children-2671783.

Giger, J., & Haddad, L. (2020). *Transcultural nursing: assessment and intervention* (8th ed.). Elsevier.

Kübler-Ross, E. (1969). *On death and dying: what the dying have to teach doctors, nurses, clergy and their families.* Macmillan [classic].

Kinney, M., Brooks-Brunn, J., Molter, N., Byars, S., Dunbar, S., & Vitello-Cicciu, J. (1998). *AACN clinical reference for critical care nursing* (4th ed.). Mosby.

Legalzoom (2020). What is a durable power of attorney? Retrieved August 4, 2020 from https://www.legalzoom.com/articles/what-is-a-durable-power-of-attorney.

Legalzoom (2020). What is a living will? Retrieved August 4, 2020 from https://www.legalzoom.com/knowledge/living-will/topic/what-is-a-living-will.

National Institutes of Health. (2020). *Palliative care in cancer.* National Cancer Institute. Retrieved August 2, 2020 from https://www.cancer.gov/about-cancer/advanced-cancer/care-choices/palliative-care-fact-sheet#what-is-palliative-care.

Oates, J., & Maani, C. (2020). *Death and dying.* StatPearls. Retrieved August 2, 2020 from https://www.ncbi.nlm.nih.gov/books/NBK536978/.

ProCon (2019). States with legal physician-assisted suicide. Retrieved August 2, 2020 from https://euthanasia.procon.org/states-with-legal-physician-assisted-suicide/.

ProCon (2020). Euthanasia and physician-assisted suicide around the world. Retrieved August 2, 2020 from https://euthanasia.procon.org/euthanasia-physician-assisted-suicide-pas-around-the-world/.

Renz, M., Reichmuth, O., Bueche, D., Traichel, B., Schuett Mao, M., Cerny, T., & Strasser, F. (2018). Fear, pain, denial, and spiritual experiences in dying process. *American Journal of Hospice & Palliative Care, 35*(3), 478–491. https://doi.org/10.1177/1049909117725271.

Scholten, G., Bourguignon, S., Delanote, A., Vermeulen, B., Van Boxem, G., & Schenmakers, B. (2018). Advance directive: does the GP know and address what the patient wants? Advance directive in primary care. *BMC Medical Ethics, 19*, 58. https://doi.org/10.1186/s12910-018-030502.

Stanford Children's Health (2020). A child's concept of death. Retrieved August 4, 2020 from https://www.stanfordchildrens.org/en/topic/default?id=a-childs-concept-of-death-90-P03044.

Stroebe, H., Hansson, R., Stroebe, W., & Schut, H. (2001). *Handbook of bereavement research: consequences, coping and care.* American Psychological Association.

Taghiabadi, M., Kavosi, A., Mirhafez, S., Keshvari, M., & Mehrabi, T. (2017). The association between death anxiety with spiritual experiences and life satisfaction in elderly people. *Electronic Physician, 9*(3), 3980–3985. https://doi.org/10.19082/3980.

Timm, H. (2020). *It seems people don't fear death, as much as they fear the process of dying.* Discover Society. Retrieved August 2, 2020 from https://discoversociety.org/2018/02/06/it-seems-people-dont-fear-death-as-much-as-they-fear-the-process-of-dying/.

U.S. Department of Health and Human Services (2020). *Advance care planning: healthcare directives.* National Institute on Aging. Retrieved from https://www.nia.nih.gov/health/advance-care-planning-healthcare-directives.

World Health Organization (2020). WHO definition of palliative care. Retrieved August 2, 2020 from https://www.who.int/cancer/palliative/definition/en/.

Zeng, Y., Wang, C., Ward, K., & Hume, A. (2018). Complementary and alternative medicine in hospice and palliative care: A systematic review. *Journal of Pain and Symptom Management, 56*(5), 781–794. Retrieved August 2, 2020 from https://www.jpsmjournal.com/article/S0885-3924(18)30390-7/pdf.

Online Resources

https://www.aarp.org/home-family/friends-family/info-2020/when-loved-one-dies-checklist.html

https://www.apa.org/pi/aging/programs/eol.

https://www.scholastic.com/parents/books-and-reading/raise-a-reader-blog/7-touching-books-to-help-kids-understand-death-and-grief.html

www.aacn.nche.edu/ELNEC/index.htm
www.AmericanHospice.org

CHAPTER 16 LOSS, GRIEF, AND BEREAVEMENT

American Psychological Association (2020). Grief: Coping with the loss of your loved one. Retrieved August 6, 2020 from https://www.apa.org/topics/grief.

Art Therapy Resources (2020). Case study: Using art therapy for a client who is grieving. Retrieved August 6, 2020 from https://arttherapyresources.com.au/case-study-grief/.

Axelrod, J. (2020). *The 5 stages of grief & loss.* Psychcentral. Retrieved August 6, 2020 from https://psychcentral.com/lib/the-5-stages-of-loss-and-grief/.

Bowlby, J. (1960). Grief and mourning in infancy and early childhood. *Psychoanalytic Study of the Child, 15,* 9–52. [classic].

Bowlby, J. (1980). *Attachment and loss* (vol 3). Basic Books [classic].

Bridges to Recovery (2020). What are the signs of complicated grief disorder? Retrieved August 6, 2020 from https://www.bridgestorecovery.com/complicated-grief/signs-complicated-grief-disorder/.

Centers for Disease Control (2020). Cases in the U.S. Retrieved August 4, 2020 from https://www.cdc.gov/coronavirus/2019-ncov/cases-updates/cases-in-us.html.

Centers for Disease Control and Prevention (2020). Funeral guidance. Retrieved August 6, 2020 from https://www.cdc.gov/coronavirus/2019-ncov/daily-life-coping/funeral-guidance.html.

Centre for the Grief Journey (2018). Theories of grief. Retrieved August 6, 2020 from https://griefjourney.com/startjourney/for-professionals-and-caregivers/articles-for-professionals-and-caregivers/theories-of-grief/.

Cherry, B., & Jacob, S. (2019). *Contemporary nursing issues, trends, & management* (8th ed.). Elsevier.

Erikson, E. (1994). *The life cycle completed: A review.* WW Norton.

Everplans (2020). Funeral traditions of different religions. Retrieved August 6, 2020 from https://www.everplans.com/articles/funeral-traditions-of-different-religions.

Feiler, B. (2020). *Life is in the transitions.* Penguin Press.

Freud, S. (1917). Mourning and melancholia. *The Standard Edition of the Complete Psychological Works of Sigmund Freud, 14,* 1914–1916.

Funeralwise (2020). Funeral customs by religion, ethnicity, and culture. Retrieved August 6, 2020 from https://www.funeralwise.com/customs/.

Gesi, C., Carmassi, C., Cerveri, G., Carpita, B., Cremone, I., & Dell'Osso, L. (2020). Complicated grief: What to expect after the Coronavirus pandemic. *Frontiers in Psychiatry, 11,* 489. https://doi.org/10.3389/fpsyt.2020.00489.

Giger, J., & Haddad, L. (2020). *Transcultural nursing: assessment and intervention* (8th ed.). Elsevier.

Hamilton, I. (2016). Understanding grief and bereavement. *British Journal of General Practice, 66*(651), 523. https://doi.org/10.3399/bjgp16X687325.

Kübler-Ross, E. (1969). *On death and dying: what the dying have to teach doctors, nurses, clergy and their families.* Macmillan [classic].

Legacy Staff (2019). *Sympathy and condolence advice.* Retrieved from https://www.legacy.com/news/sympathy-and-condolence-advice/.

Linde, K., Treml, J., Steinig, J., Nagl, M., & Kersting, A. (2017). Grief interventions for people bereaved by suicide: A systematic review. *PLoS One, 12*(6), e0179496. https://doi.org/10.1371/journal.pone.0179496.

Mayo Clinic (2020). Pregnancy loss: How to cope. Retrieved August 6, 2020 from https://www.mayoclinic.org/diseases-conditions/pregnancy-loss-miscarriage/in-depth/pregnancy-loss/art-20047983.

Mental Health America (2020). Helping children cope with loss. Retrieved August 6, 2020 from https://www.mhanational.org/helping-children-cope-loss.

Meyers, L. (2016). *Grief: going beyond death and stages.* Counseling Today. Retrieved August 6, 2020 from https://ct.counseling.org/2016/10/grief-going-beyond-death-stages/.

National Institutes of Health, National Institute of Mental Health (n.d.). Helping children and adolescents cope with disasters and other traumatic events: What parents, rescue workers, and the community can do. Retrieved August 6, 2020 from https://www.nimh.nih.gov/health/publications/helping-children-and-adolescents-cope-with-disasters-and-other-traumatic-events/index.shtml.

Potts, L. (2020). *What to do when a loved one dies.* American Association of Retired People. Retrieved August 6, 2020 from https://www.aarp.org/home-family/friends-family/info-2020/when-loved-one-dies-checklist.html.

Raab, D. (2019). *Creative ways of dealing with the loss of a loved one.* Psychology Today. Retrieved August 6, 2020 from https://www.psychologytoday.com/us/blog/the-empowerment-diary/201912/creative-ways-dealing-the-loss-loved-one.

Renz, M., Reichmuth, O., Bueche, D., Traichel, B., Schuett Mao, M., Cerny, T., & Strasser, F. (2018). Fear, pain, denial, and spiritual experiences in dying process. *American Journal of Hospice & Palliative Care, 35*(3), 478–491. https://doi.org/10.1177/1049909117725271.

Rodriguez-Prat, A., Monforte-Royo, C., Porta-Sales, J., Escribano, X., & Balaguer, A. (2016). Patient perspectives of dignity, autonomy and control at the end of life: Systematic review and meta-ethnography. *PLoS One, 11*(3), e0151435. https://doi.org/10.1371/journal.pone.0151435.

Schonfeld, D., & Demaria, T. (2016). Supporting the grieving child and family. *Pediatrics, 105*(2), 445. https://doi.org/10.1542/peds.2016-2147.

Schulz, R. (1978). *The psychology of death, dying and bereavement.* Addison-Wesley [classic].

Sinclair, S., Beamer, K., Hack, T., McClement, S., Raffin Bouchal, S., Chochinov, H., & Hagen, N. (2016). Sympathy, empathy, and compassion: a grounded theory study of palliative care patients' understandings, experiences, and preferences. *Palliative Medicine, 31*(5), 437–447. https://doi.org/10.1177/0269216316663499.

Smith, M., Robinson, L., & Segal, J. (2019). Coping with grief and loss. Retrieved August 6, 2020 from https://www.helpguide.org/articles/grief/coping-with-grief-and-loss.htm?pdf=13250.

St. Elizabeth Health Care (2020). Types of grief and loss. Elizz. Retrieved August 6, 2020 from https://elizz.com/caregiver-resources/types-of-grief-and-loss/.

The Dougy Center (2020). *Help for young adults.* Retrieved from https://www.dougy.org/grief-resources/help-for-young-adults/.

Vasquez, A. (2020). Situational vs. maturational loss: What is the difference? Retrieved August 6, 2020 from https://www.joincake.com/blog/situational-loss-maturational-loss/.

Weir, K. (2018). Healing the wounds of pregnancy loss. *Monitor on Psychology, 49*(5), 26. Retrieved August 6, 2020 from https://www.apa.org/monitor/2018/05/pregnancy-loss.

Wojcieszek, A., Shepherd, E., Middleton, P., Lassi, Z., Wilson, T., Murphy, M., Heazell, A., Ellwood, D., Silver, R., & Flenady, V. (2018). Care prior to and during subsequent pregnancies following stillbirth for improving outcomes. *Cochrane Database of Systematic Reviews, 12*(12), CD012203. https://doi.org/10.1002/14651858.CD012203.pub2.

Zakeri, L. (2020). *Students coping with grief & loss at school.* Retrieved from https://www.accreditedschoolsonline.org/resources/managing-grief/.

Zhai, Y., & Du, X. (2020). Loss and grief amidst COVID-19: A path to adaptation and resilience. *Brain, Behavior, and Immunity, 87,* 80–81. https://doi.org/10.1016/j.bbi.2020.04.053.

Zisook, S., & Reynolds, C. (2017). Complicated grief. *Focus, 15*(4), 12s–13s. https://doi.org/10.1176/appi.focus.154S14.

Online Resources

https://www.aarp.org/relationships/love-sex/info-11-2010/naked_truth_broken_heart.html

https://www.legacy.com/news/sympathy-and-condolence-advice/

www.adec.org

www.compassionbooks.com

www.nmha.org/reassurance/childcoping.cfm

Index

Note: Page numbers followed by *f* indicate figures, *t* indicate tables and *b* indicate boxes.